SURGEONS OF THE FLEET

David McLean is Professor of History at King's College London. His many publications include *Education and Empire: Naval Tradition and England's Elite Schooling, Public Health and Politics in the Age of Reform: Cholera, the State and the Royal Navy in Victorian Britain* and *War, Diplomacy and Informal Empire: Britain and the Republics of La Plata 1836–1853* (all I.B.Tauris).

SURGEONS
OF THE FLEET

The Royal Navy and its Medics from Trafalgar to Jutland

DAVID MCLEAN

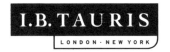

I.B. TAURIS
LONDON · NEW YORK

Published in 2010 by I.B.Tauris & Co. Ltd
6 Salem Road, London W2 4BU
175 Fifth Avenue, New York, NY 10010
www.ibtauris.com

Distributed in the United States and Canada Exclusively by Palgrave Macmillan
175 Fifth Avenue, NY 10010

ISBN: 978 1 84885 284 6

A full CIP record for this book is available from the British Library
A full CIP record for this book is available from the Library of Congress

Library of Congress catalog card: available

Typeset in Adobe Garamond Pro by A. & D. Worthington, Newmarket, Suffolk
Printed and bound in India by Thomson Press India Ltd

Contents

Illustrations

Acknowledgements

A grant from the Scouloudi Foundation in association with the Institute of Historical Research has made possible the publication of this book. Illustrations have been reproduced with the permission of the National Maritime Museum, Greenwich, and the Cambridge University Library. Above all, I am grateful to my wife, Eva Gordon, for her forbearance, encouragement and constructive advice.

Introduction

Few academic studies stand the test of time so successfully as that devised by John Keevil in the 1950s. *Medicine and the Navy, 1200–1900* remains a starting point for those who venture into the ever widening area of the history of military medicine. Keevil's contributions were published in 1957 and 1958;[1] after his death the project was completed with two further volumes by Christopher Lloyd and Jack Coulter in 1961 and 1963.[2] Histories of the armed services and of the lives of ordinary soldiers and sailors have since multiplied. Neil Cantlie produced an authoritative history of the army medical department in 1974.[3] Indeed, the care and comfort of Britain's fighting men, in both peace and war, has blossomed as a field for academic investigation. Perhaps that should not be surprising. Not only have the training, equipping and conditions for British servicemen become more publicly contentious in recent years but, as historians have increasingly discovered, for centuries the Admiralty and War Office compiled immense archives. By so doing, they not only recorded their own histories. Because they touched so many areas of life in Britain they also preserved opportunities for studying wider aspects of British society, most valuably in areas where comparable documentation has not otherwise survived.

Through supply contracts for weaponry, munitions, uniforms, victualling and in the construction of vessels and transport vehicles, the army and navy played vital roles in the growth of Britain's economy, well before the Napoleonic Wars. Large overseas expeditions, whether to Europe or the Americas, created obvious demands, but so too, albeit less spectacularly, did the steady maintenance of domestic encampments and garrisons.[4] Dockyards, along with rope and sail making, constituted important manufactures before the coming of the Industrial Revolution. But the armed forces did more than transform reluctant taxpayers into economic stimuli: they looked after pensioners, they educated children and they were notable health providers.

By the early nineteenth century, military medicine extended beyond patching up the wounded from the field or from the carnage of a gundeck. Military hospitals at home were the largest and among the most advanced of the age and reflected the nation's duty of care for those who risked life and limb for its safety and prosperity. At scenes of conflict, the army and navy supported fighting men with surgeons of varying ranks. Regiments and men-of-war all had medical officers attached, though after 1815 most of their time was absorbed by tending the victims of disease and accidents rather than the casualties of battle. The status of medics in the armed forces rose gradually from the late eighteenth century. Professional skills were enhanced as the science of healing progressed, more exacting qualifications for entry were introduced and the improved organization of centralized medical departments suggested a more coherent career structure within which dedicated practitioners might advance. As the nineteenth century wore on, the remit of medical officers at camp sites and aboard ships widened to include personal hygiene, sanitation and diet. While greater concern for the welfare of the common man was to be found across Victorian society, the army and navy, under direct government control, could be innovative both in their regulations and in the basic health education for recruits which they provided. Even where the pace of change was slow, as with the navy's attempt to reform the messing system for the lower deck and to employ trained cooks from the 1870s onwards, it was often not through lack of trying.[5]

Most of the detailed archival research into contributions made by the armed services to developments in nineteenth-century Britain has been published since the mid-1960s. By contrast, the pioneering work that Keevil, Lloyd and Coulter undertook, depending less on extensive trawls of dusty official papers, first saw the light of day a decade or so earlier in the *Journal of the Royal Naval Medical Service*. This periodical first appeared in 1915, being intended as a medium for communicating expertise within the naval medical service. It has done so ever since, though initially the take-up rate was low. Probationers and men attached to the navy's Volunteer Reserve proved to be willing subscribers at 15 shillings per annum but, as the editor ruefully reflected, the majority of regular surgeons failed to show much interest. There were only 300 subscribers compared to 1,200 for its army counterpart, which meant that costs were higher than originally planned.[6] Despite this hesitant launch, from its outset the journal inspired a number of experienced surgeons to delve into the past; it contained a wealth of memoirs, textual reproductions and historical investigation even before *Medicine and the Navy* was under way. Yet a generation after Keevil, researching among War Office and Admiralty documents still proved to be a daunting task. Examining medical provision for British forces during the Crimean War, John Shepherd remarked in 1991 that a lifetime was barely long enough to do justice to the materials at the Public Record Office.[7] For the Royal Navy in the nineteenth century, however, that vast store of boxes, files and logs housed at Kew under different Admiralty classifications forms only a part of what is available. The National Maritime Museum at Greenwich also holds an array of letterbooks, surgeons' journals and private papers – among the last is the huge, albeit still largely uncatalogued collection of correspondence bequeathed by the family of Sir James Porter.

Between Trafalgar and the Great War the navy was a sprawling institution influencing and influenced by changes at home and abroad. To focus on one facet of its activities, therefore, always risks a disconnection with essential context, and the study of medicine in the navy is no exception. As educated men with befitting expectations, and who, rightly, often saw themselves at the forefront of scientific enquiry, naval surgeons drew comfort from the rising status of the wider medical profession throughout this period. At the same time they were naval personnel – part, therefore, of a highly disciplined service where decisions were rarely made or conveyed by a process of consultation or with much regard for consensus. Newly qualified young men knew that when they joined. Complaints nevertheless abounded, although medical staff were by no means unique in that respect. Their work too was peculiar. Naval medics faced challenges between the poles and the equator both with men and in conditions often bearing little resemblance to those encountered by their brethren in private practice. And forever, it seemed, there was a struggle for collective as well as individual recognition. The public at large, politicians and the Admiralty hierarchy understandably perceived that the waves were ruled by great guns, heroic officers and fearless sailors. It was difficult to convey the message that a doctor's knowledge or the contents of a medical chest could be just as vital.

This book is largely a study of medical practice in the navy from the accounts and perspectives of those who administered it, manned its hospitals, tended its sick afloat, repaired its wounded and, especially in times of war, though sometimes young or inexperienced, might suddenly find themselves called upon to undertake unforeseen responsibilities wherein success hinged on the ability to improvise and to persevere when exhausted or with inadequate resources. Many of the archival sources consulted have been little used before. There is no matching the scope of Keevil's ambition of more than half a century ago. The following, however, spans the Royal Navy's golden age and attempts to tell the story of how the hopes, despairs and experiences of so many committed men were interwoven with its routine duties, its reforms and its various campaigns.

CHAPTER I

The Age of Cook and Nelson

It was, perhaps, an obvious point to make, but when reporting on the standard of health in the Royal Navy in 1862 Dr Gavin Milroy, a prominent epidemiologist, explained that every man who became sick diminished the navy's effectiveness as a fighting force and increased the physical burden on other sailors who inevitably assumed a portion of his duties. 'Sickness thus gives rise to sickness in more ways than one.'[1] The moral, of course, was that prevention was just as important as cure. Looking to the past, the figures spoke for themselves. Flying wood and metal had always carried men away but deaths and wounds incurred in battle ultimately paled in significance before the numbers succumbing to disease. By its nature, life at sea was hazardous. Diets were inadequate, hygiene poor, accidents common and men exposed to ailments little under-stood in unfamiliar climates. In the Seven Years' War between 1756 and 1763 the navy lost only 1,512 men to enemy action compared with 133,700 who either deserted or died from illness. A generation later, of all the seamen lost during the Revolutionary and Napoleonic Wars, 1.5 per cent died at the hands of the enemy, 12 per cent from disasters at sea, 20 per cent from accidents and 65 per cent from disease.[2] No stronger argument was necessary for maintaining a well-trained and efficiently administered naval medical service.

Fatalities did not tell the full story. In battle the wounded invariably outnumbered the dead, and during even the worst epidemics the majority of those affected would eventually pull through. Survival rates in both were determined by the availability of medical attention. This wisdom had never been questioned, though the navy had no easily identifiable medical corps before the mid-eighteenth century. Centuries earlier, chief surgeons, expert surgeons and junior surgeons had been paid by the Exchequer. In 1513 there were 32 such men in naval employment. In Tudor times and into the seven-teenth century, however, surgeons were only appointed for the duration of a particular campaign, operating at sea in the holds of vessels equipped with instruments and medical chests. Some had the status of physician though most were humbler barber-surgeons or apothecaries. But their work gradually gained acceptance as an area worthy of scientific enquiry. William Clowes, chief surgeon of the fleet that fought the Armada, published the first textbook on naval surgery in 1588, indicating how head injuries, fractures, dislocations and burns were to be treated. Wounds were irrigated and stitched, with ligatures and pressure used to minimize blood loss during amputations. Drugs were mixed aboard using pestles and mortars.[3] Best known among the early exponents of naval medicine was John Woodall who published *The Surgeon's Mate* in 1617. This was an extensive catalogue regarding the duties, training and equipment appropriate for both junior and senior medical staff at sea: Woodall even touched upon the apparent value of lemons, oranges and fresh vegetables in combating scurvy and deprecated an over-reliance on salt provisions in a sailor's diet and the low standards of cleanliness common on vessels. His work was revised in 1639 when he also published treatises on plague and gangrene. When the Corporation of Surgeons was delegated to fit out the surgical branch of the navy, Woodall was entrusted with the task. As an authority within his profession, Woodall was elected Master of the Barber Surgeons Company in 1633 and made examiner for those entering naval service in 1641.[4]

James Pierce was another prominent figure in seventeenth-century naval medicine. He served as surgeon on the flagship *Naseby* in 1658 and 1660, thereafter returning as Surgeon-General of the fleet aboard *Royal Charles* in 1665. His position ran while the fleet was active, though his responsibilities ceased once invalids were landed and thereby came under the control of the government's commissioners for the sick and wounded. A surgeon, once examined and accepted by the Company of Barber Surgeons, became responsible for providing his own drugs and equipment. This, needless to say, was open to abuse and afforded little effective check regarding quality of care; only in 1703, when a monopoly of supply was conferred upon the Society of Apothecaries, was the system brought under some measure of control. Pierce's duties included monitoring how sick and wounded seamen were treated, although his authority became uncertain after a Physician-General to the navy was appointed alongside him in 1666. He returned to sea between 1672 and 1674 during the third Anglo-Dutch War, at the same time ensuring that warships had adequate medical chests and provisions, that reserve supplies were available from the flagship and that the Company of Barber Surgeons recruited surgeons as required. His friendship with Samuel Pepys at the Admiralty no doubt played its part in making Pierce an effective administrator.[5]

James Yonge and John Moyle were also surgeons during the third Anglo-Dutch War. Aged 11, Yonge had been apprenticed to a naval surgeon and became a surgeon's assistant two years later. His knowledge of medicines and their uses developed from subsequent work for an apothecary prior to his first appointment. Like Woodall, he was a pioneer in tackling scurvy and devised his own remedies for a number of seafaring complaints. In the 1670s he tended seamen ashore in Plymouth, becoming eventually Surgeon-General of the Royal Navy as well as mayor of the town.[6] John Moyle published *Sea Surgeons* in 1668. This was an instructional work for young surgeons, giving practical advice on storage aboard and how to keep instruments conveniently packaged to facilitate rapid attendance in any part of the ship. Running a cockpit during battle was another of Moyle's invaluable tips. His treatise, re-published in 1702, also expressed reservations about the way in which some colleagues operated: amputations were undertaken too readily as quick solutions. In 1703 he produced *The Experienced Surgeon*, identifying types of wounds, fractures and sprains and recommending treatments appropriate for ulcers and tumours.[7]

How widely the erudition of Woodall, Yonge and Moyle was disseminated or practised by those most in need of it was difficult to judge. Naval surgeons did not enjoy reputations for diligence or competence, while their mates, who helped and trained alongside, frequently had no worthwhile knowledge of medicine. Aboard ship, surgeons were rated with boatswains, gunners and carpenters, although were usually paid less money. To demoralize them further, even within the medical world they lacked the status of physicians, for whom the most prestigious posts advising the Admiralty or inspecting arrangements for the fleet were usually reserved, despite the fact that a physician might never have been at sea. Some surgeons rose to be physicians but the tripartite professional structure of physician, surgeon and apothecary survived until the early nineteenth century. Other procedures established in the seventeenth century were also unravelled only very slowly. The Navy Board assumed responsibility for admitting surgeons in 1697 although candidates still had to pass an examination conducted at Surgeons Hall. When the Company of Barber Surgeons was dissolved in 1797 the commissioners for the sick and wounded became involved in recruitment. Conditions afloat, however, tended to limit the stream of applicants, so much so that on occasions in the seventeenth century impressment had to be used. The solution had to be better remuneration for naval surgeons, which was recognized in 1692 when their pay was raised from its 1626 level of 19/4d per month to a monthly figure of 30 shillings. The threat of impressment was also removed in 1692.

By the early eighteenth century a number of other grievances were being addressed. In addition to their basic stipend after 1692 surgeons received 2d per head in a ship's company. This at least acknowledged that a larger vessel entailed more work. They received a £10 grant towards the cost of drugs and instruments and an extra 15 shillings for every case of venereal disease they cured, collectable from whoever could afford to come forward for treatment. Grants were also established for the dependants of surgeons killed in battle. A bonus, known as Queen Anne's Bounty, was paid by the early eighteenth century: on a ship with 600 men this might be worth £40 a year. In 1730 a surgeon's monthly pay was raised to £5, with that for mates ranging between 30 and 50 shillings. That was certainly progress compared with levels half a century before. Those 1730 settlements, however, would not be altered for another 50 years.

A surgeon's duties were laid down for the first time in Admiralty Orders in 1731. Since 1703 they had been required to keep a journal and a record of cases, but now their daily routine was also more carefully drawn. The sick were to be visited twice daily, reports were to be kept on seamen sent to hospital and commanding officers were to be informed on the state of the sick-list. The work of mates was likewise prescribed. To them fell the menial tasks of emptying buckets, washing towels, making lint, attaching plasters and dressings, and boiling gruel. They also mustered men claiming illness for inspection. Such regulations may not have materially improved the conditions of service which either surgeons or mates enjoyed but they did go far towards identifying a permanent and indispensable medical corps within the navy.[8] Grievances continued, of course. Surgeons had no uniform and were not rated as officers. They had to provide costly drugs from their own pockets until 1805 when the monopoly of the Apothecaries Company ended and the Admiralty undertook to supply the medical service at public expense. There was no compensation for instruments lost in action or shipwrecks and pay scales were once again judged to be inadequate. A memorial to the First Lord of the Admiralty requested redress on all these points in 1780. Change, however, if at all, was painfully slow.[9]

Yet from the mid-eighteenth century the profile of naval medicine, like that of the Royal Navy itself, was steadily rising. This owed much to the voyages of Captain James Cook, whose interests went well beyond navigation and exploration. Cook's care for sailors extended to their diet and living conditions. As a young officer in the 1750s Cook knew that up to 20 per cent of a crew might die on a bad Atlantic crossing and resolved to end such needless loss of life. His three Pacific voyages of 1767, 1772 and 1776 witnessed improved cleanliness and hygiene via inspections of clothing and bedding, the removal of excessive dampness, adequate supplies of fresh water and a greater variety of food. On his second voyage between 1772 and 1775 he lost only one man from disease. Cook eliminated scurvy by ensuring the availability of fresh fruits, vegetables and meat. It was not scientifically provable how lemons and oranges cured and prevented this ancient scourge of mariners but Cook demonstrated their effectiveness, even on the longest voyages. Woodall had suggested this more than a century before, but would Cook's results now be recognized and his methods adopted throughout the navy? The experiences of the past gave no grounds for optimism.[10]

Cook was by no means the only proponent of better health for seamen. A naval contemporary, physician James Lind, made his reputation as a medical scientist by addressing the same problem. Having worked as a surgeon between 1739 and 1748, Lind experienced conditions on vessels at first hand. In 1753 he published the definitive work on scurvy and naval hygiene, and a further essay on the proper care of seamen in 1757. Lind gave prominence to the benefits not only of fresh but also of stored lemon juice and he recommended methods for effective preservation. He devised a simple system for distilling drinkable water on ships in 1761 and endorsed the use of powders and dried ingredients which, when water was added and boiled, could be turned into nutritious soups or jellies. In 1763 he published further observations on fevers and infections; his last work in 1768 was a pioneering investigation of preventive medicine and tropical diseases. In time, Lind came to be regarded as the father of nautical medicine, although the implementation of many of his ideas owed much to his successors. Being a retiring and scholarly man, he was content to write rather than to campaign. Moreover, his trials to cure scurvy, though clear in their results, were conducted with small numbers of patients, thereby making them easy to dismiss by those supporting other theories.[11] Scurvy, indeed, was not effectively eradicated in the navy until the mid-1790s. Credit for that attached to Lind's disciple – Gilbert Blane.

Blane revived and championed Lind's ideas in the 1780s after seeing the devastating effects of fever and sickness in the West Indies while physician to the fleet. He remained off the coast of North America collecting data and assessing treatments for a further year before coming home to publish his *Observations on the Diseases of Seamen* in 1785. This dealt with the most common afflictions at sea – scurvy, fevers and dysentery. Blane returned to civilian practice until appointed a commissioner on the Board of Sick and Wounded Sailors in 1795. In the same year the Admiralty ordered the use of lemon juice throughout the navy, as Lind had advocated 40 years before. Blane also promoted better ventilation and greater cleanliness aboard warships. Soap was provided after 1796 and the incidence of infectious diseases was undoubtedly reduced.[12] Blane observed in 1799 how sailors seemed to age before their time; they died younger than civilian counterparts, their constitutions broken by the privations of a life at sea. Aside from accidents and illness, the strain of arduous labour wore out their bodies: throughout the second half of the eighteenth century one in seven sailors was invalided for hernia alone.[13] Even so, statistics suggested that seamen were gradually becoming healthier. Better, though still frequently bad diet and greater attention to sanitation lowered death rates and levels of disease in the late eighteenth and early nineteenth centuries. In 1782, out of a force of 100,000 sailors and marines, about one in three were sent sick to hospital. By 1813, from a total of 140,000, the ratio was down to almost 1:11.[14]

Blane's reforms tended to overshadow the contributions of two other authorities in the field of naval medicine – Thomas Trotter and Leonard Gillespie. Trotter entered the navy as a mate in 1779, was promoted to surgeon in 1782, but left the service in the following year. He thereafter worked on slavers crossing the Atlantic where, horrified by what he saw, he took to studying the effects of scurvy and fevers. His *Observations on the Scurvy* appeared in 1786. Three years later he rejoined the navy and embarked on an investigation of its drinking water before becoming physician to the fleet in 1794. Trotter was not an innovative thinker in the mould of either Lind or Blane, with both of whom he disagreed, even regarding scurvy, and whose reputations he resented. But his own research on fevers was important, as was his promotion of better food, clothing, vaccination and more comfortable living conditions. Medical and chemical essays in 1795 preceded the completion of his most famous work, the three volumes of *Medicina Nautica* in 1791, 1799 and 1803. Trotter also urged a better deal for naval surgeons before retiring to private practice in 1802.

Leonard Gillespie served afloat in the 1790s and was in many respects a follower of Blane. He was at one time Nelson's private physician on *Victory*, although not at Trafalgar. His formative experiences were in the West Indies, following which he published *Advice to the Commanders and Officers of His Majesty's Fleet* on how best to preserve the health of their crews. Gillespie dwelt upon the usual problems of diet, ventilation, dirt, overcrowding below decks and the dangers of foul air in harbours and roadsteads. But he also warned against exposure to the sun, especially during fatiguing work, and stressed the importance of regular bathing and laundry. When sickness struck, isolating infected men was paramount; after the crisis, fumigating the vessel became essential. He also addressed the thorny issue of sailors' behaviour, particularly excessive drinking when ashore. Alcohol should be limited as far as possible. Gillespie saw it as a sign of mental dejection born of boredom, the cures for which were constant drills, gun practices, games, music and dancing.[15]

By the 1790s the navy had not only produced men capable of raising nautical medicine to new levels of scientific understanding; it had also built and ran the most advanced hospitals anywhere available. Ironically the best-known medical facility for seamen, the Greenwich Hospital dating from 1692, was not a proper hospital. The infirmary at Greenwich, built in 1763, provided only for the pensioners and infirmed resident at the establishment, of whom there were 1,000 by 1738 and almost 2,500 by the 1790s. From the early eighteenth century Greenwich was attended by the navy's senior physician, a surgeon, and one dispenser, with a matron and nursing staff in the ratio of one per 14 patients. However, as a royal charity, the Greenwich Hospital was not subject to direct control by the Board of Admiralty and it did not receive sick or wounded serving seamen.[16] The navy's first purpose-built and properly equipped hospital for officers and men was Haslar Hospital at Portsmouth, which although not completed until 1761 took its first cases in 1754. Planned to accommodate 1,800 patients, in its early decades it was seldom free from overcrowding. Exceeding by almost three-fold the original estimate of £38,000 and with an annual running cost of £14,000, Haslar was a maze of 84 medical and surgical wards with additional areas for patients with consumption and those requiring isolation on account of smallpox or fevers. Every ward had a water closet. The hospital had a bathing area for new admissions and extensive laundry provision.

Haslar was created with a medical establishment of one physician, two surgeons, a number of assistants and one dispenser. After 1795 the hospital was commanded by a senior naval officer as Governor or Captain-Superintendent, assisted by an agent and porter. Even by 1763, though, the staff had grown to include a matron and a dispensary assistant, and, on the administrative side, a steward, a butler, an agent's clerk and a cook, with labourers hired as required. In 1780 it was decided that the establishment should include seven surgeons' mates and three assistants. By 1795 its senior staff comprised three physicians and three surgeons. Many of the patients were fever and scurvy cases, among whom Lind, as physician there between 1758 and 1783, conducted much of his research; indeed, between July 1758 and July 1760 Haslar admitted 5,734 men, of whom 2,174 suffered from fever with a further 1,146 the victims of scurvy. Lind regularly had more than 300 scurvy cases under care simultaneously. In 1780 the hospital admitted a total of 8,143, 5,572 of whom had fevers and 1,457 scurvy. Mortality was high that year: the rate was 1 in 13. To conduct prayers and to comfort the sick and dying, Haslar engaged a chaplain, although this was no easy job. In the early nineteenth century and with the average patient number about 650, the Governor warned what any incumbent should expect. For those who had never visited, it was difficult to imagine the size of the building: 'the exercise of going up and down the stairs only would take two or three hours, particularly if the chaplain should not be a very young man'.[17]

The second establishment to treat sick and wounded sailors and marines opened in 1760 to serve the fleet at Plymouth. This was the Royal Naval Hospital, capable of accommodating upwards of 1,000 men by the 1790s, located on the edge of town in the adjacent parish of East Stonehouse. In 1780 the hospital housed 1,423 patients. It was built as ten blocks around a quadrangle, with each block containing six wards and each ward about 20 beds. By the 1790s its annual running cost was about £13,000, having by then one physician, one surgeon, an assistant for each and a number of administrative officers as at Haslar. Between 1795 and 1799 patient numbers fluctuated between a low of 295 and a high of 819. It had a poor reputation for nursing since many of those employed were dismissed for drunkenness or other inappropriate behaviour. Between 50 and 100 nurses were engaged at East Stonehouse at different times during the 1790s. Medical care at the beginning of the nineteenth century was also patchy. Years later Vice-Admiral Lord Dundonald recalled his experience of conducting a survey at the Royal Naval Hospital where a young sailor, admitted with a bruised shin, lost his leg after the usual application of 'infected sponge'.[18] Others were more generous in their appraisal of the medical regime. Andrew Henderson, who started his career as a naval surgeon there in 1811, reflected a quarter of a century later how at East Stonehouse he had 'gathered much which has aided me in the hour of need ever since'.[19]

Naval hospitals were never without their troubles. Relations were bad between the staff at Haslar during Lind's time when the hospital was controlled by its doctors, while at East Stonehouse tensions existed throughout the stern reign of Richard Creyke as Governor between 1795 and 1826. Corruption among those in charge of stores was not uncommon at either hospital. The accounts of the steward at East Stonehouse in 1813 necessitated an investigation in the hope that 'ultimately the whole scene will be laid before the Admiralty'.[20] Discipline, especially during the Napoleonic Wars when many patients were impressed men, caused problems too. Guards at the gates and bars at windows were designed to prevent desertion, which in places made the hospitals seem more like prisons. Whether the danger was exaggerated or the measures successful was hard to determine; with hindsight, however, only ten from among 20,895 patients at Haslar and nine from among 21,303 at East Stonehouse deserted between 1808 and 1814.[21] Admitting soldiers also caused concern. There were 46 such patients at Haslar in 1810, all of whom the Governor wanted out as soon as possible. Their costs to the navy were proving considerable, in addition to which they were 'apt to transgress the rules of the place by being disorderly, noisy and troublesome'.[22] The guards at Haslar were increased in 1815, partly again because of increasing chaos within the hospital but also on account of the admission of more than 200 French prisoners as patients. Discharge day was another occasion for disruption. Men were habitually mustered for medical survey before discharge but, given the frequent lack of sufficient executive or medical officers to examine them quickly, disorder was common among the crowd of visitors which usually gathered as both nurses and patients mingled with relatives and acquaintances, 'disturbing those ill and injured and committing other acts subversive to the necessary discipline'.[23] By 1814 this ritual at Haslar became so offensive to good naval order that the Governor decided to send cured men directly to their ships without any chance to meet with well-wishers.

Wars inevitably increased the navy's demand for surgeons. In the course of the American War their number rose from about 300 in 1779 to 450 in 1783, although numbers fell back with the coming of peace. In 1793, with the Royal Navy containing 70,000 men, the surgeons' list was 550. Not all were young enough for active duty, however; assistant surgeons (mates) were not listed at all. In 1799 the navy had 634 surgeons, rising to 720 by 1806. The first full list of naval medical officers, published in 1814, cited 14 physicians, 850 surgeons, 500 assistant surgeons, 25 dispensers and 50 hospital mates. Prolonged warfare between 1793 and 1815 raised the status as well as the number of surgeons. In 1805 full surgeons gained official uniforms, improved pay and wardroom rank on a par with lieutenants. But this was not without a struggle. When calling for a thorough reform of medical provision and in the examination of surgeons in 1790, Trotter had also wanted to improve the latter's standing, albeit recognizing it as 'a cause so often defeated'.[24] Blane urged in 1799 that although Royal Navy surgeons were probably better regarded than those of any other nation, 'it would be for the public benefit if they were still more respected and encouraged'. Old attitudes died hard. Blane complained of 'the strict and distant behaviour' of executive officers towards medical men;[25] such complaints echoed among surgeons and assistants long into the nineteenth century. Yet by the end of the Napoleonic Wars changes in the navy had impacted on the health of its seamen and the role of its doctors. Ships were generally better victualled, better ventilated and more hygienic, while accommodation aboard and treatment in the sick-bay marginally improved. Mortality among the sick had fallen from 1 in 8 in 1780 to 1 in 30 by 1812; the navy was no longer losing thousands of men annually to scurvy, typhus and smallpox epidemics.[26] Upgrading the surgeon in 1805 was designed to draw a better class of medical men into a service which would dominate the world's oceans for more than 100 years.

Credit for these developments from the 1790s has rightly been given to Trotter and Blane, both as men of science and for their influence as fleet physicians. John Harness, however, was another major figure, particularly when chairman of the Sick and Wounded Board between 1802 and 1806. Harness was both surgeon and physician, entering the navy in 1776, promoted to surgeon in 1778 and attached to Haslar in the early 1790s. He then served as physician to the Mediterranean fleet between 1793 and 1799. On becoming one of the Sick and Wounded Board's five commissioners in 1800, Harness joined the body which had overseen medical provision in the navy since 1702. This board had often been criticized for inefficiency and for frequent absenteeism on the part of its members. Under the pressures of war its accounts fell into arrears, and with much of the work devolving upon an insufficient number of clerks there was a lack of organization. As a commissioner, Blane undoubtedly effected a number of improvements after 1795 but it fell to Harness, as chairman, finally to persuade the Admiralty that radical reform was needed. Harness was thus instrumental in improving the lot of surgeons in 1805. He also changed the appointment system at the naval hospitals. Henceforth medical staff would be taken only from the list of naval surgeons, effectively making Haslar and East Stonehouse branches of centralized Admiralty administration. After 1805 no one could be appointed as physician who had not previously served five years as surgeon. When the Sick and Wounded Board was merged with the navy's Transport Board in 1806 Harness joined the new combined board as its sole medical commissioner.[27]

♥♡

By 1815 the navy had both a comprehensive medical administration and a corps of medical officers more confident than at any time before in their professional standing. Those who manned its hospitals also benefited from better conditions – manifested in 1810 by sizable salary increases for Haslar's physicians and surgeons.[28] Yet with warfare ended, the Royal Navy quickly became much smaller. In 1814 there were 713 ships in commission; by 1820 this was down to 134, with the number of seamen reduced from 140,000 to 23,000 accordingly. There were, however, new naval stations by the 1820s as West Africa and South America were added to the previous categories of North America, the West Indies, the East Indies and Mediterranean. A further administrative reorganization in 1817 abolished the Transport Board and transferred its functions, including that of medical oversight, to the Victualling Board. Dr John Weir now replaced Harness as the new board's medical commissioner.[29]

On joining the Victualling Board, Weir retained his earlier position as Inspector of Hospitals which, in practice, meant that he could never properly exercise his duties. In 1822 the Victualling Board therefore appointed a second medical commissioner, William Burnett, to assist in what was already becoming a recognizable department within the navy's administration. Weir and Burnett were supported by a chief clerk and 19 other clerks. This unit operated under an Admiralty which employed about 60 persons who were either assistants to the First Lord or who made up the secretaries and assistants for six other commissioners, their clerks and housekeepers. Beneath the Admiralty and alongside the Victualling Board was the Navy Board which had responsibility for dockyard contracts and workforces.

This organizational hierarchy owed much to Lord Melville, First Lord between 1812 and 1827. But pressure for economy, greater efficiency and the reforming zeal of the First Lord after 1830, Sir James Graham, saw many of the old sinecures, unnecessary clerkships and waste on account of excessive stores removed. The number of men employed in naval dockyards was likewise reduced, their working time shortened and their method of pay altered from piece work to regular wages. Needless to say, there was a political dimension to these Whig initiatives. The navy had long been criticized as a bastion of Tory jobbery and Graham's measures were undertaken in the spirit of other legislation regarding constitutional reform in 1832 and the overhaul of the Poor Law and municipal government in 1834 and 1835. Even Graham's critics, however, broadly conceded that in 1834 he left the Admiralty in a better state than he had found it.

Graham abolished the old Navy and Victualling Boards in 1832, replacing them with a single Board of Admiralty at Somerset House in which the First Lord presided over Sea Lords drawn from among senior executive officers, each supervising a specific area of operations. The navy was divided into five departments: those of the surveyor of the navy, accountant-general, storekeeper-general, comptroller of victualling and physician-general. Individual responsibility being held key to a greater efficiency than the previous board structures had provided, each department was to have a clearly designated permanent head who would exercise the Board's authority. Economies would also flow from this streamlined chain of command. An annual saving of £13,000 was immediately produced by a 20 per cent reduction among the 100 clerks engaged by the old Navy Board and the 68 attached to the Victualling Board. Large numbers of messengers and watchmen were also axed. In 1831 Burnett became sole medical commissioner on the Victualling Board and thus the obvious candidate for the post of Physician-General. He took over the new Medical Department on 9 June 1832. One chief clerk and nine other clerks were assigned to help him. It was their job to conduct routine correspondence, to register the qualifications of applicants for medical appointments and, if accepted, to record subsequent careers, to keep the accounts and to supervise the stores and medical supplies needed for the fleet and for naval hospitals at home and abroad. As for the volume of work, in 1834 Burnett contrasted the number of memoranda on medical affairs written for the Admiralty in the past year with those submitted in 1792: 236 compared to 25. In 1834 the Medical Department registered 4,361 letters, writing 4,699 in return. To make the post-1832 administrative structure successful would clearly require dedication, an ordered mind and an eye for detail on the part of its chief. Aged 53 when he took control, Burnett soon proved well suited to the task. He would remain in charge for 23 years.[30]

A Scotsman, like so many naval doctors, Burnett, after an apprenticeship and a brief period of study at Edinburgh, joined as assistant surgeon in 1795. He was present at the battle of St Vincent in 1797, at the siege of Cadiz and at the Nile in 1798, after which he was confirmed as surgeon in 1800. He served as a surgeon at Trafalgar in 1805. Following this, he had charge of prisoners of war in hospital at Portsmouth until promoted to be physician and Inspector of Hospitals to the 120 ships in the Mediterranean fleet in 1810. He was given much credit for his measures to combat fever there during the next four years, publishing in 1814 a medical account of the epidemics. Back home, he dealt with fevers and smallpox among prisoners held at Chatham before sailing with the Russian fleet on its return to the Baltic. With the French wars over, Burnett set up an extensive private practice in Chichester where he was also physician to the public dispensary. He remained in Sussex until joining the Victualling Board.

Even as junior commissioner in the 1820s Burnett was noticeably more energetic than Weir in attempting improvements in naval medicine. By the time he became head of the new Medical Department he was also recognized in scientific circles. His research into fevers had been expanded and was reissued in 1816; he was knighted in 1831, elected a Fellow of the Royal Society in 1833 and of the Royal College of Physicians in London in 1836. In 1841 Burnett's title was changed to Inspector-General and in 1843 to Director-General of the Medical Department of the Royal Navy, although his responsibilities remained as defined in the early 1830s. Beyond the routine tasks of recording and accounting which his clerks performed, Burnett decided on supplies and equipment, visited naval hospitals, recommended medical officers for promotion, and surveyed and invalided those no longer fit to practise. He reported to the Board of Admiralty, with whose decisions he then complied. Meticulous and with a keen interest in scientific knowledge, Burnett expected disciplined behaviour, high standards of medical work and intellectual curiosity among all who served under him.

Inevitably much of Burnett's time was devoted to the needs and requests of surgeons and assistants. Indeed in 1847 he reflected on how much trouble appointing and allocating medical officers caused: 'almost every one wanting to select his ship and station'. 'Were I to give way on such occasions,' he concluded, 'it would be impossible to carry on the duties of the Department.'[31] On occasions, too, it fell to him to confirm the worst fears of anxious families that a young medic had died abroad or that nothing had been heard of his ship for many months. He also had to judge which texts should be distributed in order to guide surgeons in their work. Doctors entering the navy would bring their own books of reference but specialist publications on particular diseases or for issue on particular stations were sometimes acquired at the taxpayers' expense. In selecting equipment most appropriate for the service Burnett likewise had to make assessments: there was no shortage of manufacturers seeking lucrative supply contracts, all making claims for wondrous potions or inventions. Those which impressed him were sent for trials on ships or at hospitals. An instrument for holding fractured bones in 1846, specimens of medicated cloth in 1847, a mechanical leech and a galvanized steel truss in 1848, a vegetable-based drug for treating gonorrhoea, and India rubber gloves for staff to guard against infection in 1852 were among the innovations which Burnett considered worthy of investigation.

Most problems with supplies, however, arose in relation to preserved foods. By tinning, bottling or powdering, meats, vegetables, juices and soups might be stored at victualling yards or issued aboard ships on long voyages or during blockade duty when nutrients were running low and crews might otherwise be living for months off salt meat and unbreakable biscuits. The value of canned food was confirmed on Arctic expeditions between 1818 and 1823. Tinning thereafter became a growing industry, with manufacturers claiming ever greater rates of success from new techniques. Not all such claims could be substantiated and it was not uncommon for stocks in yards and ships to be destroyed, so much so that as late as 1851 vast amounts of meat were condemned at Portsmouth. Not only did suppliers vary but even produce from a trusted source could become unreliable. This happened with Stephen Goldner, the foremost Admiralty contractor for preserved meat and vegetables after 1844. Goldner's displaced rivals, Cooper and Gamble, who had held contracts since 1822, thereafter disparaged the quality of his provisions and began spreading rumours and exaggerated tales of mishaps with his goods. In fact between 1844 and 1852 only 1 per cent of all Goldner's supplies had to be condemned; much of the canned food found to be unsuitable was from other contractors. Nevertheless amid this fog of commercial rivalry Burnett had to acknowledge in 1851 that Goldner's produce was not of the same high standard as when he had first undercut Cooper and Gamble, even though a parliamentary committee in 1852 did eventually clear him of any neglect. Captain Rochfort Maguire, wintering aboard *Plover* at Point Barrow in 1853, noted that Goldner's meats 'are rather strong for our tastes'. They were, however, 'relished by the Esquimaux uncommonly'.[32] In the 1840s Henry Jones patented a self-raising flour suitable for baking and D. and H. Edwards & Co. developed a superior preserved potato, for both of which Burnett ordered extensive sea trials. Edward Moore's preserved milk was also widely tested, albeit with mixed results, between 1848 and 1852. The milk decomposed when examined off West Africa but survived in storage at Jamaica in 1849 and served well in the Arctic in the early 1850s. It had an odd taste and did not mix easily with water; it was, however, palatable and for feeding the sick it was generally considered to be better than nothing.

Burnett ran the Medical Department with his ten clerks squeezed into eight rooms in Somerset House. In case of doubt, Burnett told them all sternly in June 1832, 'I shall expect that no relaxation of duty will take place.'[33] There was a daily attendance register which he inspected every Monday and, whatever formal office hours might suggest, no clerk was to leave his desk until the day's work was done. Below the chief clerk, responsibility for the department's principal work of correspondence and supplies was divided among three second-class clerks. Under these broad headings came keeping the register of surgeons' appointments, service and promotions, medical stores, and supervising the accounts for naval hospitals, dockyards and infirmaries. These men were in turn supported by five third-class clerks, again with specific duties. But in busy times all should assist each other regardless of designated functions, as the Admiralty made plain in January 1834. Promotion would be based on individual merit without reference to specific responsibilities.

Ten clerks were never likely to be sufficient and within a year Burnett had persuaded the Board that he needed another. With the House of Commons calling for ever more accounts after 1832 and with a backlog of business slowly building up, the strain on his staff was evident. That the department functioned as well as it did owed much to the devotion of the Fossett brothers, Benjamin and William, as second-class clerks, and to that of the diligent William Crandell who had been a third-class clerk in government service since 1811 and who additionally acted as Burnett's private secretary. By 1838 Crandell and a junior helper were in the office until 8 or 9pm on many evenings but even their best efforts were hampered by inadequate filing facilities. The Admiralty grudgingly allowed an extra clerk, but only for two months until the arrears of business had been cleared. But things got worse. The temporary clerk was kept on for two years until he found a better job, after which Burnett informed the Board of representations 'so strongly urged upon me by my clerks, setting forth the utter impracticability of carrying on the duties in a proper manner with the present establishment'. Yet when money was allocated for two extra clerkships at the Admiralty the Board assigned them both elsewhere. 'No other department can more require them,' Burnett pleaded in vain.[34]

In May 1841 Benjamin Fossett succeeded as chief clerk, which both raised the efficiency of the department and put in place a man whom Burnett had known for 20 years and in whom he had the utmost confidence. Fossett had worked for the old Victualling Board prior to 1832 and had more than 30 years' experience as a government employee. Crandell was now promoted to second class, remaining in post until his death in 1846. These moves completed the Fossett brothers' control of the office which had already been considerably increased in 1834 when William's son, William King Fossett, had been transferred from the old naval hospital at Deal to be a third-class clerk at Somerset House. This hierarchy survived until Benjamin Fossett's retirement in 1852, by which time the Board had finally accepted that the Medical Department was understaffed. Not only that, as a parting shot Fossett impressed upon the Board how poorly the department fared with respect to pay and grading in relation to other divisions within the Admiralty.

The burden of work was indeed taking its toll on efficiency by 1852. Burnett noticed that there was difficulty retrieving papers from the repository, only to be told by the Fossetts that there was no way in which the system of storage or conveyance could be improved. The only additional tool which the chief clerk could suggest was to keep a précis book for important documents, 'if there were sufficient clerical force in the Department'.[35] In 1830, 297 documents had been registered at the old Victualling Board. The corresponding number for the Medical Department in 1850 was 1,053. Given these pressures, Burnett lobbied for William Fossett to succeed his brother as chief clerk. His plan was then to promote William King Fossett from third- to second-class clerk. He was not, however, successful. The Board awarded the chief clerkship to Benjamin Hobart, the most senior second-class clerk, despite the latter's reluctance to assume any extra responsibilities. The department was reorganized internally in 1853 whereby its clerks, now 12 in total, were arranged into four divisions covering medical officers, hospital and ships' accounts, correspondence, and medical stores and supplies. Hobart did his best to cope but the workload continued to grow. Between April 1853 and April 1854, 6,269 letters were registered; for the following 12 months the figure was 8,576. Outgoing letters rose correspondingly from about 3,000 to almost 4,000.

When Hobart retired in 1854 William Fossett was at last given the chief clerkship. By then, however, the backlog of work was substantial and in 1855, when Sir John Liddell replaced Burnett as Director-General, it was obvious that much of the arrears could never be recovered. Regarding medical expenditures, Liddell concluded that 'we cannot clear off the current accounts, which to be worth anything ought to be closely examined'. Medical statistics were 12 years in arrears. As for the often unique returns made by many surgeons about topography and medical science from around the world, these had either become untraceable in the archive or 'consigned, after a hurried perusal, to the dusty shelves of the Department never again to be referred to or turned to any practical account'. Illness and accidents exacerbated such problems, as in 1856 when Edward Ede, a third-class clerk, 'fell from the top of an omnibus while (it is supposed) in a state of intoxication' and could not return to work for ten weeks.[36] But the fundamental issue remained chronic understaffing for the work expected. Towards the end of his career Burnett reminded the Admiralty yet again of what he had been saying for more than 20 years: although his department was not large its duties were 'not less important than those of any other'.[37]

Burnett's initial supply budget covered medical stores and victualling, drugs, instruments, charges arising from sick quarters at a number of ports in Britain and overseas, and the temporary hospital establishments at Cork and Deal. In the accounting year 1832–33, stores amounted to £12,000, medicines and drugs to £3,500, instruments to £700, victualling to £7,000 and sick quarters to £2,000. For the following 12 months the costs at Deal and Cork were set to double, with an additional £2,000 needed for provisions and stores. Within a year of the department's creation, therefore, outgoings had jumped from £25,000 to around £30,000, although reduced to about £28,000 in 1835 after the hospital at Deal was closed.[38] Most contentious among these costs were medicines and drugs; it was a significant area of expenditure yet opportunities for saving money always had to be set against the need to ensure quality. The Admiralty inherited this dilemma in 1805 when surgeons were relieved of the need to purchase their own medicines. Yet while this was convenient for the navy, it was always felt that insufficient checks on contracts existed. One of Burnett's tasks as second commissioner on the Victualling Board after 1822 was to inspect the Apothecaries Company's charges and accounts, and soon many suspicions about overcharging were confirmed. After nearly ten years of peace the Apothecaries Company was still billing at wartime prices: 'More than 50 per cent (and on some articles 100 per cent) was charged beyond the prices paid for supplies to the army,' Burnett revealed.[39] Not only that, the Company was about to implement a further hike of 10 per cent for its products. In 1833, therefore, the Medical Department introduced a tendering system whereby five or six principal druggists might compete for annual contracts requiring six months' notice of termination. Agreements were duly made with Messrs. Beckwith, Barron and Harvey and subsequently with J.J. Hodgkinson and with Messrs. Howard and Kent of Stratford. As far as Burnett was concerned the problem was solved.

Aggrieved at its treatment, the Apothecaries Company did not tender. Having supplied the navy for over a century it pointed out indignantly how its prices guaranteed the quality of medicinal ingredients because the Company checked on its importing wholesale merchants. The Company also worked to standards laid down by the Royal College of Physicians, as contained for many years in the *London Pharmacopoeia*, which further increased the cost of some compounds; it was therefore impossible to compete with suppliers who felt no such constraints. As for past sales, when one of the victualling commissioners inspected 60 items in 1830 all were judged excellent and even where some of the gums, roots, barks and cloves had been broken or externally disfigured their medicinal qualities were unimpaired. The Apothecaries Company was clearly not prepared to go quietly. Worse still for Burnett, within two years it was back.

In 1834 and against Burnett's wishes the Admiralty once again changed the supply system for medicines, chemicals and stores. The Apothecaries Company was re-engaged to provide medicinal stores at a fixed rate of £11-10-0d for every 100 sailors voted on the annual naval estimates. Howard and Kent continued to provide chemicals under a separate arrangement while surgical equipment and apparatus for naval hospitals came from specialist instrument makers. Resentful at the way in which his tendering system had been discontinued, Burnett could barely contain his glee in 1839 when the Apothecaries Company complained that the arrangement was working to its disadvantage. Quite possibly it was, Burnett reported to the Board, but the £3,476 which the Company had received in 1838 was according to the arrangement and prices which it had asked for in 1834 and which the Board had sanctioned. Research revealed that some drugs had risen in price since 1834, others had fallen, and that the army was paying 9 per cent more for some materials. The Apothecaries Company had only one just grievance: the Admiralty had arbitrarily changed the payments so that £11-10-0d was now calculated per 100 men actually borne on the books rather than approved by parliament. In 1838 the Royal Navy employed 30,227 sailors – 1,738 fewer than the 31,965 voted. This alone meant a loss to the Company of £180. With increased wholesale prices included, its loss on the 1838 contract came to £350.

The Admiralty thereafter reverted to paying per 100 sailors voted and allowed for a 5 per cent increase in the price of drugs. But while conceding this to the Apothecaries Company, Burnett could not refrain from expressing disappointment at the manner in which the Board had acted behind his back in 1834. 'More complaints have during that time been made respecting the qualities of the supplies from the Apothecaries Company than was the case during the contracts,' he observed. Although he would continue to treat the Company fairly, 'they must not expect that a return to the inordinate prices they charged the navy after the conclusion of the peace in 1814 will be again tolerated'.[40] When the Company claimed again in 1842 that it was losing money on its naval contract Burnett persuaded the Board to give notice of termination as of April 1843. This, as he had suspected, forced the Company to ask for renewal, obliging it to quote a precise price for every article. Able now to make detailed comparisons as never before, Burnett felt confident, advising the Admiralty to enter into a new annual contract with itemized prices, subject, as before, to six months' notice. Thereafter relations between the Medical Department and Apothecaries Hall became less troubled. When William Fossett checked the price list in 1854 he concluded that overall it fairly reflected market value. Whether for 30 years Burnett had been overly wary of the Apothecaries Company while showing unmerited tolerance towards other suppliers was difficult to judge. In November 1855, however, Liddell pressed Howard and Kent to account for the costs of their chemicals in a way which Burnett had never considered appropriate, whereupon Alfred Kent acknowledged that his prices were higher than those charged by wholesalers. That was because Howard and Kent made their own chemicals to specification, unlike other suppliers who simply bought and sold the cheapest available from unregulated sources. True or not, it was a further indication of how monitoring costs was an anxious and time-consuming preoccupation among staff at Somerset House.

Procurement was bad enough. Storage and provisioning the fleet posed a further set of difficulties. Medicines from contractors were initially delivered to a store at Somerset House from where, twice weekly, one of the department's trusty messengers, acting as bargeman, took them down to the victualling yard at Deptford or occasionally to Woolwich as required. Bedding, clothing, hospital stores and items in bulk for use both at home and abroad were delivered directly to Deptford where accounts were kept and returns made regarding receipts and expenditure. It was estimated that the department seldom held less than £5,000 worth of property at Deptford – enough to supply 3,000 men afloat. But as with the Apothecaries Company, Burnett's relations with the victualling yard had a troubled past. Since 1823 all medical supplies at Deptford had been supervised by a naval surgeon acting as medical storekeeper who was usually helped by an assistant surgeon assigned to the yard. The surgeon was also expected to attend the families of employees at the yard, dispense medicines and deal with any accidents arising. It was also his duty to check the instruments of, and returns of supplies from surgeons aboard convict ships, and, when required, to test the quality of preserved meats, lemon juice, vinegar, peppers and other nutrients intended to survive months or even years at sea. James Brydone held the post in the early 1830s, having been previously assistant surgeon at the Deptford dockyard. By 1828 medical stores had become an exclusive section within the victualling yard and all overlapping duties with the dockyard were discontinued. When Burnett visited in 1833 he concluded that the stores were managed as well as the cramped conditions allowed. The problem of space was eased a little in 1834 when supplies for ships fitting at Chatham and Sheerness were transferred to Chatham.

But other problems persisted. Prominent among these were the soured relations between Brydone and his assistant, Isaac Dias. By 1833 the hatred between them was so great that the Captain-Superintendent in charge of the Deptford yard announced that he was unable to keep the peace any longer and, with the medical section of the yard becoming dysfunctional, dumped the problem on Burnett's desk. Brydone insisted that Dias was rude. Dias retorted that Brydone was incapable of giving any clear directions and resorted to accusations of insubordination in order to disguise his own shortcomings. No one at the yard was prepared to testify against Dias, although one employee did overhear Brydone 'threaten to knock

Mr. Dias down'.[41] Even when the Captain-Superintendent and Burnett persuaded Dias to offer a vague apology, Brydone would not be appeased and demanded an Admiralty enquiry. Burnett removed both men in 1834, replacing them with John Brown, a senior assistant surgeon. Brown was never promoted to surgeon but he proved to be a good administrator. The secret of his success was that after 1834, on William Fossett's recommendation, he was allowed to keep apart the stores destined for ships from those intended for the hospitals; confusion was thus avoided by allowing different accounting systems whereby returns on ships' stores could be made quarterly as opposed to the weekly returns demanded for supplies to hospitals.

Brown's only flaw was that he had a tendency to hoard, and after his death in 1851 stocks were found to have accumulated at the yard vastly surplus to requirement. The Deptford yard periodically held sales for old stores but by 1852 the quantities of medicines, acids, wood and charcoal were such that Howard and Kent were invited to offer for these, while the Medical Department's principal instrument maker was despatched to sort out the equipment. The sale in August 1852 raised more than £100 but further stock had to be destroyed at a loss to the navy. Brown's successor was William Gunn, who found his duties at the yard onerous and who could not cope without help from a dispensary man whom Burnett transferred from the naval hospital at Chatham. Work at Deptford was never exciting, but its efficiency mattered not only to Burnett's ability to control his department's budget but to ships and hospitals around the world wherever a seaman's health might be in jeopardy.

CHAPTER 2

Surgeons at Sea in the Early Nineteenth Century

Medical officers were plentiful as the navy was scaled down after 1815; indeed, no assistant surgeons were recruited until 1822 when 19 joined the service. The admissions procedure required candidates to produce a certificate of competence from one of the Royal Colleges of Surgeons in London, Edinburgh or Dublin and then to undergo an oral examination lasting up to two hours at Somerset House. In 1840 a one-year probationary period was introduced during which entrants bore the title of acting assistant surgeon. A medical education was strictly defined. Twelve months of general and six months of comparative anatomy, 18 months of surgery, 18 months on the theory and practice of medicine and 12 months of clinical lectures were all required; so too were six months' study of chemistry, *materia medica*, midwifery and botany. An apprenticeship or practical knowledge of pharmacy was stipulated, along with 12 months' attendance at a hospital whose average number of patients was in excess of 80. This last qualification was raised to two years at a hospital with an average above 150 in 1839, reduced to 100 in 1853. The maximum age for entry was lowered from 26 to 24 in 1839. Finally, candidates had to be unmarried and produce good testimonials.

Medical schools, not unnaturally, compared the navy's entrance requirements with those of the army. Considering the difference in 1837, Burnett noted that the army asked for less surgery, less theory and practice of medicine, less pharmacy and less *materia medica*, midwifery and botany. The army did, however, require more hospital attendance, more anatomy, more chemistry and some knowledge of natural history. One thing the Royal Navy certainly did not do was advertise. That would only encourage men from 'among the vast herd' who could not find a position in civil practice, most of whom would already be too old and their qualifications unsuitable.[1] By lowering the age bar to 24 the navy doubtless lost some good men who simply failed to complete their studies on time, but Burnett wanted them young enough and sufficiently robust to be moulded to the hardships of sea life and to have years of work still ahead of them when later promoted to full surgeon. With the expansion of private medical schools and an abundance of university graduates in the early nineteenth century, the number of doctors seeking a living had never been higher. Hard as the regimentation of the armed services might appear, it offered a chance of employment.

Although entrance requirements were strictly applied many applicants believed that patronage was still essential. Some claimed political favours on account of voting patterns within their families – dependent, of course, upon which party was in government. Others stressed the military service of fathers or uncles in the Napoleonic Wars, or how their mothers were daughters of naval officers through whom the claims of faithful servants of the crown might be transferred. Some pleaded the circumstances of a large family wherein the meagre resources of a half-pay officer or clergyman father had been set aside for the medical studies of a son now eager to repay the sacrifice by seeking a career in public service. Government ministers, members of parliament, senior naval officers and aristocrats, if available, were used as conduits for favourable consideration. Burnett was seldom swayed, although he did assure one much valued friend, the Duke of Richmond, in 1833, 1842 and again in 1843, that the latter's protégés had passed with flying colours and been assigned at once to warships. Regarding another man due for interview at Somerset House in 1841, Richmond was informed that 'I have given him marching orders to come at double quick time.'[2] Even in cases requiring delicate handling, however, Burnett's stock response was that regulations were determined by the Admiralty and that it was not within his competence to depart from them. Only once did he blatantly waive the rules. That was for John Brown in 1852, son of the recently deceased medical storekeeper at Deptford. Young Brown was of 'a very superior character'. As a special case 'not to be hereafter quoted as a precedent' he needed a dispensation for being married.[3]

While a few entrants had the benefit of patronage, all shared a common experience of years spent as medical students. Burnett, in fact, was generally sympathetic to those who had struggled through an impecunious education; it indicated the commitment and self-discipline so essential for practice in the navy. When the suggestion reached him in 1832 that new recruits should be required to work six months unpaid at a naval hospital as a precondition for appointment he protested that this would add too much to the cost of an education which in most cases had already put a strain on family finances. Young men commonly entered the service in debt. Henry Willan, for instance, his father long dead, was fortunate to have an aunt who not only stood surety for the advance with which to buy his outfit in 1841 but who also persuaded the naval agent Thomas Stilwell to allow her nephew each quarter's pay in advance during his first year. Michael Cowan had even worse financial problems when he joined in 1854. He had recently paid out four guineas to take his MB, £10 for his diploma as a surgeon and a further four guineas for the privilege of hospital experience. He owed an uncle £60 and now needed £26 to take his MD, he hinted to his brother in Australia. Fitting out, instruments and other essentials would cost another £100. He subsequently borrowed £50 from a second uncle and would now need years on an assistant surgeon's stipend to clear a total debt of £170.[4]

Roughly a third of the 452 entrants between 1822 and 1834 held their surgical diplomas from the Royal College of Surgeons in Edinburgh, with a similar proportion so qualified among the 334 admitted in the eight years after 1 January 1840. Half the Scottish intake also held degrees from either Edinburgh or Glasgow universities; in fact, the navy could never be in any doubt that Scotland provided a heavily disproportionate percentage of its surgeons. Scottish institutions were touchy about their status, both with respect to each other and to their counterparts further south, and Burnett had to handle their occasional representations sensitively. The senate of Aberdeen University complained in 1839 that its graduates did not receive the same consideration as those from the lowlands or the English universities, while the large Aberdeen infirmary was not even recognized by the Admiralty as a training hospital. Burnett persuaded the Board to amend regulations accordingly, though in 1846 the university was back with another grievance. The Navy List did not print the letters MD after the names of its graduates whereas it did so for those of Edinburgh, Glasgow, London, Dublin, Cambridge and Oxford. St Andrews had unsuccessfully raised this issue five years earlier; now the navy conceded the point. In 1850 the Faculty of Physicians and Surgeons in Glasgow insisted that its licence should have the same status as those of the Royal Colleges. Since the army had agreed to this Burnett felt that the navy had to follow suit. Meanwhile Aberdeen asserted that its academic standards were higher than those at Glasgow while St Andrews pointed out that its students underwent a rigorous *viva voce* examination which made its degrees at least as good as those of any university. Amid a bewildering barrage of appeals against entrance regulations which admittedly on some points took little account of changes in the nature of medical education in Britain in recent years, Burnett tried to be as open minded as circumstances allowed. By the 1840s hospital practice had become even more difficult to assess than the standards of degrees and licences since many British towns and cities now boasted large hospitals about which the Medical Department acknowledged it knew very little. By 1853 Admiralty regulations listed 22 hospitals qualifying for ward training, with some also recognized as medical schools. Soon after, Burnett abandoned the notion of approved hospitals, accepting that there would always be requests for justifiable additions. The important criteria were that clinical experience should be at an institution which was both large and provided a wide range of medical and surgical cases.

By the 1840s the surplus of medical graduates appeared to have ended and recruitment had become more difficult. 'Parents have of late been unwilling to place their sons to a profession which seemed already over-stocked,' Burnett mused in 1848.[5] He urged the Board to improve the conditions of service which would surely help to make the navy a more attractive career. In 1853 the maximum age for entry reverted to 26 and Burnett changed the procedure for interview so that, instead of being called separately, candidates would come to Somerset House on a specified date each quarter. Other minor modifications were with a view to dispelling the idea that joining the navy was more forbidding than joining the army. Yet even with this laxer approach admissions remained a hit and miss affair. For the quarterly selections in November 1853 ten candidates had been called to London. Two did not appear, two more requested additional time to prepare and one failure was allowed three extra months for study. Only five were suitable for entry as acting assistant surgeons.

Those successful joined, on paper, a large medical establishment. When the Medical Department was created there were 720 surgeons and 339 assistants. Yet among the 720, only 215 were actually employed; the remaining 505 were on half pay. This was understandable in the context of naval reductions. At its wartime peak more than 700 ships had carried a surgeon; in 1831 the navy had only 143 sailing ships and seven steamers. Age was also crucial. Ninety-seven surgeons were above 55 years old and a further 86 between 50 and 55. Among all these, about 40 were fit to work at shore establishments but, Burnett ruled, hardly any would be able to cope with the strain of going to sea again. Even among the 322 surgeons under 50, only 179 declared themselves sufficiently healthy to be called up. Assistant surgeons, among whom the average age was much lower, presented a less confusing picture. Of the 339 listed in 1831, 248 were working, 91 were on half pay and only 45 were unfit for sea duties.

A surgeon's pay was ten shillings a day, rising in steps to 18 shillings after 20 years. Yet in 1831 only 43 men had clocked up 20 years of full-pay service; most surgeons had drawn a full salary for fewer than 15 years. Half pay and pension rights were determined by length of full-pay service: until 1840, however, only three years' time as an assistant could be carried forward for such calculations. Assistant surgeons earned 6/6d a day and had no half-pay entitlement until, after two years, two shillings was allowed. As a new assistant, Michael Cowan confided what he thought of that in 1856: 'I am almost ashamed to write 2/- it is so disgraceful.'[6]

In an attempt to reduce the surgeons' list, in 1833 Burnett proposed a commutation scheme whereby the Admiralty would offer 164 half-pay surgeons, who were unlikely to be needed again, a moiety of their half pay for life in return for the navy releasing them from any call to duty. This would leave them free to set up openly in private practice, though Burnett knew from complaints received from some civil practitioners that a number of half-pay surgeons already worked privately, albeit in breach of regulations. The Board deferred a decision. It did, however, support Burnett's wish to tighten the rules on incapacity by requiring all surgeons claiming ill-health when appointed to a ship to appear for medical examination. In May 1834 Burnett returned to the Board with his commutation scheme, enquiring why the navy maintained a list of around 400 surgeons fit for duty when only 177 were needed. At this point he was allowed to send letters to try to gauge how many half-pay surgeons would agree to the deal. The answer, he reported in January 1835, was 54 – a potential annual saving of £3,000. His scheme was eventually adopted in 1838.[7]

When salaries were reviewed in 1840 no significant increases were allowed. The basic pay for surgeons rose to 11 shillings a day but 18 shillings remained the upper limit. At the most senior levels, Inspectors received £1-11-6d and Deputy-Inspectors £1. The rates were slightly higher when working at naval hospitals; there were also small revisions for those afloat approved in 1843, although not implemented until 1848. In 1846 Burnett counted 184 surgeons employed with a further 50 available. There were also five Inspectors and 13 Deputy-Inspectors on active service. These were sufficient numbers for peacetime, Burnett assured the Admiralty, although the Board should bear in mind that between 30 and 40 surgeons were always seconded to emigrant or convict vessels. The problem lay with assistant surgeons, of which, Burnett argued, there should never be fewer than 25 in reserve. This, however, appeared an almost ridiculous aspiration: in 1846 he had four assistants unplaced and only two applicants awaiting interview. Pay was poor when contrasted with what those fortunate enough might earn in successful private practice, while even students contemplating public service would reflect on what the army had to offer.

The army had long suffered a grim reputation among medical students – and justly so. Army surgeons and mates were treated more like servants than professional men, while conveyance and treatment of the wounded at the hands of often poorly trained staff cost many lives. Warfare in the late eighteenth century had exposed those flaws. Thousands of soldiers died from fevers in the West Indies in the 1790s and at the time of the disastrous Walcheren Expedition to the Low Countries in 1809 students from the London hospitals had to be sent across the Channel as emergency dressers.[8] Yet the army proved capable of reform and its medical service was gradually overhauled during the Napoleonic Wars. In 1810 a specific army medical department was created with a permanent Director-General to replace the previous medical board with its part-time members. The old array of surgeons, apothecaries, purveyors and mates was replaced by standard ranks of Inspector, staff surgeon, regimental surgeon and regimental assistant. By 1831 disparities between army and navy pay were obvious. Whereas a naval surgeon of less than six years' standing earned ten shillings a day his army counterpart received 13 shillings. At almost every level army pay and half pay were higher and an army surgeon could count all time as an assistant towards his half-pay and pension calculations. Attached to permanent regiments rather than being dependent on commissioned ships, army surgeons were more likely to be constantly employed. They were also usually promoted sooner. Despite an Order in Council in 1840 recommending parity within the armed forces, even by 1855 nothing had happened.[9]

All this was common knowledge. 'There is not the same degree of stimulus in the medical schools for the naval service which formerly existed,' Burnett warned the Admiralty in 1837.[10] He warned again in 1846 that the dissatisfaction felt by many recruits was 'communicated to the professors and students of the schools by former students after they have entered the navy'.[11] But it went well beyond pay: although the 1805 Order in Council promised parity of rank between army and naval medical officers this had not been implemented. Lethargy, parsimony and the sheer size of the navy combined to make change a slow and halting process. Entrenched attitudes among admirals and many captains also contributed. Sir Thomas Hardy, who dominated the Board in the early 1830s, was certainly felt to be one case in point. 'Hardy I have reason to believe is a great enemy of the Medical Department,' Burnett reflected in 1838.[12] Another prominent example was Rear-Admiral Thomas Cochrane, who in 1841 took exception to 'the airs the army medical men give themselves' and seemed resolved that such behaviour should not spread.[13] Surgeons were not fighting men. It therefore went against the grain for many captains to respect them as officers.

Assistant surgeon William Bayne expressed his frustration at all this in 1837. He had just helped to suppress an outbreak of fever aboard *Madagascar* off Jamaica, for which he had been widely complimented. He loved the navy yet was tired of having to mix with those aboard so much his junior and railed against 'the arrogance and imbecility of men holding the power of granting promotions to us'.[14] Burnett urged the Admiralty to enforce the 1805 regulations and give assistant surgeons the same wardroom status as full surgeons had acquired. This general lack of regard meant that too many medical officers found themselves the butt of pranks and insults. Robert Guthrie, even as full surgeon in 1828, recorded how he nearly suffered a serious accident when a boisterous midshipman tried to push him off the poop deck. 'I reproved him severely, though, in presence of the captain, who took no notice.'[15] The most visible sign of a young medic's lowly status was his lack of proper accommodation. By the 1830s surgeons would usually have their own cabins where they could retreat from rowdy youths and perhaps continue with their studies. In 1846 ships were ordered to fit up an area to which mates, second masters and assistant surgeons could retire, and where they might mess together with midshipmen and cadets, but still no individual cabins were provided.

In fairness to the navy, accommodation on cramped vessels was seldom easy. Other grievances, however, merely required a change of regulations. Principal among these in the early nineteenth century was the lack of a proper uniform for assistant surgeons. This had also been stipulated in 1805 but again without result. For want of such display, medics sometimes suffered the indignity of being mistaken for engineers 'and persons of that description'.[16] With a distinctive uniform came respect and a salute, such

as even the most junior army doctor received. Uniforms were still a topic
for representation in 1855 when the Admiralty was asked if some gold lace
could be added to sleeves commensurate with the stripes worn by executive
officers. Nevertheless these standing complaints regarding pay, pensions,
status, accommodation and uniforms could be eclipsed at times by the
more immediate aggravations built into the day-to-day terms of employment. Many of these stemmed from the erratic nature of sea service whereby
no ship might be available when work was needed, yet at other times an
appointment was given with immediate effect when personal circumstances
made a spell on half pay desirable. Prolonged absences from home and
family were part of any sailor's life. The medical corps, however, also risked
material losses disproportionate to their modest stipends if costly books
and equipment were lost in bad weather, accidents or shipwrecks. Where
there was no neglect and where proper documentation could be produced,
compensation was allowed: £36 and £15 respectively for the instruments of
surgeons and assistants was paid until 1842 when Burnett switched to a
system whereby the Medical Department provided replacement sets, since
the cost of a surgeon's tools had fallen to £27. The Board enquired in 1843
about appropriate cover for books lost or damaged. Burnett avoided a direct
answer on the grounds that no two surgeons would probably ever agree
what constituted sufficient works of reference but thought that up to £12
might be allowed. This was increased to £20 for full surgeons in 1849.

Assistant surgeons started to become anxious on another issue after
about five years at sea – promotion. For this, passing a further examination
at the Royal College of Surgeons was the *sine qua non*, but thereafter chance
had a role to play. A good service record and the Director-General's timely
recommendation at the Board were crucial; how to acquire the Director-
General's favour was, of course, the difficulty. Support from commanding
officers was important; indeed, station chiefs could raise a man to acting
surgeon, pending referral to London. Needless to say, favouritism might
play a part. Rear-Admiral Phipps Hornby, for example, was clearly a valuable sponsor. The First Lord, Sir Francis Baring, assured him in 1849 that
'I have just directed the promotion of assistant surgeon Anderson, of whom
you have spoken highly.' Baring had plucked his name 'from among very
many very deserving competitors'.[17] Most young medics worried that their
efforts would not attract attention and that they would remain unknown at
Somerset House, save as names on the payroll and on ships cruising peace-
fully on the other side the world. The fate of John Palmer in 1854 was every

assistant's nightmare: 'Who is Mr. Palmer?' Burnett enquired on receiving a
letter.[18] Palmer was by no means alone. Assistant surgeons, after passing the
examination and years of reliable service, understandably became demor-
alized when held at a grade beneath that merited by their experience. In
consequence, some left the service just as they were becoming most useful.

One thing guaranteed attention at the Admiralty and would single out
any young man – distinguished service under enemy fire. Unfortunately
there were few opportunities for this between Trafalgar and Jutland.
Some medics nevertheless found themselves in the right place at the right
time. Promotions followed Navarino in 1827. In 1840 all five of the eligible assistants at the capture of St Jean D'Acre were elevated, with three
more promoted as soon as they returned home and passed the examination.
Serving in the River Paraná in 1845–46 was another opportunity: under
Argentine cliff-top batteries at Vuelta del Obligado, James Gallagher in
Dolphin was wounded while performing surgery. The ship's clerk, who was
helping him, was killed by his side, yet Gallagher went on calmly with his
operations regardless of the danger. Two other assistants were promoted for
work that day. William Dalton was promoted in 1846 when he rescued a
sick boy as *Lizard* was sinking. George Goldwin was commended in 1850
for his coolness and gallantry while on boat service at Sumatra, 'he being
several hours under the enemy's fire', the citation ran, 'and also as to his
kindness to the sick'.[19]

To ensure such recognition many assistant surgeons were neither slow
to bring heroics to the navy's notice nor to try to get a posting where
fortune might smile upon them. John McIlroy, for instance, did not want
to go to the South America station in 1830 'where promotion rarely occurs'.
'Appoint me to a station where promotion is more certain,' he protested.[20]
John Murphy sent in a glowing testimonial from the president of a local
board of health in Jamaica extolling his work during the island's 1851 cholera epidemic. External praise was one indicator of merit. Another was the
promotion of executive officers in any action where an assistant surgeon had
been present. William MacLeod pressed his claim on this ground in 1853.
Sent in with marines and gunboats to attack pirates on the coast of Borneo
six years earlier, MacLeod noticed how two lieutenants were subsequently
raised to commander, two mates to lieutenant, a senior second master
promoted and even the senior clerk aboard upgraded. Why not the assistant
surgeon too? After the engagement he had to help upwards of 400 officers and men affected by fever. Burnett acknowledged that MacLeod had

a strong claim, as did John Hamilton who had served in the same expedition. Hamilton pressed his case in 1855 when he reminded the Admiralty
of his subsequent three years on the West Africa station, his presence at
Bomarsund in the Baltic in 1854 and then at the capture of Sebastopol. As
it was, his papers were already before the Board. Hamilton was among a
good number of young medical officers, however, who apparently lacked
confidence in Admiralty procedures.

For the majority, graft and volunteering for arduous duties remained
the order of the day. Helping out amid epidemics on tropical stations, such
as those at Bermuda in 1843 and 1853 and that at Jamaica in 1855, covering for ill or exhausted colleagues on a sickly ship, and just having the
stamina to keep going when ships or hospitals were crowded with cases
of fever or contagious disease, all denoted commendable commitment.
Similarly enthusiasm to join expeditions into the great rivers of West Africa
or voyages of discovery in Arctic waters indicated a spirit of intellectual
enquiry and a wish to explore the limits of medical science. Humanitarian
work was also well received at the Admiralty: careful nursing beyond the
norms of medical treatment, stepping forward if at home to assist local
boards of health while cholera or smallpox raged in naval towns and when
famine took its toll in Ireland, or, most impressive of all, tirelessly tending
the unfortunates liberated from slavers captured off the coasts of Africa or
Brazil. Yet nothing was foolproof and Burnett acknowledged that his own
failure to recognize the efforts of some men had dogged their careers. When
Valentine Duke applied for progression from surgeon to Deputy-Inspector
in 1849 Burnett advised the Board apologetically that this case should have
come before it earlier. 'That Dr Duke has not received the promotion he
now craves, I must take some blame to myself in not before recommending
him.'[21]

Many of the same difficulties, then, bedevilled attempts to rise above
the rank of surgeon as frustrated efforts to join it from below. To ease the
bottleneck between surgeon and Deputy-Inspector, Burnett tried in 1847
to introduce a new grade – staff surgeon. This title would be conferred on
surgeons in charge of dockyards or the Portsmouth and Plymouth marine
infirmaries, those who were surgeon and storekeeper at naval hospitals
at home and overseas, those who were surgeons on flagships on foreign
stations and those in charge of hospital ships. They would all receive one
extra shilling per day, justified by the additional duties of gathering statistical data. This would only cost £529 a year, Burnett argued. The Board,

however, deemed the moment inopportune for such changes. Eight years later, the pressures of war emboldened Burnett to resurrect his idea and in 1855 it was approved. But whatever rank or position a medical officer aspired to, he generally had to work at achieving it and that might include lobbying at Somerset House. John Robertson subtly warned Burnett about his method of seeking new work if moved from his comfortable post at Pembroke dockyard in 1853: 'I have a great dislike to be obliged to be again about town canvassing for a further appointment and plaguing yourself and the Admiralty again on the subject.'[22] Michael Cowan gave thanks for his good fortune to be assistant surgeon aboard the impressive *Royal Albert* destined for the Black Sea in 1854. 'There were four who went up to the navy board when I went,' he confided, 'and they got appointed to small, scruffy vessels.' Cowan quickly learnt the ropes and therefore took matters into his own hands in 1862, in consequence of which he landed the plum position of assistant at the Portsmouth marine barracks where his wife could join him. Reading of the vacancy, he had rushed round to Somerset House and 'went to my friend Admiral Keppel who would have done anything to forward my prospects'. Then he contrived to bump into the Director-General. 'There were several candidates for the appointment,' he wrote to his brother, 'and had I not got wind of the situation from the newspaper I should have been done out of it.'[23] Cowan was lucky to be in London when the Portsmouth job arose. There had been little chance for his contemporaries stuck in men-of-war with growing sick-lists in the West Indies, the Bight of Benin, at Hong Kong or off Rio de Janeiro.

Yet the obvious qualities of many medical officers and their struggles for preferment could not conceal the fact that others were not up to the job. William MacDonald's service record in 1852 described him as being 'of weak intellect'; a year later he also had to be disciplined when 'his dirty appearance and absence of mind' required that he be withdrawn from his ship. William Graham kept his notes and journal tidily, Burnett observed sympathetically, 'though they do not show much ability'. Douglas Tucker was 'a very poor medical practitioner', the Director-General remarked in 1856, 'and he keeps his surgical journal like an illiterate man'.[24] Basic errors in either diagnosis or surgical procedures sometimes came to light. A sailor on *Viper* died in 1847 because his lung disease had not been recognized. 'I did not examine the back of the chest,' the medical officer later admitted. In 1852 Andrew Lithgow was reproached for taking no precautions to prevent debilitating shoulder stiffness after treating a fractured arm, while

Thomas Layton was cautioned for bungling a straightforward amputation. Layton's cut was poorly chosen, Burnett explained, since it was too far from the knee joint and left a long projecting stump. 'It was also wrong to leave the tourniquet screwed on the upper part of the limb which could not fail to lead to gangrene as it did – and the second operation was too long delayed to give a chance of saving the patient's life.' These were fundamental points in surgery and Layton should do all in his power 'to make yourself master of them'. The same was true of Samuel Webb on *Retribution* in 1854. Having lost a sailor after a delayed amputation, Webb was rebuked by way of Burnett's 'wish that Mr. Webb had been better grounded in surgical principles'.[25]

Other failings, even if less dire, might be accompanied by a string of semi-plausible excuses. Executive officers embarrassed or over-zealous in their duties and sailors indifferent to their health refused to report sick, or else delayed so long that remedy had become impossible. Vital information about the patient's condition and habits was withheld. Noise on board made the use of stethoscopes difficult. Supplies of medicated wine promised in London arrived too late on distant stations. Ships collecting invalids refused to embark the medications and comforts necessary for the long homeward voyage. Surgeons themselves had been too ill to attend to patients as they would have wished. Though many such explanations were genuine, not all were convincing. It was easy to express surprise at the sudden death of a seaman, which was why details of symptoms and treatments were always required. Modern science might also create problems. When the gunner on the troopship *Atholl* died from the effects of chloroform during a simple finger amputation in 1850 the two doctors aboard indignantly insisted that there was nothing wrong with their supply. There must have been something wrong with the patient's lungs.

Deficient as clinical treatment might be on occasions, carelessness could equally endanger the lives of seamen. Surgeons had to decide not only how but also where to treat a patient once a ship was in reach of a naval hospital. The purser from *Devastation* died in 1844 because he had not been sent ashore at Malta, despite the urgency of his case being communicated by the hospital to the ship's surgeon. The carpenter of *Nimrod* was likewise kept aboard too long before being transferred to the hospital at the Cape of Good Hope in 1847. Ships in the Tagus in 1850 were guilty of the same neglect. In their defence, ships' surgeons would invariably point out that moving sick or wounded men was always fraught with the dangers arising from rough handling or bad weather. When the hospital ship *Belleisle* admitted several serious cases at Hong Kong in 1859 its surgeon had no doubt as to why two of them had died within hours: 'the fatigue attend-ant on moving these men from the one ship to the other accelerated their end'.[26] Moreover naval hospitals themselves were not beyond reproach. Eager to discharge men once invalided, they sometimes bundled them on to a convenient warship and sent them home from warm climates when a few weeks' delay would have increased the chance of survival.

If ailing seamen could be neglected then there was little hope for medi-cal stores. In 1852 Burnett noticed how medicines were being returned from ships at Portsmouth; most had deteriorated 'from want of proper care'.[27] Difficult as storage conditions were on ships, rates of breakage and spoilage were sometimes unacceptably high. Problems also arose when stores and medicines were surveyed on being transferred from one surgeon to another. Junior medics could be imposed upon to sign for receipt without first checking. Frederick Crellin's experience on the South America station in 1846 revealed just how sloppy such procedures could be. It transpired that the squadron's supplies had just been passed on without question from one surgeon to the next for as long as anyone could remember. The result was 'indescribable confusion'. Jars and bottles had lost their labels, some were only half full, and other stuff was simply missing with the accounts fudged accordingly. Crellin's predecessor attended the British legation at Rio de Janeiro and many of the missing supplies had probably finished up there.[28]

But it was not just maintaining standards of medical practice and administration within the service that Burnett had to worry about. Medical officers also got into trouble for a variety of reasons. Some went missing. Christopher Schumacker, for instance, was eventually struck off the assist-ants' list in 1842, 'he not having been heard of since 1831'.[29] Constantine Conyngham jumped ship at Montevideo in 1839, excusing himself on the grounds that he had inherited an estate nearby. 'Yet I strongly suspect that he has entered into private practice,' Burnett remarked.[30] Edward Staples was refused employment in December 1852 because in 1851 he had left his previous position unannounced and sailed to New York with his family. William McClure wrote from Maidstone's debtor prison to apologize for any delay in his availability. He hoped to be out in a few weeks. James Henry, surgeon of *Britomart*, was visited by a sheriff's officer while a patient at East Stonehouse and subsequently taken into custody for debt. Augustus Preston faced a claim of £1,600 in the early 1850s and was warned by his

solicitor that the creditor 'will arrest you before you sail'.[31] Preston was eventually released from Brighton gaol in 1854.

Behavioural problems were often induced by alcohol. Drink not only
impaired medical duties but involved medics in activities which brought
discredit upon the service. Aboard ship it was easy to fall into bad habits.
Discipline for drunken doctors was, in fact, routine. 'Nothing new here,'
Captain Alexander Milne reported to the First Lord in 1851 when the assistant surgeon from *Helena* was court martialled for drunkenness.[32] First
offences were usually overlooked or mildly chastised but most captains
considered that persistent inebriation required sterner action. A court
martial might dock a medical officer one year of service time, remove
him from his ship and put him on the lowest rate of half pay, or place
him at the bottom of the list for employment. Or it could expel him from
the navy. Disorder ashore risked the worst punishments. Sidney Bernard,
not even one year in service in 1849, over-indulged at Port au Prince and
became involved in a local brawl. A crowd gathered and he was then set
upon with sticks until soldiers appeared and led him away. Bernard pleaded
self-defence but neither the British consul-general at Port au Prince nor
the court martial saw it that way: he was dismissed from the service for
being drunk and disorderly. David Campbell, ashore from *Racehorse* at the
Cape in 1854, was another embarrassing case. He had become so legless
that friends left him lying in the road, following which he later urinated at
French officers who discovered him. Campbell got off with a severe repri-
mand, subject to a satisfactory conduct report in six months' time.

Punishments for drunkenness were usually out in the open. Those for
immorality were less commonly so and cases might be dealt with more
discreetly. Hospitals recorded the numbers of surgeons either dying from
or under treatment for syphilis. Contracting venereal disease was not
an offence but a cure at Haslar or East Stonehouse would take a medical officer off the duty list for up to six weeks. Syphilis and gonorrhoea
were usually contracted in the same locations as applied to ordinary seamen
but surgeons did sometimes have particular opportunities. Convict ships,
especially those for females, provided a temptation too far for some. Even
if prisoners were not involved, other women on the ship might distract a
surgeon from his duty – as emerged at a court martial in 1854 when Harvey
Morris was accused, while repeatedly drunk, of attempting 'to seduce the
wives and daughters of some of the pensioners'.[33] Morris was barred from
further work on convict or emigrant vessels. Other cases required even

more delicacy. James Booth was dismissed as surgeon in 1832 'for frequently spending his evenings in the midshipmen's berth & etc'. He was later rein-stated, albeit downgraded to assistant, in 1836. Burnett took a worldly view: the punishment was 'sufficient for his fault'.[34]

Whether courts martial were fair to medics was a matter of opinion. Many felt that in any dispute involving executive officers the latter always found in favour of each other unless overwhelming testimony could be produced. James Campbell certainly believed this in 1850, appealing that 'my conviction was entirely prejudiced, nor was there the slightest attention paid to the evidence in my favour'.[35] Medical officers resented charges of insubordination which arose when executives behaved in a high-handed or even preposterous manner. Courts martial could also be trying experiences for junior men when called as witnesses to the alleged shortcomings of their seniors. Richard Picken protested in 1856 that he was given a bad report by the senior surgeon at the Hong Kong hospital because of his unavoidable participation in various enquiries into the way in which the establishment had been run.

On a routine basis, surgeons caused Burnett most anxiety over the way in which their journals were kept and over the irresponsible issue of, and sometimes fraud concerning, medical stores. Fraud was hard to prove even when accounts did not add up. Surgeons were good at excuses for why their ships required extra allocations of preserved meat, quinine wine and band-ages – all items, of course, with commercial value. Inadequate accounts would be questioned, such as those for the Jamaica hospital in 1845. Who had recently ordered 20lbs of arrowroot, Burnett enquired, when 461lbs were already in store? And why had this 'amazing surplus' been accumu-lated?[36] In the same year William McDermott on *Albion* was asked to account for six bottles of fever drops when he had reported so few cases. Fysher Negus's returns in 1853 likewise showed no correlation between the illness recorded in his sick-book and the large amounts of wine dispensed. The same applied to John Crawford's accounts while cruising in Australian waters in 1849–50: considerable quantities of 'good porter' were expended yet the comparatively few cases on his sick-list suffered from nothing for which this item was appropriate.[37] Confronted with the same disparity in 1854, James Harvey attributed everything to unfortunate breakages and to the need to administer it to all new recruits in the tropics. James Taylor on Ascension Island put his abnormal losses of wine down to evaporation. Casks nominally containing six and one-eighth gallons had only one and a

half gallons, he protested. 'I disbelieve entirely that it could have been occa-
sioned by evaporation,' Burnett retorted.[38]

Surgeons' journals and case histories being essential not only as naval
records but as contributions to the advancement of science, Burnett took a
dim view when these were poorly presented or contained insufficient detail.
A good surgeon, needless to say, added to his journal throughout the voyage
and recorded the topography, climate, natural history and culture of the
places visited as well as detail about the physical qualities of the inhabitants
and their common diseases. Some journals were impressive investigations;
for an assistant, good journals could weigh well in the balance for promotion. Most surgeons, though, either took a few notes occasionally or left the
whole exercise until the last minute. 'Wonderfully idle,' Alexander Mackay
noted as his ship prepared to leave Montevideo in 1858. 'Have not done a
thing to my journal, which is now overdue. I shall have it all up, however,
on the homeward passage.' Mackay could afford to be confident: he had
recently won the Blane Medal, awarded annually since 1832 for outstanding journals, for meticulous study during his years in the Antipodes. But
even so accomplished a performer could not always tie loose ends together.
'Find that my quarterly nosologicals very much disagree with my annual
accounts,' he observed: 'Can't be helped.'[39] A full record of all that had
happened since a ship had been commissioned might serve a medical officer
well in another respect. So thorough had the assistant surgeon's account of
fever aboard *Sidon* been in 1851 that Burnett was able to convince the Board
that the commanding officer's complaint about measures taken to contain
the disease had been 'unfortunate'.[40]

഼

A surgeon went to sea equipped with a variety of differently sized jars and
bottles, all containing the powders, tinctures and other ingredients necessary for compounding medicines and providing comforts for the sick. Jars
were numbered according to an established coding and were packed into
layered medical chests made up and stored in the home hospitals. Chests
came in four sizes. A number one chest contained sufficient for 300 men.
Number two was for crews above 150, number three for a crew of 75 and
number four for small vessels with a complement of 40. The ship's destination would determine which ingredients would be most in demand and the
incidence of sickness and rate of mortality to be expected. Between 1825
and 1845 mortality from disease on the South American station averaged

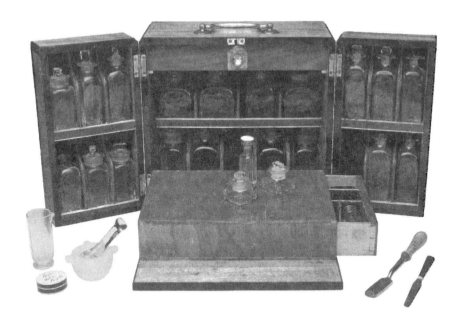

1. Medical chest: *c.*1801.

7.7 men per thousand. In the Mediterranean it was 9.3, in home waters 9.8, in the East Indies the figure rose to 15.1 and in the West Indies to 18.1. Off the coast of West Africa, however, it was 58.4 per thousand; in 1829, 202 men died there from total crews of 729 on just seven vessels, with 110 deaths among a crew of 160 on one ship alone. Individual ships might also gain reputations for being unhealthy. Surgeons speculated why, but in the early nineteenth century the reasons frequently lay beyond the limits of scientific knowledge. Disease might stem from filth in the hold or from the bilge water. In the tropics, mosquitoes breeding in the tanks holding drinking water as likely as not explained the prevalence of sickness on many warships.[41]

After 1815 the naval medical service perforce became increasingly preoccupied with tropical diseases, diet, venereal afflictions, alcohol-related illness and with general issues of health, hygiene and physical comfort afloat. In some respects this represented a reversion to the concerns of surgeons a century earlier. Indeed most ailments and even many treatments would have seemed familiar to doctors in the age of Cook. Even scurvy still appeared from time to time, as in the River Plate squadron between 1845 and 1847 and in the Black Sea off Varna in 1854. Lemon juice was known to be the answer but a surgeon was only as good as his supplies and the means of distribution. When the Admiralty sent samples made a year apart for analysis at Apothecaries Hall in 1837 and 1838 it was discovered that the juice was only two-thirds the strength it ought to be. For decades the Royal Navy had acquired its lemon juice from Sicily, where the crop was grown and its manufacture undertaken in accordance with supply contracts made at Malta. By the 1840s, however, a noticeable decline in quality was attributed to two failings. First, contrary to directions, the juice was casked and not bottled. Second, the dispenser at the Malta naval hospital had some years previously ceased to visit Messina to conduct inspections. A surgeon sent to Sicily in 1851 reported how 'the system between master and workman was radically bad' and that stipulating clean receptacles was regarded as interfering in the ways of local people.[42] Even so, Sicilian lemon juice was better than the cheaper limes from the West Indies used in the 1860s. Until then polar voyages had been comparatively free from scurvy; the 1875 Arctic expedition paid the price for the navy's attempt to economize.

Shorter voyages on steam-powered vessels also played their part in eliminating scurvy, and with transportation ended by the 1850s the last opportunity for the disease to show itself effectively disappeared. Alcohol, by contrast, continued to wreck the bodies of sailors and marines as it had always done despite efforts to control the problem. Limited experiments to substitute tea and cocoa for a portion of grog were conducted in 1823; within two years the daily rum ration was reduced from a half to a quarter-pint throughout the navy. Issuing beer was abolished in 1831. In 1850 the rum ration was again halved to only one-eighth of a pint; it was no longer distributed in the evening and money was paid in compensation.[43] Nevertheless, post-mortems frequently revealed organs destroyed by years of abuse. Seamen returning aboard might dump a senseless messmate on the deck in the hope that the surgeon could revive him, but as John Carruthers recorded on *Virago* at Piraeus in 1844 the revival sometimes never came. Carruthers used his stomach pump before administering aromatic substances and a restorative camphor mixture to one case. In desperation he applied friction and heat and then inflated the lungs with air. Carruthers could do no more, except to regret that 'I had not an electro-magnetic apparatus to assist us in rousing the nervous energy of the system.'[44]

Not only were seamen in port usually out of control but even on duty chance encounters with alcohol could cause problems. When boats from *Gladiator* captured a Brazilian slaver in 1850 two men from the boarding party disappeared below, having discovered the vessel's wine store. There they drank so much that when later exposed to the sun and wet they contracted fever and died. Most medical officers considered alcohol to be at the root of many cases on their sick-lists, either because it weakened resistance to other complaints, impaired the mind and moral character, led to knife-fights ashore or else caused accidents and brawls which even the discipline aboard ship could not always prevent. Maurice West was called to tend a man injured in a fist fight on the lower deck in 1842. Blood was erupting in jets from a severed artery inside the mouth which West could only stop by applying nitrate of silver and packing the wound with lint.[45]

Accidents with weaponry were routine for surgeons. Practice at great guns was a particular danger since a false discharge while loading could take off an arm. Men also crashed down from sails or rigging, fell overboard, or sometimes jumped when trying to desert. They were injured by heavy equipment and they tripped into holds where hatchways were left open. Paddle wheels were another death-trap. A stoker on *Hydra* in 1853 was struck while standing on a beam on the outside of the wheel and bending over to inspect it. No witness came forward, but the surgeon was in no doubt that this fatality was caused by 'the skylarking humour of the party in the port wheel who continued to turn round rapidly after the order was given to desist'.[46] Sailors impaled themselves on boat hooks or equally sharp objects; they might be crushed when casks in the hold or items on deck moved in rough seas, or when the wheel spun wildly in a storm, smashing the arms or faces of those trying to hold it. John McIlroy on *Persian* in the River Congo in 1841 was brought a man whose ankle joint had been torn open when the ship's pinnace went down. Several burly sailors had held him to prevent him being dragged under. McIlroy took the leg off straight away but the patient's suffering had been so great that he was too weak to save. On an otherwise uneventful voyage a surgeon might be able to devote long periods to tending unpromising cases – as when Charles Brien on *Cambrian* in 1848 saved a leg which had been so badly broken and lacerated that amputation seemed inevitable. Having reduced the swelling, he brought bone parts and tissue together using sutures, splints, plaster and bandages. After nearly three weeks he reported triumphantly that 'the distance between the fragments of bone is less than one inch and there is every prospect of the patient ultimately having a very good, if not perfect use of the limb'.[47] Most surgeons would have taken the easy option.

Steamers, of course, increased the incidence of burns. Fire and powder had always been hazards on men-of-war but exploding boilers and ruptured pipe-work were new and terrifying. Robert Clarke, surgeon on *Conflict*, rushed to one such disaster in 1852. Four stokers died when engulfed in steam and boiling water, but not, he regretted, quickly enough. Clarke watched the men dragged from the engine room: 'they stood howling and writhing with agony. They were literally boiled alive.'[48] Other deaths involving burns might be less harrowing but no less graphic. Charles McArthur on *Rodney* in the Mediterranean in 1838 had two men killed by lightning at the masthead. 'The electric fluid appeared like a ball of fire,' McArthur explained, 'like the bursting of a bombshell.'[49] Other emergencies seemed more mundane. David Finlay on *Minden* at Plymouth in 1838 was presented with a carpenter who had just chopped off most of his hand. Tom Pepper, a krooman serving on *Actaeon* in 1846, collapsed from a blow to the abdomen during boxing training. Gloves had been worn, the surgeon noted, but death followed soon after. Seizures or apoplexy were frequently recorded. Lung complaints were usually phlegm, bronchitis or the onset of tuberculosis, while rheumatism, ulcers and itch had always been and remained common. Scrofula was another disease often seen among seamen, although glandular swellings were sometimes plague. Cholera likewise might be brought aboard in any warm climate. Mental disturbances posed problems when violent patients needed restraint or constant observation. Others might be simply deluded, as was the purser's steward on *Lily* in 1843 who believed he had been called as a prophet and healer. When threatened with punishment he embraced it as evidence of God's purpose that he should suffer for the sake of all. Even true men of God were not spared. The chaplain on *Melampus* in 1846 professed his own madness while sinking into a state of incoherent sobbing, convulsed with fits of maniacal excitement. These were admittedly tell-tale signs, the surgeon concluded, but what clinched the diagnosis of insanity was seeing the chaplain cast his own sermons into the sea. Whether they were bad sermons or not, there was no telling what he might do next.

Digestive disorders, generally listed as dyspepsia, along with dysentery and diarrhoea also featured regularly in the returns of surgeons afloat and from those at naval hospitals. As with cholera, bowel complaints were often brought on to a ship with the water supply, although many explanations of these diseases laid emphasis on climatic conditions and on sailors being constantly wet. Poisonous fish, excessive or unripe fruit and cucumbers also came in for criticism. Although dysentery and cholera took the lives of many seamen, most cases, after being kept warm and given calomel, opium, castor oil or enema, were expected to recover. Far more worrying was an outbreak of fever aboard, though with so many varieties to choose from medical officers could be forgiven for not knowing exactly what to diagnose. There was jungle, coast, bilious, brain, ardent, intermittent, remittent, and yellow fever, and no consensus about the causes or whether fevers were infectious or contagious. In 1847 the Medical Department ended this confusion by allowing only the three headings of remittent, intermittent and yellow to be used. Miasma from rotting vegetation up rivers or along a swampy shoreline were usually cited as locations of origin, while arduous boat duty in the tropical sun or the heat of an engine room made men particularly vulnerable. New arrivals on tropical stations were believed to be most at risk. A yellow fever epidemic, above all, was every surgeon's nightmare. The most notorious episode was on *Eclair* in 1845, carrying 146 officers and men bound for West Africa. Yellow fever eventually killed 74 of her crew.[50]

Faced with an epidemic, a ship could either try to outrun the disease or evacuate ashore. Vice-Admiral Sir William Parker reluctantly prepared his Mediterranean squadron for sea in September 1849 after eight men had died from among 60 afflicted. 'The change of air will be I trust favourable to our fever cases,' he wrote to the First Lord. 'The medical men are of opinion it is not contagious.'[51] Rear-Admiral Barrington Reynolds likewise took his ships to sea after yellow fever appeared while they were at anchor at Rio de Janeiro in 1851. By sailing south fatalities had been limited, he reflected, and many of those ill were clearly rallying. Alexander Woodcock, surgeon on *Dauntless*, advised evacuation at Barbados in 1852. Seventy-seven men had already died and while the remainder of the crew were on dry land the bilges could be cleaned and stoves used to remove dampness. This often involved a thorough aspersion with disinfecting lime or a solution of zinc chloride and then keeling the ship five or six degrees each way before pumping it out.

Syphilis and gonorrhoea brought many seamen to the sick-bay. Advanced syphilis invariably led to invaliding as men became no longer fit for duty. Normally, however, sores and eruptions were washed and dressed with a diluted disinfectant, iodine or caustic lotion. The standard treatment was mercury-based calomel – indispensable in the minds of most early and mid-nineteenth century doctors, although already questioned by some as being a cure worse than any disease. Mercury, to the point of salivation, was widely held to purge the body. It was also widely used in fever cases, although again not without dissenting voices. One of those was Alexander Bryson, whose opposition to mercury was based on his experience off West Africa in 1831. Of 37 men treated, 27 died and all but two of the remainder had to be sent back to England. 'A more dismal result could hardly have taken place if "bark and wine" had been employed from first to last, or even if the patients had been left to nature,' Bryson lamented.[52] Charles Linton, in charge of the naval hospital at Jamaica in 1838, however, swore by its benefits. So too did John Sole, cruising off the coast of Brazil aboard *Express* in 1856. Despite having 100 cases of yellow fever aboard he had lost only 13 men. Eleven others went to hospital. By using calomel he had cured 76.[53]

Treating the diseases of sailors and marines was often difficult enough. The health of commanding officers, however, could present surgeons with particular problems. Too much wine, poor diet and anxiety about their reputations as natural leaders often underlay the nervous and digestive afflictions for which captains commonly summoned the doctor. Lieutenant Edward Harvey, commanding *Wizard* in 1838, knew that he was ill but when advised by assistant surgeon William Methven would consent to nothing which made him appear unfit for promotion. 'I was obliged to give up treatment,' Methven reported apologetically: 'I can only say that I could not force a man against his will.'[54] Harvey's case was not exceptional. Lieutenant George Fortescue died from fever in 1838, his condition exacerbated by ignoring his surgeon's protest that he should not walk the deck. Vice-Admiral Charles Paget also died of fever in the West Indies in 1839 after ignoring entreaties to take sufficient nourishment; his surgeon concluded that he thereby 'threw away the only chance left'.[55] Captain James Polkinghorne died at Barbados in 1839 and Captain Thomas Eden in Central America in 1850, both ignoring their surgeons' pleas that they were too weak to venture ashore. Commander Charles Bell was so ill as to fall overboard and drown off New Zealand in 1844. Reporting the case, assistant surgeon John Veitch assured Burnett that 'nothing that I could urge would prevail on him to invalid'.[56] Not only did officers frequently refuse guidance; station commanders too could be reluctant to send home a good captain who wished to stay with his ship.

Awkward as many commanding officers might be regarding physical afflictions, a surgeon's position was even more uncertain when mental faculties were questioned. Commander George Wolrige was understandably agitated when his ship ran aground in 1853. Indeed he was so distressed that he began taking all sorts of potions for a range of imaginary illnesses, subsequent to which, and unable to rest or eat properly, he died from fever. But Wolrige was never unfit to command, despite fits of crying and occasional hysteria. Lieutenant Nathaniel Knott in the River Plate in 1845–46 likewise became anxious and eccentric, reading out his private letters to all who could not escape in time. But at what point was he certifiable? One indication, assistant surgeon Robert Clarke judged, was when Knott decided that his orders to enforce a blockade at Buenos Aires meant that he was to sail into the port. Knott was duly invalided for insanity in March 1846. The captain of *Harrier* died at sea in 1839 having first suffered from imbecility. Commander Roger Curtis on *Locust* manifested madness by turning on his surgeon in 1851. The senior officer agreed that Curtis's mind had completely gone, but so violent did Curtis become at the sight of the doctor that all treatment and advice had to be conveyed via junior officers or the commander's servants. Curtis was eventually removed from his ship by the Commander-in-Chief, South America, just a few days before he died.

Whereas a captain would be prescribed for in his cabin, ordinary seamen would make a visit to the cockpit if they wished the benefit of medical opinion. There the surgeon would receive and nurse the sick, keep his stores and instruments and maintain his dispensary. Cockpits were often hot and crowded; in the tropics they could be unbearable. William Aitken, on *Atholl* in 1827, described how it was impossible to make up mixtures or pills 'without the perspiration falling on the medicine'.[57] Robert Guthrie, in the Indian Ocean in 1828, was likewise drenched in sweat every time he entered while the sick were fainting as they waited his attention. Events at Navarino in 1827 suggested that not much had altered since Nelson's day. When midshipman Henry Codrington, son of the Commander-in-Chief, was wounded on *Asia*, he soon discovered the horrors of battle. In intense heat he had to grope his way in the dark to an unoccupied spot to wait his turn. Mess tables were laid out on top of chests and then covered with bedding. All around him men lay groaning or crying out for the surgeon.[58] *Asia* had 75 men killed or wounded. *Genoa* was another ship in the firing line at Navarino where sailor Charles McPherson also witnessed conditions below as he conveyed a wounded officer. The surgeon and assistants amputated and bound up wounds amid 'a horrid scene of misery'. In the dim light he could see the figures of medical officers 'their bare arms and faces smeared with blood, the dead and dying all around'.[59] Even in a gale or with the lurch of a ship in heavy seas, lives might be lost while medics scrambled around to retrieve their instruments and find their bandages because cockpits were not adequately fitted. Proper facilities arguably mattered more on a ship than in a hospital, since a surgeon at sea could not turn elsewhere for professional advice. He had to be more self-reliant than other medical men; his cockpit was vital for making that possible.

Naval surgeons were certainly required to be ingenious. Maurice West recorded how he saved a man whose legs were almost taken off by a shark while bathing off East Africa in 1844. West and his assistant struggled to secure blood vessels by the evening light on the quarterdeck, adding candles as required. 'The breeze caused the candles to flicker,' West later remarked, 'notwithstanding the erection of screens.'[60] Edward Cree, with *Vixen* fighting pirates off the coast of Borneo in 1845, had to remove an arm at the shoulder joint. The deck was crowded with excited onlookers while he and two assistants worked by the light of half a dozen candles. The patient survived, though small thanks to the circumstances in which he had been treated: 'One had no choice,' Cree recorded.[61] Robert Bankier, on a hospital ship at Hong Kong in 1846, was called upon to operate in similar adversity. A sailor whose thigh had been deeply gashed and who had lost much blood was carefully bandaged; hours later, however, it became obvious that the source of the bleeding had not been discovered, which Bankier deduced must be an artery retracted into damaged tissue. Pressure on the groin failed to staunch the flow, and, with a sturdy assistant's thumb alone standing between life and death, Bankier realized that he would have to open the leg and look for the leak. By this time swelling had made a tourniquet impossible to apply, while damaged nerve endings were in danger of being sewn into his repair. With a dying sailor and with night approaching, Bankier gambled on extending his incision to the groin where he finally found and tied the artery. 'It was necessary to remove him from one side of the hospital deck to the other, in order to gain light enough to perform the operation,' Bankier wrote to Burnett. Though an awkward and eccentric individual, Bankier justified his reputation as a brilliant surgeon. The patient returned to duty within a month and with 'complete power in left lower extremity'.[62]

Beyond their craft as practitioners, surgeons had a preventive role to play. That, after all, was the surest way to keep down the sick-list. Yet while an initial survey at the quayside might weed out those demonstrably unfit to enlist, the threshold for fitness could be low. The wretched backgrounds of many recruits brought up with low standards of diet and hygiene meant that medical officers spent much of their time trying to overcome deficiencies brought into rather than acquired during naval service. Not surprisingly, therefore, many sailors benefited from the navy's discipline, regular times, physical work and medical supervision. William Jones, surgeon of *President* in 1848, explained that by going to sea they could escape the foul air which so much of Britain's population breathed. The stinking alleys and polluted workshops where the poor lived and laboured contrasted with the bracing, pure air which filled a sailor's lungs: 'it is for them, not for us, not for the fortunate and free, that sanitary laws are needed'.[63] Perhaps Jones exaggerated but he was by no means alone. William Guland, surgeon on *Victory* at Portsmouth where new men were held in 1853, witnessed a transformation within weeks of enrolment. Boys in particular underwent a noticeable change 'and from a thin, sparse appearance soon become stout, healthy, robust lads'.[64] Executive officers ensured physical activity and the daily routine but diet was more within the remit of the doctor.

Surgeons at sea were regularly required to conduct trials of preserved foods. It was likewise for them to advise whether men had been too long on salt rations or about any other deficiency in provisions. They were also expected to be vigilant for more mundane hazards. When this involved scientific enquiry to discover why men had fallen ill, most were happy to oblige. But merely checking that pots and pans were washed required no professional judgement and medics usually objected to being used as elementary cleaning supervisors. A surgeon's duty was done when the medical implications of filthy galleys, infested water tanks, excessive damp, inadequate clothing and unwashed bedding were pointed out to executive officers. It was a captain's responsibility to enforce regulations. Indeed there were limits to what any surgeon could say, as William Kerr, surgeon on *Hound* at Port au Prince, discovered in 1849. When his captain ordered lime juice to be issued to flagging sailors Kerr presumed to contradict him by stating that the men were not ill but needed water on account of dehydration. He was promptly confined to ship until a compromise was struck whereby both liquids would be distributed.

Captains or admirals who interfered in medical matters were an

occupational hazard and Kerr's experience was by no means unique. In
1827 William Aitken objected to the draught of salt water prescribed for
every man by his commanding officer on the grounds that it could bring
no benefit 'but would only create thirst, headache and griping pain of the
bowels'.[65] Thereupon he was humiliated before the whole ship's company
by being ordered to stand by the tub and dole it out. Vice-Admiral Francis
Austen refused William Graham permission to land five smallpox cases in
the St Lawrence in 1847 because he believed medical officers had overstated
their severity and ordered that the men be treated aboard instead. In the
cramped accommodation set up below deck to isolate the disease one man
died soon after. The Commander-in-Chief, South America, when inspecting a febrile boy on *Madagascar* in 1859 diagnosed him not so ill as the
surgeon had said. The boy died a few hours later. Captains and other officers moved sick and injured men to suit their own convenience and often
made no effort to preserve tranquillity around the sick-bay. Surgeons were
sometimes made to feel like nuisances, always looking to upset a ship's
routine. Robert Mungle, assistant surgeon on *Myrmidon* in 1852, made the
mistake of asking his commanding officer not to interfere with arrangements made for the care of men on the sick-list. Next time Mungle stepped
ashore he was arrested for leaving the ship without formal permission.

Whereas in northern climates it was essential to keep a vessel dry, in
the tropics good ventilation was just as essential to keep it cool. Yet the free
flow of air so necessary for health and comfort was frequently obstructed
by lockers, bins and fixtures, or by bulkheads which took no account of
air movement. Thomas Spencer Wells gave a graphic account of his time as
surgeon on *Modeste* in the Mediterranean in 1852 where 130 seamen lived,
cooked and slept on a lower deck 54 feet by 29 feet at its widest point and
with headroom of six and a half feet only between the beams. Chests,
mess-stools, tables, lengths of rope and the galley all vied for this area too.
Breathing space was thereby 'less than is secured to felons condemned to
imprisonment in any gaol' and officers who descended were seen to hurry
up again covering their mouths.[66] Hatchways on ships were often tied shut
against the weather, wind-sails were either useless or not regularly used,
ventilation funnels were too few and air pumps insufficiently employed.
When oppressively hot, and on a well-run ship, one watch might sleep
below while others messed under an awning on the upper deck. And what,
for every surgeon, was a well-run ship? John Goodridge on *Herald* in 1847
defined it as one where 'every attention had been paid to my suggestions'.[67]

Those suggestions might extend to curtailing shore leave, especially in ports where disease was rumoured to be rife. They might also include limiting corporal punishments, which by the 1830s were increasingly being condemned. A surgeon might put in a good word for a man known to be dim or otherwise meaning no harm by his offence in the hope of getting the number of lashes reduced. He had a right to intervene if a man was being flogged to death but otherwise a captain's authority, as always, could never be questioned. Experienced surgeons tended to believe that corporal punishment remained essential for naval discipline; in any case, liberal views soon vanished when there were thefts from medical supplies. Henry James, a young executive officer on *Wolf* in 1836, went further, asserting that firmly disciplined ships usually had the shortest sick-lists.[68] Surgeon Alexander Mackay watched a man 'very deservedly flogged' as late as 1858.[69] But Mackay was convinced that the navy had become more humane than in Nelson's day. In so far as doctors played any part in making it so, a great deal depended on the relationship established between an approachable commanding officer and a diplomatic practitioner.

Robert Guthrie hated his commander on *Seringapatam* and avoided him as much as possible. Called to the captain's cabin to perform an extraction in 1830, Guthrie recorded gleefully how he broke the tooth 'and put him to some pain'.[70] Robert Bankier was put under arrest and confined to the gun-room after a disagreement with the captain of *Herald* in 1842. Mackay, however, was much more fortunate. His captain threw a champagne party when news arrived that Mackay had won the Blane Medal; it was a generous gesture which Mackay later regretted with his splitting headache throughout the following day. But whereas the state of a crew might be the better maintained by a captain's sympathy, the state of the ship itself was not so easily altered. Newly built vessels often put to sea without their holds being properly cleared of debris, boiler rooms were breeding grounds for disease, while odours escaping from decomposing matter in the bilges could poison the air and prove difficult to overcome. On old vessels ports and hatchways no longer kept out bad weather and fittings were sometimes beyond repair. John Carruthers, on *Colossus* in 1855, had to tend men in a sick-bay awash from a water closet so defective as constantly to leak its contents on to the floor. Many ships were also overcrowded. In 1827 William Aitken found his medicines 'lying in the wet on the main deck' for want of anywhere to put them. As for his medical chest, he found people 'laying their clothes as they scrubbed them on the lid'.[71]

Predictably surgeons were quicker to express grievances than to offer thanks but some did acknowledge the help of executive officers and an appreciation of medical requirements. *Wasp* changed course in 1833 at its surgeon's request so that sick men could be taken off at Lisbon. When John MacLeod reported a fever case to the captain of *Hermes* at Rio de Janeiro in 1850 and recommended a cruise at sea the ship immediately broke off coaling and left port. Charles Anderson wrote with evident satisfaction from *Gorgon* that all his suggestions for clearing stores, moving water tanks, emptying holds, ventilating decks and using stoves had been attended to by an enthusiastic captain. Tact, personality, mixed with well-chosen and timely observations could usually achieve more than emphasizing naval regulations; the latter, after all, were for commanding officers to interpret and, for the officious among them, any implication to the contrary was but a short step from mutiny. When William Jones looked back on his many years at sea he recognized that the conditions in which medical officers worked, and even the successes which they might enjoy in keeping their rates of sickness and mortality low, owed as much to human qualities as to medical science and Admiralty orders. He had served on *Orestes* in the 1830s with a commander who seldom punished or spoke harshly and who attended to the needs of his crew regarding leave in port and entertainments by means of singing, dancing and theatre when at sea. He also sent comforts for those in the sick-bay. His crew was well behaved, worked well and was generally in excellent health. Was Jones just fortunate or had he been instrumental in bringing out the best in an old sea captain? Writing in 1847, Jones expressed no opinion about his own merits other than to say that fully two years had passed since any man had died whose life had been entrusted to his care.

CHAPTER 3

Opportunity and Adventure

W hen it came to recruitment, the service undoubtedly relied upon the restless spirit of many young men. Alexander Bell was one: 'a sea-going ship is what I desire most where I may have an opportunity to see something of the world'. Charles Prentice was candid in his application: 'I cannot contemplate without disgust the probability of being a mere provincial practitioner all my life, devoted to the comparatively trivial duties which such a position requires.'[1] Yet the navy was not just a chance to travel the globe; the world was a reservoir of scientific phenomena which might satisfy even the most voracious appetite for knowledge. Burnett encouraged contributions to mineralogy, geology, botany and climatology; indeed, when reporting on far-flung lands it was common for enthusiastic medical officers to excuse prolonged accounts for that reason. William Jones's survey of the Pacific island of Juan Fernandez in 1840 owed much to Burnett's 'anxious wishes of encouraging a degree of emulation and scientific lore among the medical officers of the Royal Navy'.[2] John Andrews's extensive investigation of agricultural opportunities on Ascension Island in 1849 was similarly inspired, as was Richard Mason's report on the climate, diseases and economic potential of Nicaragua ten years earlier. When possible, Burnett would extend periods of home leave for the completion of scientific work. He eagerly endorsed an offer from the Royal College of Surgeons in London to create two studentships in human and comparative anatomy in 1839; the College hoped that recipients, when properly qualified, might be found places in either the army or navy and expected its scholarships to produce good naturalists and botanists as well as good practitioners.

Collecting, identifying, depicting and preserving the wonders of nature became integral parts of many naval surgeons' careers. Meredith Gairdner exemplified those captivated by the intellectual opportunities on offer. He knew French, German and Italian, he assured Burnett in 1832, and was

devoted to research in natural science: 'One of my chief objects in wish-
ing to enter the navy is to have an opportunity of studying it with more
effect at the different foreign stations to which I might be sent.'[3] Benjamin
Bynoe was an avid naturalist while assistant surgeon on the survey vessel
Beagle during its voyages between 1826 and 1836, spending nine days on a
Galapagos island in 1835 studying rocks, lizards, tortoises and vegetation
with Charles Darwin.[4] John Robertson, surgeon on *Terror* in 1840, spent
much of his time collecting birds, animal skins and geological formations
in the Pacific and in Australian waters, all of which he sent home for exhi-
bition. William Chartres, on *Philomel* in 1843, undertook a study of life
on the bleak Falkland Islands. Lack of sufficient preserving materials had
curtailed the season's work, he noted disappointedly, but since the ship
would return next summer he hoped to finish the ornithological part of his
work. The hardy grasses of the Falklands might well thrive in more temper-
ate climates, Burnett wrote to Richmond: might not voyages and expeditions to the ends of the earth yet produce benefits for agriculture at home?[5]
Assistant surgeon William Alexander assembled a remarkable collection of
ferns and mosses while his ship was charting the China coast in the mid-
1840s. Surgeon James McWilliam's detailed account of the weather patterns
of Boa Vista in the Cape Verde Islands in 1846 was a meteorological tour de
force. Archibald Sibbald collected and examined mummies from the plains
of Arica when *Niaid* was off the coast of Chile in 1847. John Simpson,
surgeon with *Plover* in 1853, was a keen ethnographer who compiled a careful record of Eskimo culture and society in north-western Alaska. Seeds
and cones, stuffed creatures and natural relics of all descriptions made their
way home from around the world. And even when Burnett was not expect-
ing scientific curiosities, friends and colleagues frequently were. Sorting out
the fruits of his investigations during the long voyage back from Australia
in 1855, Alexander Mackay remembered that 'my scientific friends are looking out for all sorts of fine things from me. All I can say is I wish they may
not be disappointed.'[6]

   For the most dedicated, publications were the key to scientific recognition. In this respect, Sir John Richardson's record was remarkable.
Richardson became the navy's most renowned naturalist and an international figure following his North American travels and voyages of discovery
in polar seas between 1819 and 1849. His publications began with contributions on meteorology and solar radiation to the narrative of Captain John
Franklin's Arctic explorations between 1825 and 1827 and progressed with

four volumes describing the fauna of British North America between 1829 and 1837. He compiled the section on mammals for *The Zoology of Captain Beechey's Voyage* which appeared in 1839 and produced his two-volume *Arctic Searching Expedition* in 1851. In 1854 his study of North American vertebrae and fossil mammals formed part of *The Zoology of the Voyage of H.M.S. Herald*, while in the following year he was a major contributor on natural history to *The Last of the Arctic Voyages*. His final book, *The Polar Regions*, was completed in 1861.[7] Joseph Hooker, who went as assistant surgeon and botanist on the three Antarctic voyages of *Erebus* between 1839 and 1843, wrote a summary of the expedition for the book which followed.[8] Richard Hinds, attached as surgeon to Captain Sir Edward Belcher's explorations of Central America and Pacific waters on *Sulphur* between 1836 and 1842, edited the works on botany and zoology which appeared in 1844. Hinds established his academic credentials with text and illustrations for the second volume relating to molluscs.[9]

Outstanding as Richardson's career was, others in the medical service also acquired national reputations. Thomas Huxley, assistant surgeon from 1846 until resigning in 1854, was encouraged by Richardson during his initial appointment to Haslar and subsequently pursued research on molluscs, jellyfish and a variety of other sea life while on *Rattlesnake* in the Pacific and off Australia between 1846 and 1850.[10] William Baikie entered the navy in 1848, publishing a natural history of the Orkney Islands in the same year. He assumed overall command of an expedition aboard *Pleiad* in 1854 which explored 340 miles up the River Niger, a scientific account of which he published two years later.[11] This success led to another expedition in 1857, following which he remained in Africa as a trader and anthropologist until his death in 1864, acquiring thereby a considerable knowledge of local languages and cultures, the fruits of which he published in 1861. Yet, though attracting less public acclaim, for few young men did scientific dreams come true as for Arthur Adams who was allowed three years' leave in order to complete the copious plates and illustrations for the research conducted during Belcher's 1843–46 voyage aboard *Samarang*. The final work was expected to cover several volumes. Adams was assistant surgeon to the expedition and in 1847 reported enthusiastically that seven new genera and 52 new species of crustaceous animals had been registered at the British Museum – a larger addition to such scientific knowledge than attributed to any previous voyage. New species of fish and unknown mammals in Borneo had also been discovered. The project would probably involve production of monthly parts before the eventual appearance of a quarto edition which 'will do credit to the science of this country'. There were separate parts on fish, by Richardson, and on vertebrae, but beyond organizing so much material Adams wrote extensively on crustacea and molluscs while compiling a 150-page appendix on the natural history of the voyage and producing upwards of 300 drawings. He also kept up his medical studies, passing the examination for surgeon in 1848. Belcher's *Voyage of the Samarang* was published in 1848 although Adams's larger project continued. Not until July 1849 did he see light at the end of the tunnel, yet with undimmed enthusiasm and in appreciation of Burnett's indulgence he wrote to assure the Admiralty that he was more prepared than ever to accompany any further scientific expedition. By early 1850 Adams's comprehensive edition was being delayed only by the publisher who still awaited confirmation of a Treasury subsidy. At the end of the year Burnett noted Adams as being 'a most meritorious officer'. His work was at last out 'and is highly valued for its correctness'.[12]

When most surgeons or assistants wrote up their research pursuits, medical aspects tended to dominate. John Rees's account of the Sandwich Islands in 1839 touched on topography, climate and social customs but soon became an enquiry into the diet and health of the population, with an attempt to explain the gradual decrease in population by examining infanticide and abortion practices and the prevalence of syphilis. Robert Bankier collected considerable detail relating to the incidence of diseases among both sailors and the Chinese population when *Iris* was cruising between Hong Kong, Amoy and Chusan in 1844 and 1845. In 1848 Thomas Stratton reminded Burnett of his contributions to medical knowledge: he had published 27 essays and papers in the *Edinburgh Medical and Surgical Journal* in the past decade. In the 1840s Thomas Dunn and John Jenkins each reported extensively on diseases prevalent in Africa, while in 1864 Frederick Dickens, equipped with some knowledge of the language, used his time while assistant surgeon at the Yokohama sick-quarters to enquire into the incidence of smallpox among all sections of the Japanese population. Others were more opportunistic. One naval medic ashore at Chusan in 1842 diagnosed the high fever in an eight-year-old girl as originating with the ulcers and inflammation caused by foot-binding. He removed the bandaging on more than one occasion but every time it was replaced. Finding the girl one day dead in an unattended coffin, he quickly removed the feet in the interests of clinical study.[13]

When it came to bizarre experiences in the cause of science, few could hope to match those of William Kay while assistant surgeon on *Tyne* in the mid-1840s. Kay was a scholar and his *Rambles in Europe and the East* was a meticulous journal of his travels from Ireland to Gibraltar, Malta and Cyprus and then minute observations of society in Cairo and Jerusalem. His records of the topographies, climates, histories and cultures of the eastern Mediterranean were extensive. His tours in the Holy Land, his visits to the pyramids of Egypt, his careful sketches and paintings and his efforts to acquire linguistic skills to facilitate his pursuits were but part of the quest for learning which also led him to investigate the dangers to public health in Alexandria and the reasons for the epidemic fever which had swept Beirut in 1844. In 1813, he discovered, plague had carried away almost a thousand from among the city's then 15,000 inhabitants. Even so, the squalor and health hazards of Beirut were not to be compared to the appalling conditions he found on the Nile. The oddity of Kay's work, however, arose from a chance visit to the Emir of Brumana, who, after receiving him and exchanging the customary pleasantries, confided his fears for a beloved daughter and asked whether Kay could help. The assistant surgeon was at once ushered into the harem. 'Our approach was announced by a slave calling out in Arabic: "make way, make way",' Kay recalled. 'On entering I found some of the slaves exceedingly beautiful and engaged in various pursuits,' he continued. 'Here, one was embroidering a headdress; there, another was playing on a species of guitar and singing, accompanied by a third on the darabookheh, and all the rest clapping their hands and singing out a chorus of "Allah".' The girl was bed-ridden with chronic dyspepsia and anaemia but Kay sent her some medicines which he found in Beirut, advised on diet, and when he visited again a fortnight later found her much recovered and walking about in the harem to her father's obvious delight. It was all in a day's work for the Royal Naval medical service. Two months later Kay's patient was married to a local sheikh.[14]

For those enterprising, or perhaps just fortunate, secondment could open up opportunities that went beyond the limits of scientific curiosity and might even influence the conduct of public policy. When the Colonial Office needed a geologist for exploration in New Zealand in 1847 it turned to the Admiralty in the hope that, at little expense, a medical officer versed in mineralogy might be provided. None was to hand, though Burnett assured the Board that 'there are several distributed about in different ships who have some knowledge of the science'. Charles Forbes, an assistant surgeon of six years' standing, was eventually approached and seized his chance at once. Forbes was soon collecting the most favourable testimonials from naval captains and executive officers. His expertise, Burnett noted in 1848, 'will give him a good claim for promotion'.[15] Others acquired prominence, and Burnett's favour, for their interpreting skills. John Ternan, assistant on *Harpy*, was of great help with his Spanish when in the Paraná in 1846. Henry Johnson had been invaluable in the Pacific, speaking both French and Tahitian languages; it was a great pity, Burnett mused, that his name had to be erased from the assistant surgeons' list in 1849 on account of his having 'fallen into disgrace from intemperance'.[16] Much of the information concerning the prospects for an embryonic Australian settlement at Port Essington came from reports compiled by naval medical officers in 1839 and 1845, ultimately leading to the decision to abandon the site in 1849.[17]

Andrew Sinclair was seconded for colonial service for so long after 1844 that on his return to London in 1856 records had to be checked in order to discover what procedures had been agreed regarding his salary. Sinclair had dropped off the surgeons' list while acting as colonial secretary in New Zealand. Another unusual assignment arrived from the Foreign Office in 1857: could a surgeon be spared for attachment to the newly established consulate in Bangkok? The terms on offer from the Treasury were half pay plus £400 per annum; there might be accommodation, depending on when the building work in Bangkok was finished. Five surgeons were asked. Four declined, while James Campbell accepted on condition that his years in Thailand should be counted as sea service rather than secondment. That was too much for the Director-General to agree: the Treasury offer was already sufficiently generous. Campbell accepted anyway. For better or worse, it was probably the chance of a lifetime. Edward Irving realized his ambition of evangelical work when allowed to attend for three years a missionary expedition to the African coast in 1854. Edward Cree, surgeon from *Vixen*, though never formally seconded, clearly enjoyed his quasi-official role in 1843 when invited to make up the British party attending celebrations after ratification of the treaty of Nanking. Cree relished the late-night food and entertainment and roared at the spectacle of inebriated senior naval officers and Chinese mandarins spontaneously exchanging songs in a nascent karaoke session. It was not perhaps in the best traditions of the service but it was a great deal more exciting than his medical routine.[18]

Many young medics were drawn to the armed services by the same dangers and the chance of action so irresistible for their executive counter-parts. James Ayerst was so anxious for war service in the Baltic in 1854 that he tried to conceal his weakened health after seven years constantly at sea. A friend nevertheless advised Burnett that, though popular and respected aboard *Algiers*, Ayerst was in no state to work as the only assistant surgeon on a vessel carrying 900 crew. Off the Australian coast on *Fantome* at the end of 1854, Alexander Mackay cursed his luck on receiving news of the capture of the Russian forts at Bomarsund and victory at the River Alma. There was a great demand for surgeons in the Crimea, he noted, 'and I must say I yearn to go there'.[19]

Scarce as opportunities were in the early nineteenth century, one chance to see action was by attachment to marines put ashore from Commodore Lord John Hay's small squadron on the coast of northern Spain. With the death of Ferdinand VII in September 1833 Spain entered an era of constitu-tional conflict and civil warfare in which the crown was disputed between Ferdinand's infant daughter, Isabella, and his brother, Don Carlos. Isabella's authority was exercised through her mother, Christina, who effectively ruled the country as Queen-Regent, broadly supported by liberal opinion and constitutional bodies. The British government was sympathetic to the Queen's cause and was determined to resist efforts by the adherents of Don Carlos to re-establish royal absolutism in the Iberian Peninsula. In June 1835 Christina was allowed to recruit in Britain a 10,000-strong volunteer legion under Lieutenant-General George de Lacy Evans to fight in Spain. These were not regular soldiers: officially Britain was not intervening in the civil war. Yet after the first detachment arrived at San Sebastian in July 1835, and as it reached full strength in the weeks which followed, it became obvi-ous that the Royal Navy would render these British auxiliaries ashore both moral and material assistance.

In the months that followed Hay employed his warships to interdict supplies destined for the army of Don Carlos, transporting both Christino forces and units from the British legion and defending their sometimes precarious positions with naval gunfire and garrison duties. After a disas-trous winter during which the legion suffered greatly from illness and inad-equate supplies Hay's most ostentatious support came in April 1836 when 150 marines were landed to protect the harbour at Portugalete. Cooperation between Hay and Evans soon saw San Sebastian and Bilbao secured for the Queen's forces and in May the port of Pasajes was captured from the Carlists. The marine battalion increased to over 400, reinforced by more than 200 men, with guns, from the Royal Artillery, Royal Marine Artillery and Royal Engineers.[20] George Dabbs and James Browne were the two excited surgeons sent ashore with the marines, their first task being to set up medical facilities at the base in San Sebastian. 'We were, of course, both anxious to go out with the troops,' Browne reported in June 1836, 'but it was requisite one should remain at the infirmary.' Dabbs, as senior, had the honour, while Browne stayed in San Sebastian to receive the sick and wounded whom Dabbs sent back for hospital treatment. Within days of going ashore, however, Browne was immersed in the details of the campaign, writing enthusiastically about the battalion's engagements and the deployments of Evans's force and those of his Spanish allies. After the marines had helped capture Pasajes the British expedition had a stronger base in northern Spain. Browne judged that Evans now occupied a six-mile front between the supply ports of San Sebastian and Pasajes, behind which were several large, fortified houses and two or three villages. The marines were dug in on a hill about two and a half miles inland where Dabbs too was in his element. 'He rather likes the bivouac,' Browne observed – understandable in fine weather, though in the wet being back at base had its compensations.

But if Browne had any romantic notions about warfare the reality was brought home sharply on 6 June when the Carlists launched a counter-attack. Taken by surprise, the British auxiliaries were temporarily pushed back and the entire front threatened. 'As soon as I heard of it I bundled up my instruments, tourniquets, dressings &c and started for the field in all haste.' By the time Browne arrived Evans's men had regained lost ground but soon they were under fire again from two artillery pieces, sustaining further losses in a vain attempt to capture them. Meanwhile the Queen's Spanish forces were hard pressed to hold a fortified house nearby and as their position deteriorated were in danger of being cut off from Pasajes. 'The marines were called on for support and arrived at the crisis,' Browne observed. As their Spanish allies fell back in a disorganized retreat and all seemed lost, 'our men marched up as cool and regular as if going to a morning parade, their fingers itching for the trigger'. Steady volleys of musketry, with howitzer from the marine artillery behind, turned the tide and as the Christinos regrouped and returned to the fray the Carlists eventually broke, leaving behind 1,000 dead and wounded. The Christinos suffered about 300 casualties with Evans's legion incurring close to 100.[21]

Dabbs was caught up in a prolonged action on 11 July 1836 when the marines were sent as part of a force of 5,000 men from Pasajes to assault the old walled town of Fuenterrabia. The idea was then to move on to capture Irun nearby, the point at which many Carlist supplies were smuggled across the frontier from France. First, though, a bridge which controlled the road running between the two towns had to be taken. Evans took no artillery with him and the attack was a disaster. 'In the heat the men were exhausted before fighting began since they had climbed a steep hill beforehand,' Browne recorded, having received Dabbs's account of events.[22] The Carlists at the bridge drove off a charge by Spanish lancers and then repelled the marines with concentrated fire from behind impenetrable cover. 'Never was anything so badly managed under the sun,' one disgusted marine officer noted.[23] Two marines were killed. Dabbs had to collect six others wounded, all of whom were sent back to the infirmary at San Sebastian. Hearing of the shambles, Browne questioned whether the bridge had any strategic value; had Evans advanced directly to Fuenterrabia the town would probably have surrendered. By 16 July Browne had 45 men on his infirmary list while Dabbs had a similar number, mostly with bowel ailments, in a temporary hospital at Pasajes. By mid-August the campaign had ground to a halt with 'the legion in a disorganised state and everything apparently tending to anarchy'.[24]

Browne witnessed the marine battalion leaving San Sebastian again in December 1836. This time 58 men with artillery were needed at Bilbao where the Christinos were holding out against a Carlist siege. The six 24-pound howitzers expected to tilt the balance in the struggle at Bilbao went by *Comet*. Meanwhile so small a marine force was obviously vulnerable given that the Christinos had already lost 900 men trying to raise the siege. John Watson, surgeon aboard *Ringdove* off Portugalete, despaired of efforts to relieve Bilbao, seeing soldiers loyal to the Queen retreating back into Portugalete even as *Comet* with her artillery arrived. Two of *Ringdove*'s guns and all the guns from *Saracen* had been landed earlier but with the campaign apparently collapsing these had needed to be re-embarked quickly. Watson had been with the landing party trying to fix the guns into batteries prior to their undignified withdrawal. One marine had been hit by enemy fire but had died before Watson could examine him. With coordination at last established between Hay and the Christino commander, however, the Carlist lines were eventually breached and Bilbao was relieved on Christmas Eve 1836. Victory at Bilbao owed much to the Royal Navy.[25]

The marine battalion, with Browne now accompanying it in the field, was involved in further heavy fighting on 15–16 March 1837 when it joined the Christinos and Evans's legion as they advanced inland on the Carlists holding Hernani. After a struggle, a hill overlooking the town was captured and guns brought up to command the ground below. All seemed under control, Browne recorded, until about 17,000 Carlist troops, unexpectedly reinforced, counter-attacked. They soon outflanked the marines whose position became increasingly dire as Spanish allies started to abandon their positions to the right, while to the left other regiments, including two from the auxiliary legion, began to panic. Browne was caught with the marines at their howitzer battery as the rout became widespread. 'It was *sauve qui peut*,' he recalled with horror, even though the marines around him proved determined to hold their ground. 'We had barely time to limber up and get to the top of the hill when the battalion opened their fire and put a check to the progress of the Carlists,' Browne noted nervously when watching the chaos to their right. Encouraged by the marines' stubborn resistance, however, one of Evans's regiments then rallied and managed to drive the enemy back from an elevation which had allowed easy firing at the marines' position. But to the left Browne could see that things were becoming hopeless: 'As the marines and our guns had scarce any support we were compelled to return, the Spaniards not being able to rally a single regiment.' With one man lost and 14 wounded, the naval contingent withdrew to the safety of San Sebastian. But for the cover provided by the Royal Artillery and Royal Marine Artillery present it would not have escaped so lightly.[26]

Dabbs and Browne were not the only medical officers ashore in northern Spain in 1836: the assistant surgeon of *Tweed* was also assigned to duty with marines stationed on the heights at Pasajes. Later James Philips, assistant from *Salamander*, was given charge of the San Sebastian infirmary when, in May 1837, Browne was moved with 100 men of the battalion to Fuenterrabia. This was in support of Christino forces and the British auxiliaries' renewed attempt to take Hernani. Evans had 10,000 men drawn up in 14 battalions, with artillery, at Hernani. The town capitulated on 14 May. This was followed within days by the legion's capture of Irun and Fuenterrabia. At Fuenterrabia, however, Browne became thoroughly disillusioned with the cause for which the marines and artillerymen were fighting. The Christinos were unreliable, fractious, and proved to be so obstinate in their behaviour 'as to harbour Carlists spies and marauding parties even under our guns'.[27] There, too, Browne heard at first hand about the horrors of Spanish warfare as local people recounted harrowing tales of the cruelty practised by Carlist forces on any peasant family which resisted boys being dragged from the countryside for military service. It was fortunate that this location was healthier in summer than San Sebastian, Browne observed to Burnett, since he had been able to take only a small supply of medicines in a portable chest strapped to his horse. Dabbs, now at Pasajes with half the marine battalion, was also fed up with his part in the expedition – in his case largely because medical supplies were running low. Stores sufficient for only 600 men had been provided; in November 1837 he urged the navy to ship out at once enough medical provisions for a further 300 men.

The pessimism which permeated the correspondence of both Dabbs and Browne after mid-1837 proved, in the end, to be misplaced. Although the original British legion was disbanded in June 1837, to be replaced with a much smaller volunteer force, the war gradually began to move in favour of the Queen's armies once it became clear in October 1837 that the Carlists could never capture Madrid. His challenge for the crown collapsing, Don Carlos finally fled to France in September 1839, after which most of the towns still held by his troops surrendered in the early months of 1840. The last marines and Royal Engineers were withdrawn from northern Spain in the summer of 1840 where they had remained for uneventful garrison duties. Dabbs and Browne had certainly seen their share of action. The latter, indeed, amid the defeat and chaos at Hernani in March 1837, had been lucky to get away.

Charles Wilkinson, assistant surgeon aboard *Benbow*, was another who relished action. He found it on the eastern Mediterranean coast in 1840 where an international crisis which had been developing throughout the 1830s finally came to a head. Revolting against Turkish authority in 1831, the Pasha of Egypt, Mehemet Ali, had sent his army northwards into Syria, crushing the Turks at the battle of Konieh in December 1832. Securing his new domain, however, was a different matter. An uprising against Egyptian rule broke out in 1834 and Mehemet Ali's occupying forces were defeated in 1838. At this point Turkey re-entered the conflict in support of the Syrian resistance and a Turkish army crossed the Euphrates in April 1839. But the outcome proved to be another disaster for the Turkish empire. Commanded by Mehemet Ali's son, Ibrahim, an Egyptian army routed the Turks at Nezib in June 1839, following which the bulk of the Turkish navy defected.

Fearing the collapse of Ottoman power and an ensuing destabilization in international affairs, the British government reinforced the Mediterranean

fleet and decided that the Egyptian advance should be halted. By the
early months of 1840 there were 12 ships of the line, seven frigates and ten
steamers in the Mediterranean: by November this had been increased to
16 ships of the line, with three more arriving in January 1841.[28] Mehemet
Ali had assurances of French support. The French government, however,
soon appeared to be outflanked by British diplomacy after the other major
European powers joined Britain in presenting Mehemet Ali with peace
terms which confined him to the southern part of Syria. Nevertheless, still
confident of assistance from the large French squadron in the Mediterranean
and with up to 80,000 soldiers defending his newly acquired territories,
Mehemet Ali rejected the ultimatum. 'The old fool Mehemet Ali will not
listen to anything,' Wilkinson wrote in August 1840. 'Oh for the shoot-
ing. ... Fancy it will all end in smoke.'[29] He was not to be disappointed.
Faced with the prospect of war against a combination of European powers,
French support soon evaporated, at which point the Royal Navy began to
implement blockades and to capture Egyptian positions. With eight ships
of the line, four steamers and five lesser warships off the coast, and with
the support of a few Austrian and Turkish vessels and about 6,000 Turkish
soldiers, the navy swiftly completed its work. In September *Benbow* was
preparing for its part in an assault to drive the Egyptians out of Beirut.
Meanwhile Egyptian shipping was seized and sentries put aboard to guard
their crews. Wilkinson had to be ready for action at any time. On suspicion that the crew of one captured vessel had revolted during the night,
Wilkinson was summoned on deck where 'tourniquets, bandages and plaster were in immediate requisition and I was ordered immediately away
in the boats'.[30] *Benbow* led the bombardment of Beirut's fortifications on
9 September 1840 in anticipation of landings by 1,400 marines and 5,000
Turkish troops. Thousands of Egyptian soldiers began evacuating the city
on the following day.

Benbow was moved along the coast to where her guns could command a
valley through which the Egyptian army had to pass. Again Wilkinson saw
the prospect of some fighting. But as news from other ships made plain,
putting men ashore was fraught with difficulties. Attacking a fort north of
Beirut at Djebail, marines from *Cyclops* had found its three defensive walls
unbreachable, despite a prior bombardment, and had been initially forced
back to their boats with 27 killed or wounded. But the fortitude among the
casualties made a deep impression on Wilkinson who recorded some of the
surgery performed on *Cyclops* after the withdrawal. 'Off with it doctor!' one

young marine demanded, pointing to a shattered arm as he was carried into the cockpit. He would have no one hold him, merely grimacing as the bone was sawed: 'Doctor, this is warm work!'[31] On 25 September another boat party, including *Benbow*'s marines, was sent against the fort at Tortosa. This also experienced a setback after many boats ran aground on rocks and 19 men were killed or wounded. Wilkinson was not with the landing parties but took a keen interest in all details of the coastal campaign.

Not until 20 October did Wilkinson feel that events had taken a decisive turn, despite the earlier capture of Sidon against an Egyptian garrison of 3,000 men and the arrival of many irregular fighters from the Lebanese mountains to join the struggle against Mehemet Ali. Next an Egyptian army was decisively defeated about five miles from Beirut and a marine column supporting Turkish troops entered the city. Tyre had likewise been captured. Wilkinson was at Lattachuo when it came over to the Turks. But amid this excitement normal duties still had to be performed. 'We are again on salt beef,' Wilkinson recorded gloomily. Arriving off Beirut again on 25 October, he now had more than 80 men on his sick-list. He could also see for himself the devastation caused by bombarding the city. 'Ships have done a great deal of damage'; going ashore, he witnessed the many defenders killed.[32] Meanwhile, as rumours abounded about what would happen next, marines aboard several warships were coming down with bowel disorders. Acre, it transpired, was the navy's next destination. The garrison there would not surrender and its impressive fortifications made any attack a daunting prospect. To Wilkinson's obvious delight, though, *Benbow* would lead the firing line.

At the start of November 1840 Wilkinson watched as Turkish troops were taken aboard for the assault on Acre. 'Very unpleasant the Turks being on board,' he considered. 'They make every place in such a mess.' On the following day things became even worse as the ship prepared to go under the guns of the town's defences. 'We are all in a damned mess. Bulkheads all down and screens up. It is now every man for himself', he observed, while eagerly making his own preparations: 'chests etc. laid out in cockpit'. *Benbow* drifted into position on 3 November and the surgeon came up on deck as the captain addressed the crew. 'I hope you will take steady aim, do not throw away your shot. You have always behaved well when firing,' the gunners were told. Wilkinson knew what to expect when the captain warned the assembled company that 'I have no doubt we shall have a return.' It came as soon as the warning was uttered. 'By God, they've begun already!' the captain hastily concluded: 'Go to your quarters.' In a state of great agitation Wilkinson noted how *Benbow* tried to respond, yet 'many of our guns we could not get to bear, as we were sailing end on'. Only after some time could the ship get broadside on, at which point she, and those in line behind her, began to pour shot into Acre's defences. Three hours elapsed before the Egyptian guns were silenced. 'Many of the ships suffered by the firing, particularly about the masts and rigging,' Wilkinson observed. No one was killed on *Benbow* although her hull was hit 16 times, with one shot passing through the ship without causing a scratch. It could have been a busy day.

Yet just as Browne was brought to face the realities of battle at Hernani in 1837, so Wilkinson, landing next day, witnessed the carnage at Acre. 'The scene on shore was dreadful,' he confided. 'Bodies of men, women and children, animals of all kinds were strewn about the ruins. We all congratulated ourselves on getting off so well.'[33] A magazine had exploded in the town killing not only many inhabitants but also a marine nearby and wounding five others. By the end of the month Egyptian forces in Syria were in full retreat and Wilkinson was back in Beirut in charge of a temporary hospital which had been set up there. With a large sick-list and with other medical officers away elsewhere on the coast, Wilkinson's energies now had to be devoted to regular work; he was still tending fever patients back on *Benbow* in February 1841, leaving the scene a month later when his ship sailed for Malta.

Wilkinson was not the only medic in the fleet to see action on the coast of Syria. Assistant surgeon Joseph Plimsoll was wounded aboard *Edinburgh* during the bombardment of Acre, while another, Peter Niddrie from *Princess Charlotte*, was landed with marines on 18 September and served at their camp as principal medical officer. Four other assistants were landed with him; most were out each day on marches with the troops. Burnett later recorded 35 assistant surgeons alone who had served in the eastern Mediterranean in 1840. When recommending promotions he stressed how 'many of these young men were not only present at Acre, but have also undergone some fatiguing service on the coast of Syria where fever and dysentery have prevailed in an unusual degree and where their best energies were required and displayed'.[34] Niddrie, who by April 1841 was surgeon to the marine battalion, recalled his arduous work at Acre after its capture. In just 48 days, 32 among the 338 marines and 40 sailors quartered there died. A total of 261 had been attacked by fever. Niddrie himself had been ill for three months.

Dodwell Whipple and James Patrick were both exposed to enemy fire in 1845 when participating in an extensive engagement against a pirate stronghold in Borneo. They were away in boats with marines and subsequently caught up in fierce hand-to-hand fighting. Eight marines died and 13 others were wounded. Some of the boats were raked with shot even before the marines could land and the two medical officers had to take the scant cover available. Amid all this, Whipple had to perform an amputation.[35] Richard Carpenter, surgeon on *Penelope*, likewise witnessed his colleagues working under fire at the capture of Lagos in December 1851. To overrun the stockades and slave compounds and to spike defensive guns, 222 officers and men went off in boats. *Penelope* lost 14 men with 65 wounded. Carpenter stayed aboard, but his assistants, Michael Walling and Robert Sproule, landed with the force. Their conduct under fire was beyond praise, Carpenter reported to London. Reflecting on the entire action three days later, Captain Henry Bruce assured the First Lord that 'in this very severe affair the medical officers came forth in a way worthy of the brightest days of chivalry. Wherever they had a shipmate,' he concluded, 'there they were to be found, and the fighting men could not look round, at the storming or in the boats, that a medico was not by his side.'[36]

Danger came in many forms. Even just standing on the deck of *Fox* in the Irrawaddy in 1847 assistant surgeon Frederick Morgan was struck in the chest by a large splinter broken off the spar by a shot fired unexpectedly from the shoreline. The surgeon from *Sampson*, going in at Lagos in 1851, was thrown from his boat as it capsized crossing the bar and had to be saved from encircling sharks. Surgeon John Buchan was lost when thrown out of a gig in 1839. Colin Browning, surgeon on a convict ship bound for New South Wales in 1840, was examining a sickly child when a water cask broke loose and crushed his right leg. Henry Kelsall was surgeon aboard the convict vessel *Waterloo* which foundered while carrying 220 male prisoners off the South African coast in 1842: 189 lives were lost, including 14 sailors and 15 soldiers. 'I narrowly escaped with my own life, which is all that I have saved', Kelsall reported. The ship was 'villainously rotten', he added, and broke up within minutes. Many of its timbers had separated into flakes like the decaying trunk of a hollowed old tree.[37] Henry Brock had to be invalided in 1843 some years after his stool gave way on a rolling ship while he was cleaning his amputating knife. He never recovered the use of his right hand. James Steele, surgeon, and Bernard Delaney, assistant, went down with *Avenger* in 1847. Amid the confusion and panic which reigned in times of peril, however, medical officers sometimes displayed the utmost bravery. Kelsall saved the lives of some of the convicts from *Waterloo* before having to save himself. William Culhane, assistant surgeon aboard the most famous of all Victorian naval losses, *Birkenhead* in 1852, agonized over one man helpless in the sick-bay even as the ship was rapidly sinking. 'I could not get to the cockpit to rescue him as that was the part that filled immediately,' he reported apologetically to Somerset House. Books, accounts, everything was lost: his efforts having failed, Culhane had finally to take his chance and swim from the ship 'when the poop was on a level with the sea'.[38]

Unpopular a posting though it generally was, as the capture of Lagos demonstrated even the West Africa station had its exhilarating moments. After 1816 the navy maintained permanent coastal patrols in the hope of suppressing human traffic, which meant, for the most part, a cat-and-mouse game with Brazilian, Portuguese, Spanish and American slavers combined with repeated attempts to cajole or coerce African rulers to cease their supply. Months of inactivity and cruising in unhealthy waters could suddenly erupt into pursuit when a suspicious vessel was spotted. If full, the slaves would be liberated, usually at Sierra Leone. If empty, but fitted out for an obvious purpose, the ship would still be seized as a prize and the spoils, once determined by a Court of Admiralty, apportioned among the warship's crew. There was, therefore, every incentive to do the work well; even medical officers received a share of the prize money, though not as much as many felt was due. When *Harpy* seized a Portuguese vessel carrying 280 slaves off the Mozambique coast in 1837 her assistant surgeon, Morris Pritchett, complained bitterly that his share of the prize would not be equal to that of the mate, second master or even clerk. In any fight to make a capture, a doctor's skills would immediately be required. Furthermore, it was the medical officer who had to inspect and treat the captives in their wretched state and upon whom responsibility for their health devolved. 'Yet', he observed, 'I find myself sharing with the corporal of marines, the caulker, sail-maker &c, in fact with the common seamen.'[39]

Demoralization was compounded by relatively low success rates and the knowledge that New World and Arab slave markets still conducted lucrative business. International agreements designed to end slaving, even where they existed, were seldom enforced: an estimated 150,000 Africans were exported annually for much of the early nineteenth century. The navy's rate of interception was about 5 per cent. As late as 1848, 60,000 slaves came to Brazil despite the extension of naval patrols to the South American coast. Off East Africa the annual trade from Zanzibar to the Persian Gulf, Cuba and Brazil averaged around 20,000, at least until the 1860s. Regarding his achievements between 1832 and 1837 while Commander-in-Chief, West Africa, Rear-Admiral Sir Patrick Campbell boasted 19,129 liberated slaves; his captains had taken 18 loaded craft in 1835–36 alone with a further 26 empty, fitted vessels.⁴⁰ But such commitment could not disguise the fact that the squadrons were small in relation to the task at hand. By the 1840s there were sometimes 30 warships assigned to the West Africa station although in previous years the total had usually been fewer than a dozen. The Cape station, which covered the East African coast, was the smallest among the navy's eight foreign stations. It had an average of only nine ships between 1845 and 1860, few among which could regularly be spared for slave patrol duties.

Fevers, dysentery and fatigue all took their toll on the African coasts. Between 1822 and 1826, 200 sailors died from disease aboard vessels off East Africa. More than 500 officers and men either succumbed to fevers or were killed in action off West Africa between 1839 and 1845 while a further 500 were invalided. Medical officers often spent their time tending men whose constitutions were broken beyond the point of recovery. Pritchett, off West Africa in 1842, observed how 'it too frequently falls to the lot of practitioners in tropical climates to find all their efforts avail nothing, the disease speedily destroying vitality'.⁴¹ Nevertheless he still took the chance to discern patterns amid his casework, noting how, in similar conditions of exposure, some men seemed more disposed to disease whereas others were better able to resist it, and also how black men, when entered as ship's crew in England, had no more resistance to disease than anyone else, despite the obviously higher levels of resistance which negroes accustomed to the climate of West Africa enjoyed. James Gordon, surgeon on *Wanderer* in the Gambia in 1841, also collected data on the incidence of fevers among men out for a sustained period on boat duty in search of slavers. At night, he reported, the boat-keepers who slept in the boats never seemed to contract fevers whereas among those who slept just a few yards away on shore many succumbed. Surely such diseases could not therefore be contagious? After months on patrol, ships would interrupt their commission at Ascension or St Helena. Matthew Burton, surgeon on *Penelope* in 1853, noted 'the altered and improved condition of the crew of an African cruiser after a sojourn of eight or ten days there'. Death rates among the crews of ships off West

Africa had come down by about two-thirds to roughly 16 per 1,000 men by 1852, the Commander-in-Chief gratefully recorded. Quinine wine and the care taken to ensure high standards of sanitation aboard all helped, he continued, but credit was also owing to 'the skill of the medical officers'.[42]

Amid constant danger from the climate and disease, the West Africa station could also prove contentious as commanding officers manoeuvred for the most lucrative stretches of a 2,000-mile coastline to search. Slavers were small and increasingly fast, the pick-up points numerous and their skippers well practised in slipping in and out of ports and rivers to collect waiting cargoes. Warships were usually slower and larger: they had to be so, the Commander-in-Chief explained in 1850. A small naval ship carried neither executive officers nor sailors sufficient to board and sail a prize. Not only that, their boats would not be large enough to despatch adequate numbers of men if fighting had to be done. Then there was the problem of medical officers: a small ship carried only an assistant surgeon, which meant that none would be available to accompany boat parties. If a capture was made, the pressure on medical facilities became even worse, with hundreds of liberated Africans now needing attention.[43] No wonder West Africa was an unpopular assignment, surgeon Alexander Anderson reminded Burnett in 1853 when requesting a transfer. Nevertheless 'if two years' service of medical officers on this unhealthy coast were considered equal to three there would then be some inducement and pleasure to serve'.[44]

Yet, as John McIlroy described enthusiastically in 1841, West Africa certainly could provide the excitement of the chase. As surgeon on *Persian*, 25 miles up the River Congo, he watched as boats went off to investigate a suspicious vessel. Suddenly a 12-pound gun and musketry opened fire. Two sailors were killed and one wounded as the boats rowed swiftly in the hope of getting boarders astern. With a prize in their grasp and their blood up nothing could stop the sailors and, sensing that all was lost, some of the defenders jumped overboard, being either drowned or, as McIlroy believed, taken by sharks. Others tried to escape by lowering some boats, but before most could get away the British had boarded. 'When our men entered the vessel they cut down everyone they met with,' McIlroy recalled. The lieutenant with them 'had great difficulty in saving the lives of those who cried out for pardon'.[45] Soon after, *Persian* came across an American trader whose crew quickly abandoned her as the warship approached. At St Helena three months later McIlroy watched *Fantome* bring in a prize containing 450 slaves. When taken, there had been more than 600 below deck but many proved too sick to be saved.

Back in the River Congo in 1842 McIlroy witnessed the action against the slave barracoons at Cabenda undertaken by men from *Madagascar* and *Waterwitch*. The factories there were owned by Spaniards and it was to these that the African chieftains brought their prisoners for sale and shipment. Everything was burnt. Over 1,000 slaves had been freed and were on their way to St Helena. This was the way to stop the trade, McIlroy insisted: destroying the coastal settlements where the commerce was conducted meant that there would be no rendezvous for slaving vessels. For him, Lagos was the obvious target. Cruising off the town a few weeks earlier, McIlroy had learnt of 800 captives imprisoned by the local ruler. In 1842, however, taking the town was not an option and McIlroy, like the rest of *Persian*'s company, spent his days at sea 'lamenting our ill fortune in having seen so few slavers'. Then his luck changed. A craft was spotted which, although too fast for *Persian*, was followed at a distance. When the wind dropped three boats were sent out in a final pursuit. 'We had marked her down as a prize,' McIlroy later recalled.[46] After a ten-mile pull at oars the three boats caught and boarded the vessel without a struggle; she was trying to get into Lagos to pick up 700 slaves bound for Havana. It was a job well done, but, as McIlroy was well aware, while any warship was pursuing a prize others slipped in and out of port. Even worse, perhaps, slaves left uncollected in the barracoons would probably just starve, since their captors would soon lose interest in them once the navy had thwarted the chance of a sale. It was distressing work. Yet as Robert McCrae, surgeon aboard *Growler,* recounted, being at Sierra Leone as the survivors arrived was often no less so.

At Sierra Leone those rescued from slave ships were offered passage as free emigrants to British Guiana. In 1847 McCrae and his assistant, Herbert MacKarsie, were given the task of examining volunteers for this experiment in order to make sure that they could withstand the voyage. 'We found a large proportion of them to be boys and girls, some of them of very tender years, and many of them much emaciated and feeble,' McCrae informed Burnett. In fact many were in no state to board a ship. But the medical officers were told that children could not be left behind, since their parents might not embark without them. *Growler* was duly loaded on 25 July 1847 with 62 men, 102 women, 183 boys, 118 girls and seven infants, and arrived at Demerara a fortnight later. The crossing was as McCrae and MacKarsie had predicted. Eager to leave Sierra Leone, some passengers concealed symptoms of dysentery until *Growler* had sailed and widespread sickness soon developed. Four adults, 13 children and three infants died at sea, for which McCrae knew some explanation on his part would be required. With no interpreter, he wrote apologetically, it became impossible to organize the sick and to isolate them from the rest of the ship. Many became confused or despondent and appeared to lose the will to live, while others, unfamiliar with the notion of medicine, refused treatment. But it was not just the spectacle of so many malnourished and ill-treated souls being brought to Sierra Leone or the hardship which they might endure *en route* to their next destination which sometimes made work with the West Africa squadron so depressing. It was also strenuous, and McCrae soon made his own sufferings and those of his assistant plain. Their duties among liberated slaves had been of 'a most arduous and exceedingly unpleasant nature, embracing nearly our whole time and attention, and could not have been continued much longer without serious consequences to our health'.[47] West African duty was for those whose lives sought moral purpose and who relished a small part in the great struggle of their generation.

The remaining areas of physical and intellectual challenge were the polar regions. Until the 1850s, indeed, the centuries-old idea of a North West passage to the Pacific still haunted the imagination. With the Napoleonic conflict ended, the navy embarked on polar exploration with the voyage of Sir John Ross in 1818, those of Sir Edward Parry between 1818 and 1821 and again between 1821 and 1823, and Sir John Franklin's early expeditions of 1819 to 1822 and 1824 to 1827. Sir James Ross likewise explored Antarctic waters between 1838 and 1842. Franklin's disappearance in the Arctic after sailing from Britain again in 1845 prompted extensive searches in 1848–49 and again between 1850 and 1854. The hazards from ice were obvious, yet no expedition ever lacked medical volunteers. Frozen wastes, fossil remains and the effects of controlled diet and privations on the human body could all be studied by an eager surgeon-naturalist, and at the first rumours of ships being fitted out applications to accompany them would arrive on Burnett's desk. Trapped aboard or camped in extreme conditions on an icy shoreline during the darkness of an endless winter, officers and men were brought together in a shared struggle for survival. Healthy exercise, theatricals, fancy dress, concerts and a strict routine for issuing rations all helped to break the monotony and to maintain vigour and morale. 'Moping below is very injurious,' Henry Piers, assistant surgeon on *Investigator*, observed in the depth of winter in 1850: 'A number of us have been playing at "rounders" and throwing and catching a ball.' David Lyall, surgeon on *Assistance* throughout two Arctic winters in 1852 and 1853, recorded how 'a house of ice was built on shore, which, being converted into a sort of skittle alley afforded both amusement and exercise to officers as well as men'. Then there was schooling and lecturing to while away the time. 'The very few amongst the men who could neither read or write were possessed of these necessary acquirements before the season returned for active operations,' Abraham Bradford, surgeon with *Resolute*, observed in 1851. 'Others more advanced by previous education made considerable progress in navigation, and the select few got deep into the mysteries of Euclid.'[48] As men of learning, the medics' role was often much to the fore.[49]

Controlling diet was a major responsibility normally devolved to the medical officer, especially when supplies were running low or sickness had appeared among the crew. *Pioneer*'s commander in the Arctic in 1850–51 complimented his assistant surgeon, Thomas Pickthorn, for enthusiastic 'superintendence of the commissariat, both public and private'.[50] To prevent scurvy, adequate stocks of good lemon or lime juice were vital. On *Resolute*, Bradford gave every man one ounce daily and issued allowances for those travelling in sledge parties. He could not prevent it freezing but no harm was done. The sailors found it always so tasty that 'almost everyone was desirous of getting more than his allowance'.[51] Admittedly the limited cuisine available did tend to distort the palate. 'An Arctic winter is certainly a good sharpener of appetite,' Piers noticed in 1851. Reindeer, ptarmigan, hares and seals could sometimes be hunted and the men were well when successful. But for much of the time polar explorers had to contend with salt provisions interspersed with the issue of chocolate and preserved meats, potatoes, carrots and soups. Cold, fatigued, not having seen the sun for weeks and usually hungry, men were never late for a meal. 'Ship's salt beef and pork, the sight of which on the table, occasionally, could scarcely be tolerated by some on our passage out from England, now quickly disappeared before them, and are found to be <u>excellent</u>,' Piers joked. 'Tripe, which used to go off the table as it was put on, is now a favourite dish.' Dry bread was devoured as if plum cake. By February 1852, however, *Investigator* had no biscuit left: men were piped at 6pm just to receive 'a small piece of dry bread and tea'.[52]

Piers and Bradford were fortunate in the quality of their preserved supplies and praised the manufacturers accordingly when writing up their journals. John Robertson, with *Enterprise* in 1848–49, had a different tale to tell. He distrusted his lime juice from the start and, when ill himself, became convinced that it was useless. The preserved milk intended for use among the sick also proved a complete failure. All his salt provisions were insufficient in both quality and quantity, while the preserved meats 'were a disgrace to the contractor'. Only his preserved potatoes were worth bringing and survived 19 months in a damp and frozen hold; otherwise, Robertson concluded, 'through a set of designing and heartless harpies the expedition was badly provided and consequently the lives of all placed in great danger'.[53] But it was not only food supplies that could put men at grave risk in such extreme conditions. Stuck in the ice for far longer than expected, coal rations for heating and cooking would also diminish, with little to spare for men sent out for days in hunting parties. Piers, in charge of a week-long hunting trip in tents in 1851, was brought the disagreeable news on waking one morning that no coals were left to prepare any breakfast and that the best the cook could do was to heat some cocoa over his remaining scraps of wood coated in grease.

Though only an assistant surgeon, Piers had in effect assumed the responsibilities of executive officer. 'I told the men to take their guns to shoot anything they might fall in with,' he later recalled; in particular, though, they were ordered 'to look after any pieces of drift wood there might be on the beach, and see if they could collect some of the dwarf willow'.[54] Enough was gathered to prepare a meagre meal of preserved meat, potato and bread before heading back to the ship with their modest haul of 25 hares and 11 ptarmigan. Bradford meanwhile had charge of six men on a sledging party searching the northern and eastern shores of Melville Island for traces of Franklin. Despite a serious fall he was away 80 days. 'For nearly a month the gallant officer was dragged upon his sledge, carrying out, thanks to his own pluck and the zeal of his men, the object of his journey,' his commanding officer commented approvingly.[55] William Domville, surgeon from *Resolute* in 1854, likewise had to exercise discretion when out with two sledges and nine dogs in the Arctic. The party kept together, as required, until Domville noticed the health of one of the men deteriorating rapidly, whereupon he announced that he would split the sledges, taking ahead two men with four of the dogs in the hope that the ailing seaman would reach help in time. Back on board, Domville and his assistant, John Ricards, took their turns as officers of the watch and were commended for so doing by a grateful captain.[56] Polar exploration was thus a chance to command. The navy rarely provided such opportunities for its medical officers.

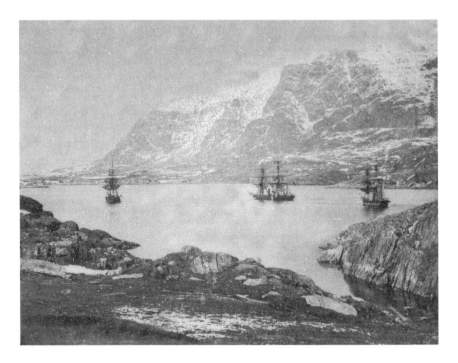

2. In the Arctic: 1854.

In fact few medics who had experienced the wonders and hardships of the polar regions never wished to return. For most, the camaraderie forged with officers and men in their daily struggle with the elements remained long in the memory. Who could ever forget Christmas dinner locked in an ice pack? 'It consisted of reindeer, which was in prime condition, fat and delicately tender, cooked as the men pleased,' Piers recalled. The meat 'was roasted or made in puddings or a sort of stew with vegetables, puddings etc'.[57] It was the last of the venison and they had saved it, frozen outside, for the occasion. Domville was delighted with his Christmas dinner in the Arctic in 1852. 'Few tables at home were better provided, if in quantity certainly not in quality,' he boasted. *Resolute* had collected fresh beef when calling at the Orkneys, while hunting excursions and fishing had provided a range of venison, hare and salmon. Next day many of the men were looking seriously the worse for the wine which had also been taken. In the circumstances, though, Domville considered, 'some little charity should be shown towards this frailty'.[58] Others recounted the lavish provisions sent out on their vessels and thoroughly enjoyed amid such bleak surroundings. John Holman, assistant surgeon on *Phoenix* in 1854, enthused about his

meats, soups and vegetables, all preserved so well, and even the excellence
of the ship's biscuit. Pickles and cranberries were daily available, preserved
milk and cocoa were plentiful, while stocks of flour allowed soft bread to
be made and issued thrice weekly by the qualified baker aboard.[59] This was
luxury indeed, but it was not unique. Ricards, assistant on *Pioneer* in 1852–
53, also praised the preserved vegetables, fruits and milk with which he had
been supplied. Allsopp's ale had also survived the perilous conditions well,
he wrote by way of scientific study; all ships bound for the Arctic in future
should carry copious amounts. David Lyall, confined to *Assistance* between
1852 and 1854, came to the same conclusion.[60]

Caring for the sick in those circumstances posed few problems. When
food and fuel were scarce, however, or when out with sledges, medical
duties were far more challenging. Medical officers tried to ensure that men
in the sick-bay received a diet conducive to recovery: 'the birds go to the
sick mess: the hares to the general stock', Piers decided as winter set in early
in November 1851. Infectious disease was not normally a problem at these
latitudes. Problems arose from exposure and frost bite. Piers discovered one
sailor in a sorry state on the pack ice in 1851. In great distress and with no
movement in his knee the man had sat down and declared himself unable
to go on. 'Knowing indeed how stupid sailors are,' Piers reflected disparagingly, 'it might even have cost him his life.' Piers got the man up but then
noticed that he had thrown away his shoes. With time running out, Piers
bullied and goaded the sailor back to the ship, 'telling him I should not
mind walking all night without resting, and what others had done'. A fortnight later Piers described himself as 'a lame duck' with such sores on his
heels and pains in a knee that he could scarcely do his job.[61] Service in the
Arctic, in the tropics or in action often came at a high price. But how many
who had survived their dangers could ever feel fulfilled by a life in country
practice?

CHAPTER 4

Home Hospitals

After 1815 reductions at Haslar and East Stonehouse matched peacetime needs at Portsmouth and Plymouth. The Admiralty nevertheless soon recognized the inadequacy of medical facilities at Chatham, where in 1828 a new hospital, the Melville, was constructed. The Melville had 15 wards, each capable of holding 14 men, contained in three pavilions. It had a further 12 beds for officers located in six separate cabins. This gave an overall capacity of 222 and allowed for wards to be isolated for infectious diseases. With epidemics of scarlatina, smallpox and measles common, Chatham had a reputation as the least healthy naval town. In its early years the hospital's highest occupancy was 167, of whom 130 were marines and 36 sailors. It served predominantly the marine headquarters in Chatham, which in practice meant that a high proportion of admissions were always venereal cases. In an emergency its basement and store rooms could be fitted up to take an additional 70 or 80 sick, though that was never an issue before the late 1840s. In fact at the end of 1839 the Melville had only 46 patients, 19 of them venereal; few ships were fitting in the Medway and many of the marines were away on duties elsewhere.

The Melville carried only a small medical establishment. While Haslar and East Stonehouse in 1833 both had an old-style physician, the Melville did not merit so senior a rank. Haslar had two surgeons; East Stonehouse and Chatham each had one. Whereas the two larger hospitals each carried what was referred to as a junior surgeon, the Melville had none. Likewise with assistant surgeons: Haslar had four, East Stonehouse three and the Melville only two. Haslar and East Stonehouse also each retained an old-style hospital mate which the Melville lacked. Together these hospitals were the pride of the Medical Department. New regulations for the home hospitals in 1830 stipulated that patients should receive baths with soap and warm water, clean bed-shirts, nightcaps, blankets, pillows, hair-mattresses and fresh linen sheets every fortnight. Surgeons were even required to sooth their charges by hearing complaints. Night nurses were to be provided, while in daytime their numbers should ensure one for every seven patients. Labourers cleaned the hospitals' surgical instruments, prepared dressings and waited on the sick where appropriate.[1] But for all this, was the exalted reputation which these hospitals enjoyed really justified?

Burnett was so certain of it that he dismissed a report in 1836 that seamen had been discharged from a naval hospital because they required surgery which could better be performed elsewhere. Any medical officer complicit in this should be instantly dismissed, he ruled. Four years earlier Burnett had specifically praised the skill of Haslar's surgeons. Admittedly hospital interiors could be rather Spartan. In 1839 Burnett persuaded the Admiralty to invest in four chairs per ward for convalescents at both Halsar and East Stonehouse so that they might recline more easily than on the existing wooden forms constructed for long dining tables. A further improvement was to ban smoking in most hospital wards: in 1848 the Board eventually confined pipe and cigar smoking at Haslar to one corner of an outdoor quadrangle and the walkway for patients within the hospital grounds. Smoking was abolished at East Stonehouse in 1852. It was a dirty habit, the Inspector explained, 'and when carried to excess I have known it induce disease of the heart and lead to the aggravation of other complaints'.[2] As Deputy-Inspector at the Melville before 1849 he had already outlawed smoking there.

The use of anaesthetic was introduced into surgical procedures at naval hospitals almost as soon as it became available. Chloroform was not commonly applied in the navy and issued as an item among medical stores until 1852, yet at Haslar fingers were amputated, teeth removed, and buboes and abscesses in the thigh opened using the new inhaler of sulphuric ether early in 1847. At the same time, the Melville performed three operations where deep groin incisions and scarification in an anthrax case were made without any pain experienced. The new equipment did not always work well but trials continued: hard drinkers and smokers seemed less susceptible to the effects of ether, while, in most instances, the amount to be administered was difficult to gauge.[3] Naval hospitals were invariably clean, well organized and provided care to the highest standards, Burnett regularly reported. The Admiralty might be assured, therefore, that the taxpayers' money was well spent.

But not all were convinced. James Veitch, long on half pay but formerly a surgeon at East Stonehouse, did not share such a complacent attitude when he wrote to the Admiralty in 1835 suggesting deficiencies in hospital management. Veitch regretted the long-established practice of dividing the wards between those of the physician, which were the medical wards, and those of the senior surgeon, which contained the surgical cases. This, he felt, perpetuated the age-old professional distinction between physician and surgeon and thereby a status and hierarchy which bore no relation to the proper working of a naval establishment. Burnett, a physician himself, would never acknowledge the validity of that criticism. Veitch was moved by jealousy and frustrated ambition, Burnett told the Board, and his observations could be safely set aside. Ironically when the Admiralty restructured the top echelons of its medical service, abolishing the title of physician and replacing it with the grade of Inspector in 1840, it did so along lines which Veitch would doubtless have approved.

A second reproach from Veitch in 1835 was that many medical officers entering the navy were inadequately educated and that, once employed, the resources of the hospitals were not made sufficiently available to them in order to perfect their knowledge. In short, he wished to see Haslar and East Stonehouse resemble medical schools to train young doctors for the rigours of naval duties. Burnett resented this implicit criticism of his failure to raise standards in the service. Haslar and East Stonehouse were and should remain hospitals devoted exclusively to the care of sailors and marines in peace and war, he advised. In any case, assistant surgeons attached to a hospital or to a nearby vessel already had opportunities for further study and practical experience. 'I have not slept at my post,' Burnett wrote indignantly.[4]

At all the inspections of Haslar throughout the 1830s and 1840s the number of patients remained small in relation to the hospital's capacity. In September 1832 the physician's wards had 41 cases, mostly consumptives and heart conditions. The surgeon's wards contained 42 men. A year later the physician had only 17 – 'the smallest number of patients I have ever found in this department in any of our great hospitals,' Burnett noted.[5] Subsequent years saw no great change: the Inspector's wards held 64 men in 1843 while those of the Deputy-Inspector (formerly the surgeon) accounted for 89. As usual, venereal cases among marines constituted a high proportion of the latter's work. Visiting again just before the Crimean War, Burnett recorded 220 patients under the Inspector, among whom 128 suffered from tuberculosis with a further 41 rheumatics. The Deputy-Inspector tended 139 inmates of whom 82 were syphilitics and 15 had severe ulcers. It was a depressing trip. All the consumptives were dying, and though Burnett approved the unsparing doses of cod liver oil administered, he, like Haslar's staff, knew that it could effect no cure.

Going on to Plymouth, Burnett's accounts painted a similar picture. Again the wards were divided between physician and surgeon prior to 1840; in 1832 the former cared for 43 patients and the latter 57. Admissions rose in 1836 when sick and wounded returned from the squadron supporting the British auxiliary legion in Spain: the physician had suddenly to accommodate 197 men and the surgeon 83, half the total being fever cases with a further 19 rheumatics, 28 syphilitics and 23 with pneumonia. By 1839, though, patient numbers were down to the lowest that Burnett could recall and would have been even lower, his old friend, physician Sir David Dickson, complained, had not newly discharged men been put immediately to such arduous duties as to cause relapses. Visiting at the end of 1853, Burnett found that numbers had not increased like those at Haslar. The Inspector at East Stonehouse still had only 55 cases while the surgeon tended 78. East Stonehouse received a glowing recommendation: its comparatively light burden, no doubt, contributed to its success.

Ignoring annual fluctuations, however, both hospitals had increased their admissions over the years. Given the gradual increase in the size of the navy from its low point in 1818 this was to be expected, though Burnett took pride in the fact that the numbers of servicemen ill had remained static. In the six years between 1816 and 1821 a total of 137,000 seamen had been raised, with 20,821 entered on the sick-list; in the six years between 1828 and 1833 the total was 175,000 but with sick-lists amounting to only 20,475.[6] But, as Burnett always stressed, naval hospitals had to be prepared for peaks in demand. By 1847 Haslar was effectively allowed one full surgeon more than its 1831 establishment. On paper, the medical staff at East Stonehouse in 1847 remained much the same as in 1831 yet that hospital only functioned efficiently because it could draw upon newly entered assistant surgeons held as supernumeraries aboard the Port Admiral's flagship. Opening the Melville inevitably relieved some of the pressures on the other home hospitals. On his visit to Chatham in December 1841 Burnett reported 81 men currently detained for treatment in its wards, though, as at other hospitals, this did not reflect the large number registered annually. More than 1,230 men passed through the Melville during 1839; in 1847 the figure was 2,230. The Melville accepted eligible residents in the vicinity suffering from seasonal fevers and dysentery, seamen from ships fitting and recruiting in the Medway, sailors from coastguard and revenue vessels and men who had incurred serious injuries while working in the dockyards at Chatham and Sheerness. Admittedly few of these would otherwise have been sent to Portsmouth or Plymouth. The Melville, though, by 1848 had established itself as an important medical facility. It contained 156 patients in March 1848 and its routine of care was considered second to none.

The daily round at Chatham was described by Deputy-Inspector William Rae in 1848 just before he left to take up his new post as Inspector at East Stonehouse. Rae had run the Melville since 1840 and was widely credited with raising medical standards. Early each morning up to 20 naval recruits had to be examined personally by the Deputy-Inspector. When this time-consuming job was done he hastened to the hospital wards where junior colleagues were already waiting. When Rae first came to the Melville he examined and prescribed for every patient each morning but by 1848 this was simply beyond him. Even allowing only two minutes for each man, which in any case he considered too short to allow a proper assessment, this would take nearly five hours on most days. The assistant surgeons therefore had to prescribe too; even so, he stressed, the morning's work could not be finished without encroaching on the lunch hour for patients, nurses and hospital labourers alike. Taking such a meal as time allowed, Rae proceeded to the office to attend to correspondence, papers and accounts and then on to the dispensary and stores to oversee requirements. Out-patients, usually naval officers or their families, had next to be visited before returning to check some of the more serious cases in the wards before the evening round. 'I have not had a moment to call my own from eight in the morning till 4pm, and soon after the evening visit was awaiting me,' Rae recorded wearily.[7]

Hospital routine took its toll on the junior staff too. Indeed prolonged duties amid the depressing atmosphere of a large hospital were not conducive to health or happiness. In 1848 Rae had four assistants who worked in the dispensary, were on call for out-patient emergencies, kept the medical accounts, helped with dressings and bandages on ward rounds, had day-to-day responsibility for issuing and receiving stores needed for 3,000 men attached to the 34 ships currently nearby, and generally supervised the wards, admitting new patients, registering their ailments and keeping the discharge book. 'The duty of this hospital is carried on, and its accounts kept as nearly as possible in the same way as at the other hospitals,' Rae explained.[8] The medical staff at Chatham, in consequence, had little time for relaxation.

The Melville, like Haslar and East Stonehouse, served as a valuable training opportunity for many new recruits to the medical service. In 1832 the Admiralty sanctioned an application from Burnett that of five assistant surgeons borne as supernumeraries on the Admiral's flagship at Portsmouth, four should be sent to the hospital, while at Plymouth two of the three assistants on the flagship should be likewise despatched. When needed for sea service they would be recalled, starting with those longest ashore. In reality the hospitals relied upon them, although Burnett was certain that the benefit was mutual. In 1833 he argued that two or three years spent in wards ashore was a better training for young assistant surgeons than ten years in any cockpit and in 1837 he petitioned the Board angrily when he discovered that supernumeraries were not being released by Commanders-in-Chief to the hospitals as required. He was also annoyed when young assistants were removed to ships without any obvious reason or notice.

While Inspectors and surgeons at the home hospitals were naturally grateful for all the help available, the procedure after 1831 whereby supernumeraries were lent from flagships masked a grievance bitterly felt by senior medics. The grievance was that senior hospital staff were barred from taking paying pupils. There were strict rules forbidding paid work outside naval service: medical officers would sometimes volunteer to work during local epidemics but in 1802 the Admiralty had made it plain that no practice or appointments of a private character were acceptable. Forbidding pupils at the hospitals was not Burnett's idea and he tried to persuade the Board to overturn this ban which had been introduced in 1825. Before 1825 pupils had been useful helpers for hospital physicians and had never got in the way of efficiency, he argued; furthermore, he had never heard any explanation of why the ban had been adopted. To appease senior hospital staff the Admiralty had initially allowed the hospitals increased establishments of assistant surgeons, though this was discontinued in 1831 on the grounds of expense. Using supernumeraries who might otherwise be idle aboard the flagships was the best deal that Burnett could get for the hospitals after 1832. The problem, however, was that it did not provide senior hospital staff with the fees which came with private pupils and effectively confirmed the significant cut in income which had been imposed in 1825.

No one expressed this more forcefully than Dickson as physician and then Inspector at East Stonehouse between 1824 and 1847. Why, he enquired in 1837, could men of his rank not take a limited number of pupils when their counterparts in civilian hospitals made a handsome living by taking so many? Creyke, when Governor, had supported the idea of the physician and surgeon having pupils; indeed he had positively recommended it in 1810. Having pupils would mean that more assistant surgeons could be made available for warships and that a training regime specific to the needs of the Royal Navy could operate at its hospitals – led, of course, by men of great experience who had themselves worked in tropical climates, seen every affliction which could befall seamen and passed through every grade of the service. Burnett felt that two pupils per senior colleague was permissible; he also wanted the sons of medical officers to be allowed to join ward rounds in the hope that it might stimulate an interest in studying medicine and joining the navy. In the end it came down to money. 'The hospital physician cannot look anywhere around him without seeing his civil brethren accumulating an ample fortune,' Dickson remarked. By contrast, a naval medic devoting his life to public service, 'finds at last that his income is becoming yearly less adequate to the education and maintenance of his growing family'. Even at the end of a distinguished career, Dickson reflected, as far as providing for his old age and his children were concerned 'he may be said almost to have lived in vain.'[9]

Despite this refusal to allow pupils, Haslar and East Stonehouse did provide more by way of training for assistant surgeons than simply clinical experience. There were lectures and surgical demonstrations to attend: at both hospitals after 1827 the physician and surgeon lectured in alternate weeks during the summer months about recent treatments, and although the schedule was modified in 1829 and the lectures not always well attended they continued to be regarded as an educative duty by senior staff. While attached to the hospitals assistant surgeons were encouraged to keep a journal of their cases as a surgeon would need to do at sea. Young men were 'taught to apply the principles of medicine and surgery they formerly studied to actual treatment of disease,' Burnett made clear.[10] When major operations were to be performed a flag was hoisted at the hospitals to alert medical officers aboard ships nearby. In the operating theatre the scene could be chaotic as the assistants jostled for position. Haslar needed mirrors above the table in 1835 so that the audience could observe the detail of what was being done without interruption. But this was not just for the benefit of the assistant surgeons. 'I have, almost in every instance, felt how much the attention of the operator is distracted by the endeavours of the students to obtain a clear sight of the sufferer,' the surgeon added to his application for

the increased expenditure. As for the hapless patient, amid his agony he was
distressed even further 'by the hisses and groans of thoughtless young men,
who, when the head of a principal assistant or dresser is perhaps necessarily interposed between them and what they very properly have an anxious
desire to behold clearly, make use of such inconsiderate and indecent means
to effect their purpose'.[11] It was education of a sort: it was, presumably,
better than nothing.

The home hospitals also accumulated important research libraries,
largely built upon bequests from avid collectors within the service. The
most substantial of these were Robert McKinnal's 1838 legacy of more
than 200 volumes and medical treatises and then the 400 textbooks left by
Leonard Gillespie in 1842. Haslar's library opened in 1827 and by 1844 had
6,500 volumes and 400 pamphlets, In order to maintain it the navy allocated £150 per annum beyond an initial grant of £400. The library at East
Stonehouse was built in 1834 at a cost of £700 and an annual grant thereafter of £100. Ironically the book money was not all spent and after 1836
the annual award of £100 had to cover purchases at both libraries. Given
the high price of medical works these libraries were valuable repositories
of knowledge within the naval medical corps.[12] After 1827 Haslar also had
a lavish museum, built up from geological exhibits, examples of flora and
fauna gathered from across the world and objects of pathology preserved
within the hospital. One of the most trusted and in time much respected
labourers was paid 2/6d a day after 1832, raised to four shillings in 1841, to
act as keeper and to prepare expertly the specimens of natural history. The
Haslar exhibits 'may vie with those of any museum in Europe,' Burnett
noted approvingly,[13] observing in 1842 that the museum had the status of
a national institution attracting many visitors each year. Attempts to create
a similar museum at East Stonehouse were less successful and Burnett's
report in 1841 made for gloomy reading. No one was designated and paid
from among the hospital's staff to act as caretaker and hence specimens
were seldom prepared. Over the years Haslar's appetite grew at the expense
of the more modest museums at other establishments, acquiring material
from Malta in 1828, from Chatham in 1835, from Greenwich in 1846 and
from Plymouth in 1911. Haslar symbolized the spirit of scientific enquiry
which Burnett was always so anxious to instil in the service. Extra rooms
were added in 1840, 1850 and again in 1903. Although much of the museum
was lost in enemy action in 1941 Haslar's historic library survived.[14]

Although the hospitals at the three major ports were by far the Medical

Department's largest shore institutions in Britain, it also had charge of four marine infirmaries at Portsmouth, Plymouth, Chatham and Woolwich and smaller hospital establishments at Deal and on the southern coast of Ireland at Haulbowline. The 1805 Order in Council which, on paper, provided for the standing of both surgeons and assistants had also directed that the naval surgeons who staffed marine infirmaries should be paid the same as their counterparts in hospitals and dockyards. But like so much else promised in 1805 this intention lapsed within five years when an Admiralty review raised the salaries of hospital and dockyard surgeons to £500 per annum but left those of infirmary men at a lower figure. For years the marine infirmaries were not even inspected. Only when the Medical Department was created did any serious interest in their work begin, after Burnett accepted that the duties of medical staff there could be as arduous as any other in the service. Infirmaries, however, were smaller than hospitals and the treatments provided were limited. Surgery was not generally performed and serious cases of injury or disease were transferred at once to the naval hospitals. Indeed, as Burnett conceded in 1832, the facilities at an infirmary were similar to those of a ship's sick-bay in that they gave rest, medicines, nursing care and sick-diet.

In 1834 the Portsmouth and Plymouth Royal Marine infirmaries each had one surgeon and one assistant while that at Woolwich had two assistants to aid the surgeon. Anxious for economy in the mid-1830s, the Board cast a watchful eye on these establishments and suggested that they might even be abolished, with all cases accommodated at the hospitals. Burnett staved this off with a variety of well-chosen arguments. The marines would still require some on-the-spot provision for minor ailments and injuries, so the saving would be minimal. The hospitals also had no secure accommodation for men under punishment, such as the infirmaries provided, and in an emergency or in bad weather the inevitable delay in getting cases to an hospital could cost lives. In any case the infirmaries were not all the same. At Woolwich and Chatham seamen were increasingly being admitted as if to proper naval hospitals; those infirmaries could handle more serious cases, as was acknowledged by 1847 when both were run by a Deputy-Inspector rather than a surgeon. Although Plymouth still had only one surgeon and one assistant in 1847 the other establishments had all increased their staff in recent years. By 1847 Portsmouth had one surgeon and two assistants while Woolwich and Chatham each had two assistants to support their Deputy-Inspectors.

Officially the Portsmouth infirmary was ordered to hold no more than 20 marines, exclusive of men under arrest. In practice, however, the number of admissions was often higher. On inspection, there were 80 in 1835: half the cases at all times were venereal. Burnett did suggest that some of the latter might be sent to Haslar but the infirmary surgeon expressed a wish to keep them all, 'being better acquainted with the characters of the individuals'.[15] Knowing that rowdy marines would not be welcome at Haslar, Burnett let the matter rest, deeming the cases to be only minor afflictions. Marine barracks were a hard life. In 1844 the Inspector at Haslar complained about the state in which a marine who had just died in the hospital had been admitted. The man had been among a number confined for five months in the garrison cells at divisional headquarters and fed a diet barely adequate to sustain life. The barracks was also an unhealthy posting for medical staff. Portsmouth barracks contained up to 6,000 men in just two buildings – ideal conditions, as the scarlatina which swept the marine division in 1854 demonstrated, for the spread of any infection.

Conditions among the marines at Plymouth were no different. Half the infirmary cases there too were invariably syphilis, though overall the numbers of patients were generally lower than at Portsmouth; in 1835 there were 18, and still only 30 in 1853. As at Portsmouth, the barracks were frequently unhealthy for inmates and medical officers alike. In 1847 its assistant surgeon had to be transferred to the purer air of a seagoing vessel due to bronchial inflammation. His successor, William Kay, who came to Plymouth after his travels around the eastern Mediterranean and who Burnett had marked down for rapid advancement, died from dysentery at the barracks in 1853. It also proved impossible to keep cholera out of the barracks when Plymouth was severely affected by the 1849 epidemic; likewise, smallpox struck down several marines when introduced from nearby towns or ships at anchor in 1852. Woolwich had a similar problem of isolating men with infectious diseases: in 1853 Burnett warned its Deputy-Inspector that more control over both the attendants and other patients entering the smallpox wards was necessary. Because Woolwich also admitted sailors, it always had more patients than the marine infirmaries at Portsmouth and Plymouth; it had its lowest ever number, 18, when Burnett visited in 1839 but held 100 patients in October 1852.

Whereas the surgeon in charge of the infirmary at Portsmouth could claim an overall responsibility for up to 6,000 men, the marine division at Woolwich was closer to 1,300. Nevertheless the Woolwich infirmary was always sufficiently stretched that almost any indisposition among the medical staff necessitated an urgent appeal for another supernumerary assistant surgeon to be sent. It also fell foul of economies regarding supplies in the 1840s whereby many articles, necessary even for compounding medicines, were frequently out of stock. In 1848 the Deputy-Inspector was reproached for providing such luxuries as fruit and jellies to the sick: Burnett grudgingly acknowledged that medical logic lay behind these extras but added for the future that 'it is very desirable that the liberal diet allowed by the scale should not be exceeded, except on special occasions'.[16] But the worst problem at Woolwich was the chronic shortage of space. This sometimes meant that officers of different ranks had to share a ward and always meant that other ranks, and stores, were squeezed together. The infirmary required more wards, a receiving room, such as hospitals enjoyed, and a place nearby for the immediate bathing of new admissions. It also lacked a cookhouse, a washhouse and a proper storage area for bedding. In fact the infirmary at Woolwich did increase in size after 1844 although not at a rate sufficient to accommodate its swelling admissions. By 1856 it seldom had fewer than 240 patients. But what made matters worse at most of the marine infirmaries were the outpatients: marines and their families, inside and outside the barracks, were entitled to medical provision.

The extent of this duty and the pressures it created were particularly noticeable during epidemics. Andrew Millar and William Kay, as surgeon and assistant at the Plymouth infirmary during the 1849 cholera outbreak, were so overwhelmed by calls upon their services amid the murky backstreets of Plymouth and East Stonehouse that an additional assistant had to be sent to help them. When the Deputy-Inspector's health broke down at Woolwich in 1852 Burnett assigned a supernumerary assistant surgeon specifically to cover the extensive duty of home calls upon marine families. Millar had to ask for extra help again at Plymouth in January 1854: it was, he appealed to Burnett, because 'fever, catarrh, bronchitis and choleraic diarrhoea prevail extensively among the women and children of marines, there being now ninety cases under treatment'.[17] In January 1855 Millar was again stressing the burden of his work, so much so that he applied for promotion to Deputy-Inspector at either the Woolwich or Chatham infirmaries should a vacancy arise. In six and a half years Millar had tended a total sick-list of 10,397 marines and examined a further 2,558 recruits. Millar failed to get away from Plymouth. In 1857 he complained that despite now having two permanent assistant surgeons the infirmary could not handle the ever growing demand. The Plymouth marine division numbered 1,859 by 1857, almost 500 of whom lived at least half a mile from the headquarters and barracks. Additional duties for medical officers had also been devised whereby men undergoing new systems of musketry instruction had to have an assistant surgeon present at firing parties and when great guns were exercised. Weekly marching in the countryside and parades in the town also required a doctor in attendance. As for calls upon the augmented numbers of women and children, up to 1,600 were eligible for this benefit by 1857, of whom 200 were already receiving treatment in their homes. Prescribing and dispensing for them alone almost fully occupied one of Millar's precious assistants. Then there was the constant call for midwifery: the Plymouth infirmary responded to more than 100 calls during the second half of 1856. Few medical officers who joined the navy envisaged this as one of their common duties.

Midwifery was bad enough for any medic: time was wasted simply waiting for something to happen. In other ways, too, delivery was unrewarding and generally unwelcome. Healthy babies and happy mothers were wonders of nature and signs of God's unfailing bounty, whereas medical complications or disasters were always likely to be reflections on the ability of those in attendance. Then there was the problem of conflict with local practitioners who, not unnaturally, could be resentful of the way in which the navy denied them so much potential employment. It certainly opened a can or worms at Woolwich in 1838 where, as at Plymouth and Chatham, marines were in the habit of paying into a midwifery pool. There had been a comparable collection in Portsmouth but that was defunct by 1838. The origin of the Woolwich fund was uncertain, though it was known to have operated since 1809 and it was officially recognized by the Admiralty. From it, assistant surgeons or any local practitioner could be paid half a guinea for attending the wives of marines at childbirth. On investigation, however, it was unclear who at Woolwich managed it and where exactly the estimated £450 collected every year had gone. The marine commandant was nominally responsible but when pressed in 1838 he merely told the Deputy-Inspector at the infirmary that the fund was empty. Surely the Admiralty had the power to call for accounts, medical officers enquired? The suspicion was that the fund had been plundered over many years to pay the salary and other costs of a higher-ranking bandmaster than any other marine division was able to afford.

Problems also arose at Plymouth after customary payments from the weekly Penny Club were stopped in 1845. Until then women of the marine corps chose where to spend their £1 midwifery entitlement. Now choice was being denied them and they had to make do with the assistant surgeon from the infirmary. It seemed that the infirmary's medical staff were intimidating the women, threatening to stop all future medical attendance for their families if they used a local doctor. The infirmary denied trying to cream off the fund for its exclusive benefit. Local practitioners were sometimes too old to inspire confidence in the younger women, the surgeon retorted; in any case, the women frequently wanted the assistant surgeon to help them apply for charity from other funds administered by the marine division or privately by officers' wives. It was difficult in London to determine where the truth lay. The Admiralty resorted to the time-honoured practice of government departments by saying that such matters were for local management and that it could offer no opinion.[18]

Smaller establishments, officially classed as temporary hospitals, were maintained at Deal and at Haulbowline. Deal dated from the early eighteenth century. In 1794 Trotter spoke most unfavourably of its facilities and it was closed at the end of the Napoleonic Wars. It re-opened for an emergency in 1831 when there was much sickness in the fleet nearby but was otherwise so little used that in 1843 Burnett could no longer resist persistent requests from the coastguard to hand over part of the building on condition that the coastguard kept the place in good repair. Deal was not used until 1854 when the navy repossessed the hospital in order to accommodate sick and wounded expected from the Baltic. Haulbowline, near Cork, was until 1843 little more than a surgeon aboard a ship at anchor and a small building on the island close by, but it was run according to hospital procedures and was in permanent use. In 1843 the navy expanded Haulbowline to accommodate 24 patients on the island, allocating one assistant to support the surgeon in his duties. By 1849 its accommodation and stores had been extended to take 64 patients, and the medical staff had experienced additional work associated with famine and disease in Ireland. It was extended further in 1852 and raised to the status of a permanent establishment in the naval estimates for 1856–57.

Beyond the home hospitals and marine infirmaries the navy stationed medical officers at its dockyards and at its major depot at Deptford. As with the hospitals, these sometimes provided posts for men too old to return to sea and occasionally for younger men for whom that was no longer physically possible but whose medical skills could still be employed. One of the assistant surgeons at East Stonehouse clearly fell into the latter category in 1851 when the Inspector reported him fit for duty in a few weeks 'when more habituated to the use of a wooden leg'.[19] Andrew Clark, an assistant surgeon in 1855, was given a thorough medical examination in London where his right lung was found to be extensively diseased. He could never serve afloat again, but 'he is fit for the duties of a hospital', the Medical Department decided, and he could be sent to Plymouth 'where the climate is considered to be favourable to persons labouring under phthisis'.[20] In the Deptford yard, John Robertson was surgeon in 1857. He had sustained a serious thigh injury by falling through Arctic ice in 1849 and though his leg had been saved it was no more than a 'dangling member'.[21] Despite such cases, dockyard posts were generally sought-after appointments and frequently regarded as a reward for family men who had already spent years in unhealthy climates. There were seven yards in all. In 1847 Portsmouth, Devonport and Chatham each had one surgeon and assistant, while the smaller Pembroke, Sheerness, Woolwich and Deptford yards were each allowed one surgeon. As with the marine infirmaries, severe injuries and illnesses were sent to the naval hospitals: the dockyard medics treated less severe cases and were also required to tend the families of the dockyard officers and labourers, many of whom lived at some distance. During working hours the surgeons were forbidden to leave the yards. Save in times of epidemics, most of their cases, as Burnett described them in 1834, were skull and compound limb fractures and lacerations, often of arteries, where immediate attention meant the difference between life and death. At other times, home visits might include checking that labourers were not absent without good cause.

Portsmouth dockyard reported 13 injury cases and 39 sick in 1833, though, as Burnett observed, the surgeon and his assistant 'have many more patients amongst the women and children than amongst the men'.[22] This workload seldom changed. In the 1849 cholera epidemic the yard's medics had the additional task of mixing compounds to alleviate the abdominal pains and nausea suffered by many who worked there, though deaths in Portsmouth were comparatively few. That was not the case at Devonport, where cholera was so extensive that 38 men died in the dockyard and a temporary cholera hospital, equipped with bedding and stores from East Stonehouse, had to be set up on site. That had also been necessary during the earlier epidemic of 1832. In normal times work at Devonport was more relaxing. The Devonport yard had 12 men hurt and 23 ill at the 1833 inspec-

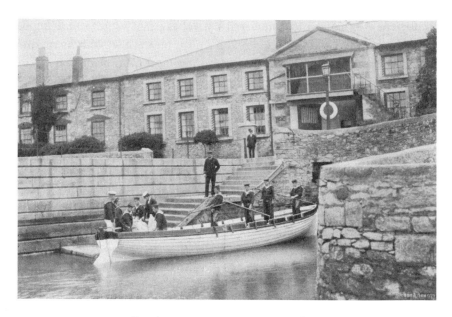

3. Landing a patient at East Stonehouse.

tion, with 18 hurt and 34 sick in 1853. Chatham dockyard registered six injuries and 21 ill at the 1838 visit. Burnett invariably commented on the good order at all three major dockyards and the zeal of their surgeons.

Where, at the smaller dockyards, there was no assistant for the surgeon, life could be more arduous. The surgeon at Sheerness, for instance, complained in 1836 that much of his time was spent on trivial cases. There were many ships fitting at Sheerness, often lying at a distance from the yard, yet in all weathers he was expected to be on call. In the circumstances, he urged, he should be spared having to make visits except to the officers, wives and children of the yard itself; all other claimants on his services, except for the most urgent, should be required to attend his surgery at stated times. The Sheerness yard had nine injuries and ten men ill when visited in 1838. Life at Woolwich was easier, with no injuries recorded in 1840 and only ten men absent sick. Burnett liked the Woolwich yard as well as any. 'I was particularly gratified to see a case where the surgeon had performed one of the neatest amputations of part of the foot I have ever beheld,' he noted approvingly in 1833.[23] Pembroke, by contrast, attracted little notice at the Medical Department except when the private practitioner who performed the duties there pointed out how much the dockyard had expanded without any commensurate increase in medical cover. Although in 1815 and again in 1827 the Admiralty had authorized a naval assistant surgeon to help out at Pembroke, the latter was seldom at his post; meanwhile, with its marine battalion, the size of the yard had grown from 400 men on the payroll in 1827 to 1,300 in 1846. Being a civilian, he was paid £50 less than the proper naval surgeons at other dockyards; he had also to maintain his private practice and, since many of the dockyard workers lived several miles away, much time was occupied in travelling with no prospect of referring serious cases to any nearby naval hospital. The supposed assistant surgeon spent his time on yacht duty and had not visited the dockyard surgery in the past six months. The Pembroke yard was clearly an unsatisfactory arrangement. Deptford, on the other hand, not only paid £500 per annum but came with an excellent house as accommodation. Not surprisingly, in 1845 Burnett felt able to assure the Duke of Richmond that a surgeon in whom the latter took an interest would be comfortable there.[24]

At yards and infirmaries it was usually the lot of the surgeon, or his hard-pressed assistant, to compound the medicines, keep the accounts and be responsible for the stores and day-to-day supply contracts. At the hospitals, however, these management burdens were lightened by specific dispensary and civilian staff. When he assumed charge of the medical service Burnett set about dismantling the old dispensary structures at Haslar and East Stonehouse whereby young men were sometimes simply questioned about pharmacy before being engaged. The Deputy-Inspector described one such interview for a junior post in the latter's dispensary as late as 1848. Admittedly the candidate had served an apprenticeship and submitted documents which suggested a good knowledge of pharmacy, but when asked to read and translate from a list of substances his total ignorance was revealed. He could not understand the Pharmacopoeia, he failed to identify many powders and he had no idea how to mix medicinal ingredients. Such men were not only unfit to dispense medicine but, owing to their lack of medical knowledge, could be of no assistance to other staff. Burnett had already persuaded the Admiralty in the early 1830s that experienced surgeons should run the hospital dispensaries rather than men of inferior talent who in the past had frequently been drawn from the ranks of hospital mates. Henceforth the position of dispenser would be abolished and replaced at the three home hospitals with the combined office of surgeon and medical storekeeper who would be accountable for everything issued both to in-patients and to those aboard ships in port. As so often, Burnett's success with the Board owed much to his judicious line of argument: by adopting his plan 'we are not only supplied with medicines which can be entirely depended upon as genuine, but also all due economy is preserved'.[25]

With the dispensaries now run by medical officers, men with qualifications only in pharmacy, if employed, assumed the role of dispensary helpers. Haslar needed a dispensary helper in 1845 when it proved impossible to find a suitable assistant surgeon. William Toon applied for the vacancy. Toon had previously worked in the Portsmouth dockyard helping its surgeon to mix compounds. He both knew the *materia medica* and had practical experience in handling the ingredients. For four months he had effectively performed the dockyard surgeon's dispensary duties, issuing medicinal wines, porter and arrowroot, and he had kept all the record books which formerly had been done by an assistant surgeon. On examination at Haslar, Toon's knowledge of the Pharmacopoeia and Latin prescriptions was impressive. Burnett was not pleased at taking a non-medical man but sanctioned Toon's appointment. Toon, however, would have no grading, being employed merely to 'assist in the dispensary'. His pay could thereby be kept at 2/6d a day whereas an assistant surgeon would have cost seven shillings.[26]

Dispensaries were usually a source of problems in hospitals not only because of the difficulty of finding suitable men but also because of the constant pressure under which their work normally had to be done. William Rae explained his anxiety when running the Melville in 1848: although its dispensary had been judged efficient seven years earlier, by 1848 it could no longer provide properly for both the hospital wards and for the warships moored in the Medway.[27] When patient admissions rose the two dispensary helpers who had been engaged had to work late into the night preparing such medicines as would not spoil for use the following day. It could have been worse. The Woolwich marine infirmary had also been allowed to take on two dispensary helpers by 1848, mostly to compound medicines for marine families in the vicinity, but the Deputy-Inspector had been obliged to discharge them for drunkenness. The Woolwich dispensary and its accounts had all but broken down, he confessed to Burnett, which must entail a waste of medical stores. Burnett tried to find him an assistant surgeon but none with sufficient knowledge to assume responsibility in an establishment of that size was available. Toon's case at Haslar had since been repeated at Greenwich and now Burnett had once more to concede that the service would have to settle for 'a person who has been educated as a dispensing chemist and druggist.'[28] The same dilemma had just arisen at East Stonehouse where the assistant surgeon who had run the dispensary was dying. Again, much of the work would have to be entrusted to someone without medical qualification.

Toon was a cheeky young man but he did his work well at Haslar and thereby demonstrated that at least some of Burnett's apprehensions that dispensary work might be slipping back into old ways were unfounded. By 1852 Toon's pay had been raised to five shillings a day, with coal and candles in his small rooms. Anything more would spoil him further, the Captain-Superintendent of the hospital remarked: the medical staff already considered him sufficiently forward. Haslar used Toon in the same way as the Woolwich infirmary used its dispensary help – to make up prescriptions required outside the wards, mostly for servicemen's families and ships in port and to distribute sago, arrowroot and other nutrients. But with upwards of 400 patients already in the hospital by March 1854, and with a further 100 daily expected, even the trusty Toon would no longer be able to cope. Already in the wards where rounds began at 6am medicines did not arrive until noon, and with assistant surgeons now urgently needed for both the Baltic and Mediterranean fleets such delays could only get worse. 'Compounding medicines might be done more regularly and cheaply by aid of two or three men from a druggist's shop,' the Inspector at Haslar wrote to Somerset House. 'I dare say such men would readily offer for a temporary engagement were the want known.'[29]

By the end of March 1854 the Haslar dispensary had engaged three helpers to work with Toon, all having served apprenticeships. Demand was such that they began compounding medicines at 7am each day, taking only a mid-morning breakfast. But even this arrangement had to be changed because the work could not be completed. The hospital assigned cabins where they could take their meals and where, in rotation, they could sleep at night in case of emergency. In practice the pharmacy became the domain of the dispensary men because the assistant surgeons remaining at Haslar would not cooperate with them, considering it beneath their station to work alongside non-medics. This demarcation dispute was ultimately referred to the First Lord of the Admiralty who, Burnett's misgivings notwithstanding, sided with those who believed it impossible to do anything other than to turn over virtually all the dispensary's functions to druggists. This was also a reflection on the medical education which assistant surgeons had received before joining the navy, one member of the Board advised Burnett privately: even when newly recruited assistants were available they were unlikely to know how to mix medicines. The best doctors in the navy had always learnt their profession by working in it rather than studying outside of it; if Burnett wanted to use only assistant surgeons in the dispensaries then it might be necessary to have appropriate training for them in the home hospitals. Otherwise, employing men such as Toon at least had the benefit of relieving surgeons and assistants from duties 'which may not be exactly suited to their rank'.[30]

Whatever frictions arose with the junior medical staff, Haslar was generally well served by Toon and his associates who remained at the hospital during the Crimean War. East Stonehouse was not so fortunate. When a suitable helper for its dispensary was found in 1854 Burnett vetoed the appointment on the grounds that the man also ran a drug shop in Plymouth and would have a clash of interests. In 1855 the hospital's dispenser, who had worked there since 1848, simply disappeared without even informing his wife and family. By the 1840s even Haulbowline had dispensary workers, the most faithful of whom had served for ten years in 1857.

Large hospitals and infirmaries inevitably employed many staff other than their medics and those who undertook pharmacy. Haslar and East Stonehouse each had an agent and a steward prior to 1831 who were effectively their chief administrators. As economies, the roles of agent and steward were subsequently amalgamated and clerical support reduced. It was the responsibility of the agent and steward to keep the financial accounts of the hospital, to advertise for and enforce the performance of contracts from local suppliers and workmen, to maintain and protect the stores, to ensure the quality of food and that it was properly cooked, and generally to oversee the employment of labourers, the upkeep of the grounds and the cleanliness of the buildings. Unlike Haslar and East Stonehouse, the Melville had no agent. 'We have only one clerk with a small salary to attend to the whole of the clerical department,' the Deputy-Inspector complained in 1848.[31] That had remained the case for at least the past decade and although the number of patients at Chatham had expanded no allowance for the extra administration had ever been made. The Melville had experienced difficulties in its early years, which had doubtless made the Admiralty reluctant to tinker with a system which at least worked, however much stress it placed upon the clerk. After opening in 1828 the Melville had employed a purveyor whose 'errors and neglects' led to his dismissal in 1835. The virtue of using the clerk, Burnett explained, was that it put one man in a position of accountability 'from which he cannot readily depart without my having the means of checking him immediately'.[32]

Haslar acquired a reputation for sound management. Two dependable men held the post of agent and steward between 1831 and 1851, where-upon the much respected John Russell was appointed. Russell had previously been clerk to the naval hospital at Malta since 1819 and now served Haslar throughout the Crimean War. He was widely regarded as an active and highly intelligent man and probably the best clerical officer in naval employment. East Stonehouse also had long-serving and competent agents. John Grant served for many years until succeeded by Charles Holworthy in 1842. The agent's clerk at East Stonehouse was also judged deserving when he asked for a pay increase in 1852. Since the clerk had been at the hospital for several years and had been allowed 2/6d a day extra for heavy duties during the 1849 cholera epidemic in Plymouth, Burnett suggested that this might be permitted again.

More mundanely, all establishments required labourers who toiled in the gardens, offices and sometimes in the hospital wards. East Stonehouse never had fewer than 16 until 1849 when the Captain-Superintendent dismissed six of them for being useless. Some labourers were more skilled than others and wanted pay differentials to be maintained – as in 1838 when the carpenters, bricklayers and other artificers who worked at Haslar requested the same four shillings per day as they believed their counterparts elsewhere received. The labourers were usually mustered for the annual visitation, which gave those members of the Board of Admiralty present a chance to be assured that all were fit for purpose. Burnett's concern regarding staff numbers at the hospitals was not simply to ensure that unnecessary costs were avoided but also to free space by moving as many as possible out of the accommodation which had increasingly been provided for them in hospital buildings in recent decades. He was, however, still trying to control entitlement to accommodation in 1853. Then there was the problem that workmen who performed specific functions wanted recognition. Henry Dawe, who tended the shrubs and flowers in the grounds at East Stonehouse, wished extra money for the care which he lavished upon them. It was a fair claim, Burnett advised the Board in 1851: the hospital gardens were a great ornament to the place. James Coffin at Haslar in 1853 was another petitioner: he had acted as postman for eight years and had the Captain-Superintendent's recommendation for an upgrading. He also wanted more suitable quarters for his family since his current rooms were too close to the soldiers of the guardhouse whose conversations and manners, he feared, would corrupt his children. Coffin was raised to skilled labourer with a weekly wage of 10/6d, with provisions, to replace the eight shillings paid before. He did not, however, get a move. Rat-catcher was another specialist position meriting additional pay. At East Stonehouse a man from Plymouth had usually been called in, but when his health failed in 1853 one of the labourers quickly volunteered for duty. Being on site and knowing how to access all parts of the hospital would be an advantage, the Captain-Superintendent ruled. The volunteer had already shown a great interest in vermin and demonstrated skill in catching them.

Hospital agents and their clerks were civilians. By contrast, at the marine infirmaries this type of work was done by men in uniform or by a purveyor in the pay office at battalion headquarters. Between 1827 and 1848 a devoted marine sergeant acted as steward, clerk and porter at the Woolwich infirmary and had become so indispensable that the problem of replacing him eventually arrived on the First Lord's desk. The sergeant had remained until 10pm most evenings after the day's other duties had been done and he always stayed well into the night before quarterly store inspections were due. Not surprisingly no one came forward and the only possibility was to sanction the cost of using two men in the future. Having an experienced sergeant in control of the infirmary's daily workings had many advantages, some of which only became obvious after he had gone. Suddenly the water closets were becoming regularly blocked and needing repair at considerable expense as patients were throwing in flannel band-ages, rags and grass: 'in fact, anything they can get hold of', the purveyor concluded. If the Medical Department would not supply paper would it at least sanction local procurement? News of this breakdown of discipline at Woolwich was received badly at Somerset House. Paper was not provided at any other establishment nor had such a difficulty ever arisen. With the old sergeant gone, tradesmen coming to the infirmary also sensed a laxer regime. The butcher, on being informed in 1849 that the quality of his meat had deteriorated in the past year, launched into a torrent of abuse, 'damn-ing and buggering the contract', insisting that he would be glad when it expired and asking who else would be fool enough to take 'such a damned buggering thing'. All this was played out in earshot of patients and labour-ers at the infirmary. The contract was not renewed.[33]

Among an agent's other headaches was the lack of adequate laun-dry facilities. This arose most acutely at Haslar after Russell took up his appointment. Haslar and East Stonehouse both employed washerwomen on a daily or weekly basis. Washerwomen earned four shillings a week; the woman who also acted as overseer received 4/8d. It was uninspiring work which fluctuated according to hospital admissions. Burnett was wary that the hospitals, especially East Stonehouse, kept on more poor women in the laundry than were really needed, probably as a surreptitious form of local charity for widows and other members of seamen's families. Judging the right number was not easy: in 1849, however, he concluded that one washer per 25 patients would be ample. Applying a similar principle to other women engaged to repair bedding and clothing, one seamstress would be adequate for every 50 men. At Haslar this whole area of operation was inefficient because the women were not trustworthy and rarely had any supervision. To raise the quality of work, in 1851 the Captain-Superintendent proposed offering a shilling a day to attract a suitable overseer and in 1853 his successor planned to create a more permanent laundry arrangement whereby 20 women would be engaged full time at six shillings a week to replace the 26 who worked erratically for only four shillings. The nine temporary seamstresses engaged at three shillings a week could likewise be replaced by six permanent employees paid five shillings. By such measures, he assured the Admiralty, 'the services of a more respectable class of people would be always obtained.'[34] But there was no sign of immediate progress: weeks later Burnett was still raising the issue of laundry work and urged a general increase for washerwomen from four to five shillings weekly.

Laundries usually functioned well enough in summer: problems were more likely to arise in winter months when indoor drying space was needed. East Stonehouse, and even the Melville, had always been better off than Haslar in that respect. Russell was disappointed to discover that not only was there no steam-washing machinery but that some of Haslar's laundry was being sent out at double the cost. A scarlatina epidemic, brought to Portsmouth aboard *Agamemnon* early in 1853, exposed real shortcomings at the hospital. By February Haslar was fuller than at any time during the preceding 35 years. In April it held 279 suspected cases; it was just as well that most remained on their feet and were able to wash their own clothes and dry them outdoors. By January 1854 the hospital was generating 1,200 laundry items every day and the system was collapsing. The indoor drying horses and their rollers were old, broken and unable to cope with more than 270 pieces every 12 hours. Early in 1854 new outbreaks aboard *Illustrious* and in the marine barracks further increased the pressure. By the end of March 1854 the Inspector had more than 350 scarlatina cases on his hands.

Badly understaffed and unable to handle disease on such a scale, Haslar faced paralysis.

Burnett knew, after many years of practice, that the only way to persuade the Board to sanction expenditure was to convince it that doing nothing would cost even more. The latest steam-powered machinery was needed, such as other large establishments in England and Scotland had recently installed and which could be found in large hotels in America and in soldiers' barracks and hospitals in France. There was a steam laundry machine in Southampton, although not the most advanced model, which could wash thousands of items daily and which required only one employee to supervise the operation alongside a few women to mangle and fold. Haslar's manual laundry employees in 1853 cost £660, with a further £203 in materials. But the old ways were not just cumbersome and expensive; fabrics wore out more quickly, thereby incurring additional replacement charges. The Board approved a cost analysis, but even though Haslar's antiquated system had been successfully patched up over many years there was, it seemed, no escaping the obvious conclusion. In any case, the issue extended beyond institutional management. Seamen were now better tended in hospitals than ever before and kept cleaner and healthier. They were all discharged to their ships with washed clothes, which was important for reducing the incidence of disease throughout the fleet and which in turn produced knock-on economies in medical provision. Russell was despatched to Glasgow to assess the latest technology.

Medical staff at the hospitals, of course, saw little of the laundries, never dealt with rude contractors or cared what labourers were paid. The group with whom they most came into contact, other than the dispensary men whom they disdained, were nurses. Nurses, male and female, were supervised by women, usually the widows or daughters of naval officers, who were paid 1/8d per day as either ward or store matrons. Home hospitals in the mid-nineteenth century tended to have matrons of long standing who, though often efficient and providing continuity, came to epitomize a nursing regime which appeared to have changed little since the eighteenth century. Mary Lawton, for instance, the widow of a marine sergeant with three children, had combined store and ward duties as matron at the Melville since it opened, and had worked since 1811 in the navy's earlier rudimentary medical facility at Chatham. Aged 74 in 1854, poor health obliged her to seek a pension which, as 'an old and faithful servant', the navy granted, based on her salary of £35 per annum with an extra 10d a day in lieu of rations.[35] Mrs Denny, retiring from her position as sole matron at the Woolwich Royal Marine Infirmary aged 70 in 1857, had served for 46 years. The marine infirmary at Portsmouth employed Julia Murphy as sole matron between 1831 and 1845 on an annual salary of £20. When she asked for a pension on the grounds of ill health there was some doubt about her entitlement as a married woman, but so well had she served, and her husband being 50 years in the marines, that medical staff at the infirmary were determined that an effort should be made. Burnett was worried about the Board's response; nevertheless, he advised how best the infirmary might press Murphy's case. There must be an official letter, he directed, 'which is not to contain anything respecting her husband but merely her own service and desire for retirement, when I will endeavour to obtain something for her'.[36]

Nearby at Haslar, Margaret Wright had been ward matron since 1838 when she had effectively inherited the position from her mother. Wright's father had been physician of the fleet for 20 years and his widow had been appointed on his death in 1822. The younger Wright, however, was never a suitable choice, as became clear when her health deteriorated in 1851 and she requested a pension. Burnett assured the Board that he had known nothing about Wright's appointment in 1838 but that on his subsequent visits to Haslar medical officers had expressed disquiet about her lack of enthusiasm, frequent absences and lady-like airs. 'I must express a hope that an entirely different kind of person may be selected as her successor,' he concluded.[37] In the end the Admiralty allowed her a small pension, taking her parents' years of loyalty into account. The diligent Ann Gregory proved to be a much better appointment as store matron at Haslar: to Burnett's surprise, she even asked his permission to re-marry in 1848. The Director-General replied that it was not for him to say whether or who she should marry, although, in the continuance of her duties, it would not be possible for him to find married accommodation for her within the hospital. East Stonehouse also had long-serving matrons, at least until 1849 when Charlotte Pearce was dismissed after many years as ward matron, her post being abolished. Mrs Weale, the widow of an assistant surgeon and store matron since 1836, was kept on to perform both functions. Paid £30 per annum, however, she received less than the hospital's policeman and less, she suspected, than some of the nurses whom she supervised, while her counterparts at large London hospitals earned £100 a year with fewer responsibilities. With her work-load increased by the pressures of war, by

1856 Weale had more than 100 nurses, washerwomen, cleaners and seamstresses to keep an eye on. The navy appeared to be letting matters slip with
respect to valuable staff.

Nursing in hospitals and infirmaries had always been of question-
able quality. Old pensioners, marines detached for ward duties, widows
of servicemen and others recruited locally constituted a motley collection
throughout the early nineteenth century. They were paid on local scales:
five shillings per week with provisions at Haslar, East Stonehouse and Deal,
£10 a year at the Melville and 1/6d a day at Haulbowline. The infirmaries
paid £10 per annum, plus victualling, to pensioners and women and £5 to
serving marines. Some were too old to work properly. Others owed their
places to the patronage of surgeons or matrons. Weale, for instance, used
her position at East Stonehouse to secure work for her friends among local
married women. Eight of them had been engaged, at the expense of more
needy widows, one of whom, it was claimed, not only had the benefit of
her marine husband's half pay but otherwise received £15 annually from
the government and was fraudulently drawing six shillings a week in parish
relief. Drunkenness had never gone away as a problem among nursing staff.
Nancy Dunn was dismissed from East Stonehouse for this as late as 1857.

The Melville tried to raise standards in the early 1850s when old pensioners and other undesirables were cleared off the wards and replaced by fit and
able marines. But while there were obvious advantages to using strong men
for many ward duties, there were even more obvious advantages to having
them back in barracks doing what they were paid for – as the marine
battalion commander remonstrated when noticing how the strength of his
division was being depleted. Soon the old pensioners had to be brought
back on the former terms of £10 per annum, with an extra shilling a night
if nightwatches on seriously ill patients were necessary. A similar experiment at the Woolwich infirmary a few years earlier had to be unravelled
too. The marines used as nurses at Woolwich 'very soon became tired with
the confinement and discontented with their wages … they, therefore, by
degrees left the establishment'.[38] Early in 1854 the Woolwich infirmary was
back recruiting the wives and widows of marines, and six women of good
character had soon been engaged. Three serving marines had been kept
on temporarily for work in the venereal wards until suitable replacements
could be found.

Haslar's plan for improvement was to recruit a smaller number of
permanent nursing staff. Haslar, like East Stonehouse, had a number of

long-serving men and women, but too many others came and went and, since replacements usually had to be found immediately, there was little opportunity for screening applicants. Haslar calculated that it needed one nurse for every seven patients. Ideally those of middle age with a regular lifestyle and still possessing physical stamina would be employed, which would improve both the internal discipline of the hospital and public perceptions regarding the respectability of its staff. In an average week in 1852 Haslar had 44 nurses working in its medical and surgical wards for a weekly average of 241 patients; the Captain-Superintendent therefore suggested a fixed nursing body of 15 men and 20 women all paid seven shillings a week. If extra nurses were needed in emergencies they could be taken on at five shillings weekly. Burnett approved the idea but concluded that average numbers could never justify 35 nurses as a fixed establishment. Burnett further suggested that rather than seven shillings a week for all, which was too generous, there should be two grades among the nurses. Each ward would have an experienced, first-class nurse paid six shillings a week assisted by a junior whose pay would remain at the current five shillings. Promotion to the higher grade would be attainable by efficient work and fitness for responsibility.

Whatever its defects in hospital and infirmary management in the mid-nineteenth century, to its enduring credit the navy maintained and bestowed much care upon a remarkable institution at Portsmouth – its lunatic asylum. This was formed in 1818 and attached to Haslar. It received 126 patients when opened, 20 of whom were still living there in 1838. In the intervening 20 years it had admitted a total of 638 men, of whom 273 had died, 236 been discharged, four had escaped and 118 remained. Admittedly, even after 20 years, the Haslar asylum still had a number of defects. Most obvious to visitors were the dilapidated state of its internal decoration and the want of repair within its bathing cellar. Nevertheless with its secure environment and designated staff it represented a vast improvement on anything preceding it.

Inevitably the asylum was a depressing place to visit and Burnett, who had first gone there in the early 1820s, was still visibly moved on several subsequent occasions. A variety of cases could always be observed. Some raged violently against humanity and required constant restraint, some were deluded and confused, while others, once fine officers and sturdy seamen, seemed content to sit all day looking blankly out across the water, their minds lost or locked in a troubled world of battles long ago and oblivious to the fate which had befallen them. The asylum had its own Deputy-Inspector after 1840 who received some help from Haslar's assistant surgeons, from those sent over from the flagship and from a dedicated body of hospital labourers. The asylum could list a succession of humane heads, the most notable being James Anderson who ran it as Deputy-Inspector and later Inspector between 1842 and his death in 1853. Anderson was a pioneering figure in caring for mentally ill patients. He transformed the asylum soon after taking charge.

At his inspections after 1831 Burnett always commented upon the care and sympathy shown by the medical and other staff. Probationary wards were established where careful observation, sometimes for six weeks, of cases referred to the institution might reveal which type of treatment was appropriate or whether, indeed, the men referred were really mad at all. This was not only to help those eventually admitted but also to ensure that 'no unnecessary stigma might attach to a person who recovered under such circumstances'.[39] For those admitted, the gardens were used as therapeutic aids; inmates tended the fruit and vegetables cultivated there with obvious signs of benefit and, Burnett quickly reminded the Admiralty, at an annual saving of up to £100 in hospital provisions. Men had sometimes to be restrained from destroying their clothing and becoming ragged; often, too, the old penny magazines which some of them read repeatedly were destroyed. The cradles in which the men slept were modified in 1837 after one patient extracted material used to commit suicide. Special convalescent wards prepared hopeful cases for eventual discharge, though cure was always a matter of definition and could prove to be only temporary. Burnett did not wish to categorize mental illness as something wholly distinct from physical disease yet undoubtedly it did need a measure of specialized training and a different attitude towards the afflicted.

For all Burnett's interest in the institution, there had been complaints in the past. Edmund Griffin, a former purser in the navy who had been confined there for 12 years, asserted in 1839 that the deaths of several patients had been accelerated by the 'brutal and merciless treatment of the keepers'. The Captain-Superintendent at Haslar duly conducted an inquiry. Burnett conceded that in the past physical restraint had been too frequent, although the surgeon in charge between 1838 and 1842, John Mortimer, argued that force was sometimes necessary. But, knowing all the attendants as he did, Mortimer believed that none was capable of the excesses to which Griffin referred. Griffin's allegations were the product of an unsound

mind. While in the asylum he had frequently needed 'the gentlest coer-
cion' and would never have been released had not his sister constantly
applied for custody.[40] Anderson made much of this debate redundant by
virtually abolishing physical restraint. He sent many patients out, albeit
with attendants, to walk in the countryside, allowed them to stroll freely
around Haslar's grounds in the same way as men from the main hospital
and even had an attended boat supplied for their amusement. Anderson's
only form of punishment was confinement in a dark room, which seemed
to calm troubled minds and make those incarcerated cheerful when their
liberty was restored. Breakages were now only half the level of those in
Haslar's main wards, Burnett reported in 1843. The asylum was tranquil,
meal times were orderly, and most men could muster in the grounds when
piped to do so. 'I was rowed across the water by them,' Burnett noted excitedly, 'and nothing could behave better than they did.' One man sent fishing became so animated on catching a whiting that he started speaking
for the first time in seven years. Men had been encouraged to construct a
mound in the grounds from which they could see the harbour and dockyard at Portsmouth and look out towards Spithead. 'The chance of recovery
at Haslar or at a private asylum is at six to one in favour of the former,' the
Admiralty was informed.[41] The only pity was that with a railway network
now existing across much of the country, cases from Greenwich and other
naval establishments were not transferred to Portsmouth sooner.

Such a liberal regime undoubtedly caused disquiet among many of the
attendants and, as was acknowledged, sometimes made their duties more
demanding. Yet Anderson was still not content. He wanted the old iron
bars removed from windows and replaced with less forbidding wire. The
staircases should be made safer to prevent suicide and injury. A kitchen
should be constructed in the asylum where patients who were accustomed
to cooking could benefit from its therapeutic effects. Attendants should be
equipped with smarter dress which would be replaced if torn or damaged
while handling patients. Daily prayers were to be read and suitable books
of a religious nature acquired. Many inmates had once had skills as tailors,
carpenters and shoemakers and these should be encouraged. For others,
bagatelle, backgammon, drafts, dominoes and restricted card games should
be allowed as distractions and entertainment. When John Wilson succeeded
Anderson in 1853 the asylum had 117 patients, only eight of whom had any
realistic chance of ever leaving.

Wilson was only two years at the asylum, yet his 1854 report was a seminal document for medical healthcare in Britain. Wilson's basic standpoint was that no case should ever be considered hopeless. The human mind was a source of wonderment and perplexity and the care of mental illness was an interesting and challenging calling, undiminished by the frequency of failure. Many minds now wrecked were once 'of uncommon depth and compass', Wilson observed; it was also a fascination for him why the incidence of lunacy should be greater in the navy than in civil society. Since Britain's naval establishment was nearly 50,000 men in 1854 the asylum saw only a fraction of those who might benefit from its care. Who looked after all the others in the service who suffered from mental infirmity? True, sailors and marines were spared some of the anxieties which men in civil life endured. They were fed, had reasonable clothing and accommodation which was kept clean, and they had regular wages, even if they did not always spend their money wisely. Many of the stresses which led to bitterness, depression and strife in civil life were also absent in the navy. At the root of the problem, Wilson insisted, was the alcohol which had destroyed the lives and minds of so many seamen. 'This is a humiliating if not disgraceful admission,' he concluded.

As late as 1854 many men confined to the Haslar asylum were veterans of the French wars. Such men had played a valiant part in the glorious outcome, but Wilson saw them now as 'wretched, broken remnants'. Much might and ought to have been done in years past for such men and society certainly had no cause to take pride in the way these working men had been rewarded. But the specific cause of their ruin was drink: 'the great bane and crippling curse of the service'.[42] Perhaps the next generation of sailors would not be so afflicted: indeed, Wilson acknowledged that some reforms within the navy had been introduced. For now, though, the Haslar asylum continued to pick up the pieces of so many lives irretrievably destroyed. In 1855 Alexander Stuart, holding the newly created rank of staff surgeon, took over the institution.

Even with so many of Anderson's principles adopted, the reality of dealing with disturbed yet sometimes wily men still posed problems which were unlikely to be encountered elsewhere in the service. The case of John Pridham, for example, a former ship's master aged 30, who was admitted in 1856 suffering severe delusion, amply demonstrated that. Pridham was an urbane and well-behaved man, in consequence of which much indulgence was shown him. He was allowed the run of Haslar and was a stalwart in the gardens. One night, however, with an adapted garden tool, he unscrewed the iron guard outside his room, dismantled the sash window and, using his bedding, escaped without creating the slightest noise. Stuart set off for Southampton, checking trains and ships, and eventually found Pridham at the railway station. But the escapee did not want to return and soon collected a large crowd around him which, as Stuart recalled with astonishment, Pridham was able to turn 'unfriendly towards me'. Fortunately for Stuart some nearby policemen dispersed the crowd and took Pridham off to the cells for being disorderly, though not before Stuart, compassionate as ever, had urged that he be treated 'comfortably'.[43] Docile as a lamb and the complete gentleman again next day, Pridham was collected and taken back to Portsmouth by two attendants. Unruffled by the irregularities of asylum duty, Stuart's priority was the physical ease of its inmates by rendering the building itself less barren of decoration and furniture. Although the gloom which hung over the institution could never be dispelled, most naval medical officers believed that those admitted were fortunate. In 1858 Alexander Mackay visited a young colleague there who had attempted suicide while serving on the South America station. Cure for his insanity was doubtful: nonetheless Mackay consoled himself on leaving, 'he is in an exceedingly comfortable place'.[44]

CHAPTER 5

Hospitals Abroad

Seamen were cared for not only at hospitals in England; around the world naval hospitals received sick and injured sailors and marines. The largest of these were on Malta, in Bermuda, at Jamaica's Port Royal, and Simon's Bay at the Cape of Good Hope. Others were maintained on Ascension Island and after 1851 at Lisbon, while in the mid-nineteenth century a hospital ship at Hong Kong served the Far Eastern squadron. Facilities were seldom comparable to those at Haslar, East Stonehouse or the Melville, but for seamen in distress in the Mediterranean or the tropics the comfort and quiet which they offered were, as John Gibson, assistant surgeon on *Protector*, observed in 1829, hugely preferable to 'the miseries, I fear I must call them, which a small classed vessel offers to the sick'.[1] Inevitably a hospital within reach tempted captains and surgeons alike to offload their sick regardless of whether such care was really required. Abroad, as at home, naval hospitals had to be vigilant about admissions.

Overseas establishments were largely exempted from the new regulations issued for home hospitals in 1830. They were also more likely to expect unpaid, light work from convalescents: under an Order of 1822, mat-making, bed-picking, work with sheets and dressings and maintaining table cloths were all prescribed as duties in which patients might assist nurses and labourers as long as there was no danger of relapse. In the tropics disease could easily overwhelm a small hospital. But even amid such crises record keeping was never allowed to slip and the origin of any epidemic, its progress and the cures attempted were to be carefully noted. In 1833 Burnett required the senior medical officers at dockyards, with marine divisions and at hospitals, home and abroad, to keep a book containing all scientifically interesting or unusual cases for the benefit of their successors at their respective institutions.

As for staffing levels, in 1834 Malta and Port Royal each had a surgeon, one assistant and a dispenser, Bermuda had a surgeon with three assistants, while at the Cape one surgeon and one assistant were allowed. Ascension Island, though not strictly classified as a naval hospital, carried one surgeon and one assistant. The size of these establishments did not alter greatly over the years. Following the new rankings for the service in 1840, Malta was run by a Deputy-Inspector, supported by one surgeon, who also acted as storekeeper, and one assistant. Port Royal and Bermuda now also had each a Deputy-Inspector, a surgeon-storekeeper and two assistant surgeons while Simon's Bay was reduced to just one surgeon, although on the understanding that he could draw upon help from the flagship nearby if need be. In practice all overseas hospitals drew on the medical staff of warships in port in times of crises: a fever epidemic or outbreaks of smallpox could be so sudden that there would be no time to get help from home. The defining feature of a naval hospital lay in the regulations and accounting procedures for supply. In 1848 Ascension was still victualled on the books of the ship stationed at the island under sick-mess fund arrangements. At a proper hospital the Deputy-Inspector or surgeon in charge contracted for provisions and, assisted often by an agent or clerk, was responsible for keeping the accounts. Nursing levels varied but in general one was stipulated per seven patients. In addition to sailors, dockyard and other naval personnel often had access. Soldiers were sometimes taken in as patients under an agreement between the War Office and the Admiralty, while merchant seamen in distress could likewise be accepted, subject to assurances about recovering victualling costs.

Serving in the tropics was always hazardous and young assistant surgeons fresh from England frequently suffered when fevers were rampant. Yet there were also obvious attractions to these locations where, in quiet times, medical officers might enjoy a great deal of leisure in tight-knit communities amid the trappings of colonial life. Oliver Evans, Deputy-Inspector at Bermuda, worried in 1847 that his three assistants liked their posts too well: all had been at the hospital for three years and although Evans had no criticism of any of them, 'I doubt that they are doing themselves much good by staying out so long.'[2] Commodore Henry Kellett, commanding the squadron at Jamaica in the mid-1850s, likewise warned the Medical Department against young doctors being left too long in the island's balmy atmosphere and advised that three years should be the maximum. It was a bad sign when assistants started to complain about allowances for personal servants – as Francis Hardinge did from Lisbon in 1857. The Director-General had a sharp reply: 'No special servant is borne on the establishments of our foreign hospitals to attend on assistant surgeons.'³

Malta was the largest of the foreign hospitals. After the island's capture in 1800 and with its obvious strategic value as a naval base in the Mediterranean, a good location was quickly discovered at Bighi. Nelson, no less, had identified the site: having a naval hospital would mean no longer entrusting sick and wounded sailors to the army. Yet nothing happened until the Admiralty finally acquired the Bighi site in 1829. Opened in 1832 and built at a cost of £20,000, the hospital could accommodate about 250 patients housed in two large and two small wards. Its central building had cabins and a mess and dayroom for convalescing officers along with a chapel, library, dispensary and ample storerooms. More than 200 steps led up from the water to its grand entrance. In an emergency the hospital could squeeze in up to 300 men, though by 1837 there had never been more than 100 patients at any time and the stores held were never more than to provide for that number.⁴

Fever among several crews in the Mediterranean in 1837, however, prompted increasing the stores to cover 200 men, although with the proviso that these were not to be touched unless really required. Loss and deterioration of stores overseas was always a worry at the Medical Department. Not only that, but expensive and carefully packed hospital stores abroad were always vulnerable to raids ordered by senior naval officers if the supplies of surgeons on their ships ran low. Burnett protested bitterly in 1838 that his authority over this vital area of both medical judgement and financial control was being interfered with by the admiral responsible for the hospital's discipline and administration at Malta; for three years the admiral had 'endeavoured to prevent that free official intercourse between my Department and the medical officers'.⁵ The Board supported Burnett although in doing so it was only really reiterating earlier orders. In general, as Burnett was well aware, the Admiralty was reluctant to reproach senior naval officers who might have acted if they felt the immediate needs of their ships required it.

Stores were not the only area of dispute. John Stewart, Deputy-Inspector at Malta between 1851 and 1855, resented the way in which he, like his predecessors, was called away twice a year from important hospital duties to attend surveys for invaliding and superannuation in the dockyard; this could have been done by any junior medical officer. The Admiralty backed the Commander-in-Chief, Mediterranean, on this issue: one of the reasons why Malta was allowed a surgeon-storekeeper as well as a Deputy-Inspector was so that an experienced medic could run the hospital in Stewart's necessary absences. Disagreements with commanding officers aside, Malta also developed problems with some of its basic facilities in the 1840s. By 1845 its laundry provision had almost broken down. Linen was sent out locally but the quality of washing was poor and theft was common. The hospital needed its own washhouse and drying area which, it was argued, would eventually pay for itself through better security under a watchful matron and lower costs per item. But economy got the better of such plans and, more than ten years later, Stewart's successor, James Salmon, voiced similar dissatisfaction. Admittedly laundry was no longer sent out, but, Salmon observed, 'the present place used as a washhouse is the kitchen of the west wing'.[6] No proper washing or drying area was ever constructed. There were no fixed washing troughs. Moveable tubs were filled with water fetched by hand from a boiler situated in another corner of the room while dirty water, for want of a proper conduit, collected in puddles where the washerwomen stood. Because drying could only occur outdoors, two or three weeks sometimes passed in winter without being able to dry the linen on account of rain.

Salmon's list of defects at Malta by the 1850s included the need for proper lightning conductors, a clock whereby hospital procedures could be better regulated and improved ventilation in the four larger wards. The grounds had been neglected for some years, a smoking building for convalescents was requested and the skylight above the operating room needed enlargement. Worst of all, though, was the plumbing. There were only two baths where six were required. Furthermore, getting water through the pipes was a slow process: a more practical system of pipes and cocks was needed. The food was awful too. Assistant surgeon Michael Cowan, confined as a patient in 1856, informed his mother: 'hospital fare dry toast and dish water!!'[7] Yet not all inmates were so critical. Cecil Sloane-Stanley, a midshipman admitted with measles in 1852, enjoyed his palatial surroundings with its well-ordered routine. He described Stewart as a kindly man who on his rounds after breakfast 'never paid us a visit without making some cheering remark and cracking a joke'. After three weeks Sloane-Stanley was almost reluctant to return to his ship.[8]

Malta worked as well as it did not only because of the dedication of its medical staff but the efficiency by those engaged in its administration. When Russell left for Haslar in 1851 his duties as clerk fell to a Royal Navy paymaster who not only kept the accounts up to date and monitored the

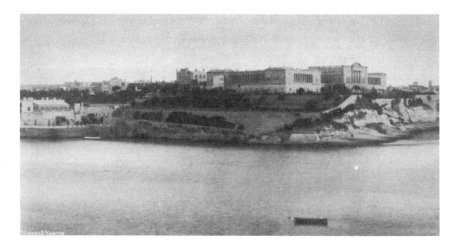

4. Malta hospital.

stores but also after the outbreak of war in 1854 had the additional worry of forwarding supplies to an expanded Mediterranean fleet and to the temporary naval hospital created near Constantinople at Therapia. Lucy Staines was another loyal employee whom Stewart commended to the Admiralty in 1855. Before leaving England in 1851 Stewart had heard of Staines's diligence as matron but had believed the stories to be exaggerated. They were not. 'I do not know that the Crown has a more devoted servant,' he reflected.[9] Exhausted after 40 years with the navy, Staines needed a pension for her old age which in 1856 Salmon hoped the Admiralty would grant her.

Patient numbers at Malta fluctuated. Fever aboard ships coming from Palermo and Naples in 1848 led to a steep rise in admissions which the hospital attributed to impure drinking water taken on at those locations. Even so, there were no more than 80 patients. There were 152 men in the wards in January 1852. Fevers were the common ailment. The hospital also had its share of the usual naval accidents, illnesses and occasional stabbings. In 1847 surgeons from several ships came to witness one of the earliest amputations performed under the effects of ethereal vapour: all were impressed that the sailor was unaware that his limb had been removed. Outside, medical staff performed duties among the families of naval personnel – as evinced in 1852 by Stewart's plea for 'the appointment of an officer possessing matured experience in midwifery and the diseases of women'.[10] Staffing was increased with the Crimean War: Salmon had two surgeons and three assistants under him in February 1856 when the hospital held 138 patients. By April 1856, though, numbers were beginning to decline. There were only 43 by the start of July. Staff at Malta could at last return to the problems of plumbing and laundry which had consumed so much energy before the outbreak of hostilities.

Malta was not considered an unhealthy posting. Jamaica, by contrast, exposed medical officers to some of the worst drawbacks of naval service. Set in a tropical paradise, there was, as its Deputy-Inspector asserted in 1854, 'no hospital in the world so sweet and pure as this is at present'.[11] But appearance masked the truth: Port Royal was a graveyard for many young men. 'Almost every medical officer (there is scarcely an exception) appointed to do duty at this hospital contracts fever,' his predecessor had observed in 1850.[12] By 1851 one in five of all the assistants posted to the hospital in the past 25 years had died there. Between 1815 and 1849 two-thirds of all admissions were fever cases, the death rate among which was one in six. Yellow fever was the principal culprit; it killed between 20 and 33 per cent of its victims. The only consolation amid such depressing statistics was that since most of its patients either died or recovered after convalescing the hospital's invaliding rate was very low. It was, in fact, less than 2 per cent.

Port Royal was described by one naval officer in 1828 as 'a dirty little village'. People only lived there because of the naval installations; merchant craft trading in Jamaica all seemed to pass on to Kingston.[13] The hospital was rebuilt after a fire in 1815 destroyed an older structure but in many ways the accommodation remained flawed. Burnett informed the Admiralty in 1841 that 'a great mistake was committed in the construction of this building'.[14] Instead of supporting the structure on piles or arches, the ground was excavated and the basement wards so low that men placed there, frequently those with ulcers and others requiring surgery, often contracted fever after admission. Moreover the capacity claimed for 180 patients was nominal. One of its six pavilions had to serve as the Deputy-Inspector's residence while another was set aside for sick officers; the number that could comfortably be taken was thereby reduced to 130. Shortage of living space was a distraction for all who worked at Port Royal, as the two assistant surgeons attached to the hospital discovered in 1849 when relocated on the orders of the station commander. Their cramped environment was not just an inconvenience, the surgeon in charge wrote sympathetically in 1852: 'the very anomalous sickness and mortality among the assistant surgeons is mainly due to the faulty quarters assigned to them'.[15] He wanted them moved again so that they might live above the dispensary. Two years later the Deputy-

Inspector was embroiled in a further disagreement with the commodore after the latter had ordered privies to be cut in sandy soil nearby. This would be injurious to the health of staff and patients alike. The public hospital at Kingston had already suffered from the proximity of cesspools: indeed, they were probably the source of cholera there in recent years. Asked to use his influence at Somerset House to protect the naval hospital, Burnett had no hesitation in so doing. There were already sufficient health risks at Port Royal without creating new ones.

Grievances over working conditions, space and staffing levels inevitably came to the fore during epidemics. In April 1835 Charles Linton, surgeon in charge, suddenly had to accommodate 129 cases when *Vestal* arrived in port with fever aboard. Within four weeks 18 men were dead, including *Vestal*'s surgeon, and the hospital was so pressed on account of sickness among its own staff that an assistant surgeon had to be borrowed from another vessel. With the weather fine, Linton was able to place cradles along the verandahs; in different circumstances, however, the only option would have been to vacate his own quarters. According to regulations the hospital had access to an old warship, *Magnificent*, moored nearby which could be used to house convalescents. But *Magnificent* had never been fitted or cleaned sufficiently and was, in practice, useless. Such periodic emergencies, however, barely showed up in the quarterly nosological returns: in the four quarters of 1835 the daily patient averages at Port Royal were 25, 37, 21 and 13 respectively, and at one point towards the end of the year there were only five patients in the hospital. When the Admiralty saw such returns it was always hard to make the case that the hospital needed more doctors or more money.

The hospital's duties nevertheless extended beyond caring for seamen from men-of-war in the West Indies. Officers and artificers at the Jamaica dockyard and their families also regularly received medical attention from the hospital, although this was not formally sanctioned by the Admiralty until May 1843. Burnett was not enthusiastic about this but had to concede that since there was no private practitioner in the town to whom the dock-yard people could turn it was impossible to withdraw a service upon which they already relied. Investigation into tropical diseases was also expected from senior medical staff, in the same way that the effects of climate, miasma and exposure to the elements were reported from the West Africa station. In 1848 Stewart, who was Deputy-Inspector at Port Royal before his transfer to Malta in 1851, had the chance to study 14 men who had been lost and short of food for ten days during boat duty on the coast of Nicaragua.

He compared their health with that of other boat parties sent into rivers in Central America. Despite their hunger and exertions, because the men never slept on shore none developed a fever – except for one, weeks later, who it transpired was subsequently ashore for other reasons. This was in great contrast to the incidence of fever among all other boat crews, Stewart observed. But, to the Medical Department's intense annoyance, these additional reporting duties did not prevent the Commander-in-Chief, North America, Vice-Admiral Lord Dundonald, deciding in 1849 that the hospital was maintained at too high a level and that although money had been spent on improvements the lower wards were still unfit to receive seamen. Examining the statistics, Dundonald noted that the average daily number of patients during the past four years was only 12. Port Royal, he concluded, required reorganization.

Meddling admirals looking to save money always spelt danger for the Medical Department but were the more irksome when they came on top of other difficulties. Port Royal, like other foreign establishments, was never entirely safe from the apparently arbitrary orders of ships' officers who, though they had no authority over hospitals, nevertheless assumed a responsibility for their men when admitted. Professional etiquette allowed surgeons from warships to visit sick sailors in hospital and to report back to captains, but in no circumstances did this entitle them to interfere in treatment, express opinions on the conduct of the hospital or attend post-mortem examinations, and, when visiting, ships' surgeons should make a courtesy call on hospital staff. The problem arose at Port Royal in 1832 when the captain of *Ariadne* ordered warm baths at the hospital for two of his lieutenants without prior reference to the surgeon in charge. Even worse, as Linton discovered in January 1836, the hospital's medical staff were regarded by some station commanders as at their disposal. Unannounced, the Commander-in-Chief, North America, removed one of Linton's assistant surgeons and replaced him with another. Linton had now had three new assistants in just 12 months, which meant that it was impossible to maintain efficient continuity. And as if this sudden change was not difficult enough, the latest assistant, it transpired, had neither worked in a hospital nor seen a case of yellow fever before. Even when the station had sufficient assistant surgeons, those not immediately required on warships were seldom left at Port Royal where they might help out at the hospital. Several young men recently sent out from England, Linton complained, who should have been temporarily assigned to help him, were 'sent on to Bermuda or Halifax in order to join the Admiral'. Part of the problem, as he knew only too well, was that the assistants usually let it be known that they were keen to go with the flagship rather than stay in Jamaica. Staying close to and being recognized by an admiral was a better career move than toiling unnoticed among febrile sailors at Linton's behest. When it came to promotion, the latter reflected ruefully, hospital service 'is considered as a drawback to their claims'.[16] Burnett, naturally, was anxious to quash any idea that Port Royal might be off the beaten track as far as preferment was concerned: the contrary was true, he wrote reassuringly, adding that a strong testimonial from Linton would enhance the prospects of any aspiring assistant surgeon.

Linton's final years in Jamaica until he retired in 1839 were also bedevilled by insubordination and incompetence within the establishment. Michael Moore, in charge of the dispensary, was a 'dead weight' on account of intemperance and consequent ill health. Linton had tried repeatedly to alter Moore's habits but to no avail; now he was understaffed because one of the assistants had to be detached for dispensary duty. Moore's replacement in 1836 was James Ballard, who proved equally unsatisfactory. Ballard neglected his work in the dispensary, at times leaving a local boy in charge whose only real competence was to sweep the floor. Meanwhile he practised privately in the town and among soldiers in the garrison despite such activities being forbidden. When Linton tried to report this he was urged by an indifferent Commander-in-Chief to deal with the problem by 'remonstrance and counsel' rather than resorting to a court martial. This had only encouraged Ballard in his behaviour; indeed, by June 1839 Ballard was quite out of control, asserting that Linton had publicly insulted him by denying him use of a stethoscope in the wards. Ballard had no idea how to use a stethoscope, Linton explained, and was making such a spectacle that in order to preserve some respect for medical officers Linton ordered him back to the dispensary. Ballard became litigious, insisting that 'he had as good a right as I had myself to go among the patients and to visit them as often as he pleased'. The man was 'unfit and untrustworthy', Linton concluded: he also failed to order supplies for the hospital on time – a failing which had already caused displeasure at Somerset House.[17] It was an embarrassing matter for Burnett to have to refer to the Board. Once again, it would not raise Port Royal's reputation in the minds of those who settled the naval estimates.

Ballard's neglect of the stores proved to be only one instance of a growing problem with supplies. Ballard had left the establishment short. In 1845

Deputy-Inspector Edward Hilditch erred in the other direction by ordering excessively. Burnett concluded that since Hilditch 'has such trifling
medical duties to perform' his chaotic ordering could only be attributed to
carelessness.[18] But the real problem regarding stores and supplies in Jamaica
came to light five years later when it was discovered that the hospital clerk,
George Knox, had long been defrauding the hospital, particularly over its
purchase of brandy and ale. In November 1856 he was also detected dealing improperly with a patient's money. Enquiries subsequently revealed that
Knox was heavily in debt to all and sundry in the town foolish enough to
advance him money or goods on credit. He was duly dismissed and thrown
into prison.

    While Knox was not representative of those who worked at Port Royal,
the need to replace him at the end of 1856 highlighted the problem of
recruitment. A man in his mid-50s with no experience of such work was
brought in temporarily at eight shillings a day but the surgeon in charge
had no confidence in his abilities. The Commander-in-Chief recommended
a junior serving in the victualling office: he was not expert at figures but
was thought to be honest. Finding nurses posed similar problems. Because
they were only taken on as required, competent nurses drifted away or
found other occupations when admissions were low and then were unavailable when the hospital filled up. Nursing was particularly important when
caring for fever victims in January 1848 and Stewart argued for a permanent engagement of three nurses on liberal wages. Burnett knew that the
budget would never allow that and asked Stewart to report again 'when
he has had more time to mature his opinions'. But Stewart was not exag-
gerating. Deputy-Inspector James Wingate-Johnston returned to the issue
in 1852, reminding Burnett that at Port Royal 'it is a well-known fact that
with good nursing and often repeated nourishment, many lives have been
saved that would otherwise have been sacrificed'.[19]

    The Medical Department's worries about Jamaica were compounded by
those surrounding its other principal outpost in the Americas – Bermuda.
Hulks and temporary sick-quarters ashore had existed at Bermuda since
1794 and were consolidated into a permanent hospital in 1818. This was a
two-storey structure to which wings for staff and additional patient accommodation were later added. In fact it was still unfinished in 1840 when
Burnett reported that it could hold 72 patients. It took the sick from naval
vessels coming into port, from the army garrison and, after 1824, from
Bermuda's large convict settlement. Built in the hills on Ireland Island,

the hospital presented an idyllic setting which belied its primitive facilities. Its drains were not completed until 1849, and until 1840 it had only one lavatory for officer patients, two outside privies for other ranks and two more for convicts. Even so, economies were always needed. The truth was, Burnett insisted, the hospital was barely adequate for the navy's own needs, let alone those of others in Bermuda.

The hospital also admitted cases from the naval dockyard which required more care than the surgeon there could provide. Given the growing pressures on the dockyard surgeon, this always threatened to become a regular intake. Thomas Jones, dockyard surgeon for many years after 1826, complained that about 700 people lived in the vicinity who, in the absence of any private practitioner, all considered that they had a call on his professional attendance. The hospital found itself in much the same position, with its services being in particular demand during the outbreaks of yellow fever which swept Bermuda in 1818–19, 1843 and 1853. Midwifery was another area where both dockyard and hospital medical officers found themselves called away from their establishments; Jones calculated 151 births attended by 1832. Even the soldiers on Bermuda, he reported in 1828, had no medical officer attached. Expenditure on stores reflected this constant demand. Jones's practice consisted of 'hundreds of persons of all colours, and totally unconnected with Government'.[20] Isolated as Bermuda was, the dockyard and hospital both found it impossible to refuse help to people who, elsewhere, would have been judged ineligible for the navy's care.

Jones, however, inadvertently performed a great service for the hospital in 1832 when he persuaded the Commander-in-Chief, North America, to change the regulations regarding dockyard workers. He had noticed how men were being sent repeatedly from the yard to the hospital to recover from alcoholic excesses. Jones's solution was that all artificers so afflicted should be required to pay for hospital expenses. Hospital admissions from the dockyard soon collapsed from 66 in 1832 to only seven in 1835. By this time the hospital's medical staff consisted of the surgeon in charge (raised to Deputy-Inspector in 1843) with two assistant surgeons. This was adequate for the long periods when there were fewer than 20 patients but never sufficient when sickly crews arrived or when confronted with local epidemics. Yellow fever in 1843 was a case in point and an example which Burnett later used to resist renewed suggestions for staff reductions. The Deputy-Inspector and a handful of assistant surgeons available from men-of-war treated 1,200 hospital patients between March and December. Among

those, 939 were eventually discharged while 110 died: 'a very small proportion indeed when the nature of the disease is considered,' Burnett assured
the Board. Yet among the 1,200 admissions only 274 were either sailors or
from the families of dockyard employees who had a legitimate claim on the
hospital. For much of 1843 the hospital accommodated twice its prescribed
maximum, with storerooms, basements and private residences all converted
into makeshift wards. Not until January 1844 did the crisis pass. Bermuda
had survived, the Deputy-Inspector informed Somerset House, probably
from the disease having 'already attacked every susceptible person and from
want of fresh subjects to act upon'.[21]

More than any other foreign establishment, Bermuda gave rise to
disputes with the army. In this respect there were parallels with Chatham,
where in 1840 arrangements had been made to accept up to 40 soldiers
from the garrison (raised to 50 in 1842) in order to stave off the idea that
part of the Melville should be transferred to army control. By June 1841 the
Melville housed 34 army patients and Burnett was becoming aware that
agreements for tending sick soldiers, both at home and abroad, were working to the navy's disadvantage. The procedure which operated at Bermuda
was that set up between the two services in 1820 whereby each admitted the
other's sick at a uniform charge of 9d per day. 'This I presume could only
be meant to apply to casual cases and not to such numbers as we have lately
received from the army,' Burnett appealed to the Admiralty.[22] Nine pence
would cover victualling costs in most naval hospitals, and even where the
daily cost was 10d, as in Jamaica, numbers were so small that the loss to
the navy was inconsiderable. But at Bermuda the cost of rations alone for
patients was 10½d per day and of the 6,428 rations issued by the hospital to
patients during the first quarter of 1841, 3,044 had been issued to soldiers.
On that calculation, in one quarter alone at Bermuda the navy incurred a
loss of £149.

Given the scale of provision for the army, overheads and other expenses
also had to be considered and could not just be ignored as was done elsewhere. When the issuing of medicinal wine, bedding, laundry costs, staff
wages and victualling for the nurses were all taken into account the real
burden to the navy of this arrangement became clear. It also had to be
remembered that naval hospitals, even Bermuda with its basic facilities,
compared favourably with army counterparts and provided fuller diets.
Men discharged cured from naval hospitals were expected to be fit for
normal duties aboard ship, where there would be no opportunity for conva-

lescence, whereas the army usually just discharged men to barracks. At Bermuda, above all places, Burnett urged that the army should acquire its own military hospital.

Burnett never solved this problem at Bermuda. After 1848 the hospital was no longer required to take convicts but army admissions continued until the mid-1870s. In fact the problem grew worse and he restated the unfair way in which this reciprocal arrangement between the services was working in 1843 and again in 1844. In 1843 the Treasury was drawn into this dispute, for the benefit of which Burnett again explained his difficulty. The average real cost of caring for soldiers amounted to one shilling a day for all home hospitals, 1/9d at Bermuda and three shillings at Jamaica. Jamaica's higher costs did not matter so much since only 40 soldiers had been treated in the 12 months to 1 June 1842. At Bermuda, however, 529 soldiers had been admitted in the same period. Given the reimbursement rate of only 9d per man the navy was subsidising the army at about £600 per annum. The best deal the Medical Department could get came into effect in April 1845: the recovery charge would be 9d for all naval hospitals while army hospitals would waive charges for sick sailors. There would still be a deficit of £200–£300 a year and Bermuda would continue to be the main reason why. The navy had at least cut its losses. In 1854 there was some relief when a makeshift hospital was created by the army regiment stationed on Ireland Island which greatly reduced the numbers going to the naval hospital. At the end of 1856 Bermuda had 33 men under care, only seven of whom were soldiers.

Bermuda remained a shabby establishment notwithstanding improvements made over the years. When Oliver Evans was Deputy-Inspector in 1845 he was struck by the poor state of the dispensary and its fittings compared with what he had seen at Port Royal. He ordered a new supply of jars and bottles to replace the existing hotchpotch in all shapes and sizes. Evans also wanted a surgeon appointed to the hospital in place of one of the two assistants currently attached. But the establishment was not increased and, as at Jamaica, Bermuda had to struggle on, often with medical officers ill or absent during busy periods. Like Jamaica, it also had problems retaining other staff. The hospital was frequently short of steady nurses. The surgeon in charge in 1847 requested three or four unmarried men to be sent for duty in the convict wards, adding that he had tried recruiting local men but that the level of basic knowledge necessary for such work was hard to find among the black community. Ex-soldier-pensioners would probably be best suited.

Like several other establishments, Bermuda relied upon, though usually took for granted, the daily vigilance of its matron. In this case it was Sarah Wells, whose husband had served the navy for 32 years as clerk both at the hospital and later at Port Royal. When he died in Jamaica in 1846 Wells returned to Bermuda with her children. When John Rees came out as Deputy-Inspector in 1855 he recognized that Wells had been badly treated in the interests of economy and supported her petition to the Commander-in-Chief for a review of her position. In London, Liddell was also sympathetic and arranged for her pay to be raised to equal that of her counterpart at Port Royal. Bermuda was, however, spared the difficulties over stores which so beset Port Royal from the 1830s onwards. The Medical Department's only worries on this account arose with Hilditch in 1850. Having previously bemused Burnett with his arrowroot mountain at Port Royal in 1845, Hilditch caused consternation again by his issue of what seemed to Burnett to be a most luxurious diet to all the patients. The hospital's diet was already 'most liberal' and nothing appeared to justify the 'enormous extra expenditure' on beef, eggs, flour, rice, arrowroot, scotch barley, sugar, bread and milk. As in 1845 this area of Hilditch's duties had been performed without sufficient attention. Even worse, Hilditch's accounts showed too much spending on coals, wood for fuel, and oil. As a check on the Deputy-Inspector's generosity, Burnett requested copies of his prescription tickets. Hilditch clearly lived in a world of his own when it came to anything except the practice of medicine. Remember that Bermuda chickens were very small and of poor quality, he replied. While naturally sorry that the Director-General should have cause for distress, Hilditch nevertheless waved off most of Burnett's complaints with assertions either that economies were being made or that the accounts did not contain anything unjustifiable on medical grounds. 'I trust that you will be pleased to reconsider and cancel that portion of your letter which directs me in future to send home the copies of the prescription tickets,' he added indignantly.[23] Even the most senior men in the service hesitated to address the Director-General so bluntly. In so hopeless a case as Hilditch, however, Burnett faced up to the fact that there was no point pursuing the matter. He would leave everything in the Deputy-Inspector's hands, adding merely that he hoped to have no occasion to make any further observations.

Burnett even found it possible to forgive so respected a medical officer for more than just his profligacy over diet. In January 1851 it transpired that Hilditch's record keeping of patients was no better than his handling of supplies. The medical details were models of scientific observation and diagnoses: Hilditch, however, had listed most of the sailors against the wrong ships in the hospital's muster book so that it became almost impossible to identify them. Burnett feigned surprise after reading such a chaotic return from Bermuda although by then must have been resigned to Hilditch's ways. In future, he rather meekly suggested, Hilditch might care to check the work of his clerk. It was almost the last occasion on which the clerk at Bermuda could be blamed for anything, as the post was abolished in 1853 and its duties merged with those of the hospital steward. Like the economy attempted by abolishing the matron's position in 1854, however, this measure was not successful and in January 1856 Rees asked for distinct clerks and stewards to be restored. There were now more vessels in the West Indies than when the 1853 staffing reductions had been devised and more work, therefore, than one hospital employee could manage.

These 1853 staff reductions came a year after a comprehensive review of government expenditure on the navy's foreign hospitals. This was no surprise to the Medical Department which had already had to deal with Dundonald's unwelcome criticisms in 1849. In fact the Royal Navy's costs had been under scrutiny for several years. In 1847 the Admiralty had alerted all dockyard superintendents to the need for economies; they employed too many men, their work was inefficient and stores were poorly maintained. A Select Committee enquiring into the 1848 estimates criticized the expense of steam factories being built at Portsmouth, Plymouth and Malta and concluded that audit and monitoring procedures were generally inadequate. Against this background, Dundonald had concluded in 1849 that reducing Port Royal's medical staff should be possible. Touring the dockyard and hospital at Bermuda in 1849, Dundonald was dismayed that so many inexpensive things were neglected while useless and expensive undertakings went ahead unquestioned. Malta's dockyard, victualling yard and hospital also came under scrutiny in 1849. Justifying all these enquiries with a view to lowering the naval estimates, the First Lord, Sir Francis Baring, ruled that 'there have been large reductions made at home, and it is but right that some consideration should be extended to our foreign establishments'.[24]

No one familiar with Malta could possibly deny that money had been squandered there in recent years, particularly with respect to the dockyard. Yet, even as more waste was uncovered, politicians began to worry that cutting back on the nation's defences was a dangerous game to play. The Governor of Malta warned Baring, as an old friend, not to be 'deluded by the cry of economy or induced to take measures which the very same men who now call for economy will be the first to condemn on the first change of public opinion'.[25] Baring duly backed away; indeed by the end of June 1849 he well nigh disowned the inspections of foreign establishments claiming that 'I never had much expectation from such revision'.[26] Annual savings in the Mediterranean were settled at £970, which Baring conceded did not go very far given that total dockyard expenditure at home and overseas in 1848 amounted to £625,273. With Malta off the hook, however, the spotlight was on the West Indies.

With the Bermuda hospital no longer admitting convicts after 1848, the Treasury wanted to know how it could still justify a Deputy-Inspector, two assistant surgeons and its current numbers of non-medical staff. Burnett responded that the Treasury's figures for Bermuda made no allowance for the losses incurred by treating so many soldiers and he fell back on the argument that both Bermuda and Port Royal had to be staffed at levels which could cope with epidemics ashore and in the fleet, citing examples in recent weeks when *Alarm* and *Vixen* had arrived at Jamaica with 45 yellow fever cases all needing hospital admission and with their own surgeons too ill to be able to assist. The nature of fever care was such that ten cases occupied as much of a medic's time as a hundred suffering from other ailments. For 20 years the Medical Department had been organized along the most economical lines. It would not, therefore, be just, he insisted, if it was now accused of unwarranted expenditure by those 'either grossly or wilfully ignorant of the whole matter'.[27] Pressed from all sides, Baring waited until the end of September 1849 before making any decision on cuts at the overseas hospitals. With Malta already safe and with Bermuda apparently immune because of its arrangement with the army, Port Royal was the remaining candidate for economies. But Burnett had done enough to save the day in 1849. Baring thanked Dundonald for his investigations in the West Indies but concluded, 'I do not feel sufficiently confident as respects the reductions you propose in the medical staff at Jamaica.' Dundonald accepted that the First Lord had been placed in an embarrassing position with respect to 'that costly institution' at Port Royal but asked nonetheless that its accounts and patient numbers should be kept under constant review.[28]

Within a year, however, epidemics on Jamaica were to justify Baring's caution. Cholera affected a quarter of Port Royal's population in 1850 and continued at Kingston until the end of the year. The naval hospital was still admitting cholera patients in November. By then a fever epidemic had developed on the island and several ships in the squadron had long sick-lists. *Persian* was the worst afflicted. Returning from the coast of Nicaragua in November 1850 she had already lost nine men, among them her assistant surgeon, and 52 fever cases were transferred immediately to the hospital. As so often in the tropics, the conditions which caused so many patients to be admitted also reduced the hospital's capacity to cope; one of the assistant surgeons fell ill again having barely recovered from his previous attack of cholera. In March 1850 Port Royal had housed only 23 seamen; at its peak in 1850 it contained 121. With the hospital short-staffed at a time of crisis, the Deputy-Inspector protested that too many men were being sent there whose cases were treatable on board ship. Burnett was sympathetic though well aware that it was precisely such influxes during epidemics that were used to justify staff numbers at foreign establishments.

When all the overseas hospitals came under renewed pressure early in 1852, after a Treasury Committee once more questioned their expense, Bermuda and Jamaica, as before, proved to be the most difficult to defend. Again it was galling for Burnett to have to do so given that the most recent annual naval estimates came to about £6.5 million. When the estimates had been around £5 million in 1837 the running costs of all the Royal Navy's overseas establishments had amounted to only £44,000, whereas home dockyards, hospitals and victualling depots had come to £527,000 a year and a two-decker ship of the line cost £80,000 to build.[29] Set against these vast sums, where exactly was the scope for worthwhile economy in the navy's medical provision? The Treasury seemed to be suggesting that the navy did not need two hospitals for the North America station. As in 1849, Burnett retorted that naval hospitals had to provide for emergencies and could not be judged on the basis of average daily usage. False economies would cost valuable lives, especially when the work currently done among dockyard families and the local population was taken into account. The Bermuda hospital, being relatively isolated on Ireland Island, had also to be self-sufficient in terms of labour and could not rely upon casual local employment or on any short-term assistance from other military or governmental institutions. Bermuda's one nurse for every seven patients, and one washer for every 20, had to be maintained, therefore, as permanent staff. Small hospitals, which for much of the time had few patients, would also have no pools of convalescents upon which to draw for free labour: everything at Bermuda and Port Royal had to be paid for.

The strategic weakness in the struggle to preserve the establishments at Port Royal and Bermuda was that well-meaning naval commanders claimed that they were essential supports for any fleet defending the West Indies in time of war. But who exactly either could or would challenge the Royal Navy, the Treasury replied? As far as Bermuda was concerned, might it not be more economical to hand it over to the army to be run as a military hospital on the understanding that sailors would always be admitted as needed? Mention of an army takeover was bound to excite Burnett who expressed the strongest opposition. To convert Bermuda into a regimental army hospital would be to downgrade it. At present seamen received the attention of an experienced Deputy-Inspector; if admitted to an army establishment they would most likely be tended only by junior medical staff unaccustomed to dealing with many of the common ailments of sailors. The food provided would also be inadequate since that available at regimental hospitals corresponded more closely to the sick-mess aboard ship than to a proper hospital diet. The hospital also acted as a depot for medicines and stores required on the North America station which could only be properly looked after and distributed if under naval control. He also appealed to the Admiralty to resist the suggestion that disruptive convicts should again be admitted to the hospital. 'Most happy was I when the convicts were removed,' he added, 'I hope never to return.'[30] Regardless of what the Treasury appeared to believe, Burnett asserted that, like the soldiers treated there, the convicts had been a financial drain on the institution: in short, it was because the navy had subsidized other branches of government service for so long that its modest foreign hospitals, especially Bermuda, seemed so costly.

Reductions were, however, unavoidable. Cutbacks elsewhere were leading to a 20 per cent drop in the workforce at dockyards, steam factories and victualling depots from 1849 levels, with the navy's overall dockyard costs down by a half from those in 1848. The medical service would have to take its share, although Burnett reported to the Board in October 1852 that Bermuda was the only place where economies would not affect basic hospital functions. Despite the expense of Port Royal, he could not countenance any savings there beyond those which would result from reducing the rations allowed to some staff, dismissing the office messenger and combining the duties of dispensary assistant with those of surgery man. This would save £187 a year. At Malta £151 per annum could be saved by dismissing two of the three seamstresses and by using convalescents as bed-pickers instead of paying 8d per day for outside labour. Bermuda's annual costs would be lowered by £740; there was no disguising the fact that Bermuda currently had only nine patients, yet 25 employees, including its three medical officers. Yellow fever at Bermuda in 1853 forced some adjustment to the planned reductions. It was a timely outbreak, reinforcing Burnett's earlier assertions that any further cuts either there or at Port Royal would leave them unable to cope with emergencies.

Simon's Bay, Ascension Island and Hong Kong were also reviewed in 1852, although all emerged unscathed on the grounds that they were maintained at such minimal levels that, apart from cutting some of the staff rations at Simon's Bay for a meagre saving of £36, nothing else was possible. Simon's Bay, with its surgeon and with one assistant sent from warships at the Cape, had a maximum capacity of 78 patients but had never held more than 63 at any time in the three years since 1849. Burnett had succeeded in getting a medical officer stationed there permanently only in the early 1840s; until then the hospital had been run, largely unsatisfactorily, by an assistant surgeon sent from the fleet. Labour at the Cape being expensive, hospital workers often had to be sent out from England and reliable nurses were hard to come by. The surgeon explained in 1843 that, having recently lost his dispensary man, a replacement could never be found in the colony for the wages on offer. Ascension also had periodic difficulties with staff: clerks, dispensary men and matrons were regularly sent out from home. Clerk and matron were usually a married couple, as was expected for the positions of dispensary man and seamstress, although, as Burnett recognized in 1853, finding suitable couples was difficult 'in consequence of the smallness of the salary'.[31] The only other staff at Ascension were the surgeon and his assistant: the latter took charge of the hospital's small mountain annex used by convalescents. The main hospital could take up to 40 patients and occasionally did so, as in 1846 when ships returned from the West African coast with sickly crews, or as in 1823, 1838 and 1865 when fever and dysentery were rampant on the island. Sometimes there were merchant vessels to tend to, particularly when prolonged poor weather or sparse rainfall curtailed the island's agricultural production and supplies had to be brought in from the Cape. But, isolated in the mid-Atlantic, for much of the time Ascension had little to do. For a medical officer with ambition it could easily become a forgotten backwater.

In light of increasing pressures for economy, by the late 1840s it seemed incongruous to set up another hospital at Lisbon. This was, however, recommended by the Foreign Office in 1849; a hospital there might serve the needs of British merchant vessels as well as those of warships in the Tagus. For several years the navy had used a hospital run by Dr J. Mackenzie, its sole agent for medical requirements at Lisbon, who had the considerable merit of performing all work 'at stated moderate payments'.[32] Such civilian provision was not unprecedented. Arrangements had been made at Valparaiso in 1824 for sailors to enter Dr Leighton's private hospital. Access to facilities ashore for British seamen was urgently needed there, John Cunningham, surgeon aboard *Cambridge*, had noted: he had lost several men who he was convinced could have been saved had there been a suitable establishment in the town. In 1849 the navy rejected the idea of stationing a hospital ship at Valparaiso in favour of another agreement, this time with a civilian hospital managed by Dr W.R. Ancram, upon whom the honorary title of surgeon and agent was conferred 'to give him additional respectability and authority'.[33] At Lisbon, Mackenzie ran a 30-bed hospital to which, Burnett suggested, merchant skippers might pay small subscriptions. It would need to be supported in this way 'as we have no funds which could be appropriated to such a purpose'. But things were not so simple. Although Mackenzie was happy to continue taking Royal Navy men into his hospital on a per capita basis without any subsidy from the British government the question arose of who was actually responsible for them. Did he have the authority to invalid them? Did naval surgeons have the right to an opinion on how his hospital treated men from their ships?

Using a civilian establishment at Lisbon also had implications for discipline. Rowdy seamen were not likely to be controlled by Mackenzie who, in any case, lived at some distance from his hospital. Reservations were also expressed about Mackenzie's facilities. His building had no courtyard; convalescents were often turned out to exercise in the surrounding streets where, all too regularly, they were discovered drunk. The idea therefore gained ground that since the navy maintained a squadron in the Tagus it might be better to set up a separate institution. This would be expensive although the overall cost would doubtless be partially offset by a naval hospital discharging its patients more quickly than a private one, there being no commercial incentive to retain them. This seemed an even better suggestion when the commodore in the Tagus, William Martin, reported in 1851 that some of Mackenzie's bills in the past had been excessive. Mackenzie had been charging eight shillings a day for accommodation and treatment; in its own establishment the navy could do the same for only three shillings. The annual saving would be £450. The facility would be under naval discipline at all times.

A naval hospital would have the additional benefit that patients, ill or convalescing, could receive the prescribed sick-mess diet administered via the purser of the flagship. Stores, bedding and other supplies would all need to go out from Deptford, Burnett observed, and an experienced surgeon would take charge. These arrangements would place Lisbon on the same footing as Ascension Island. Plans were well advanced by the time Mackenzie discovered that his services were to be dispensed with in August 1851 and he protested that the care which he provided for British seamen in no way justified such an apparent loss of confidence. He had cured many otherwise hopeless cases and, since he had never had more than 24 patients in his hospital, was at a loss to understand why the navy claimed it needed larger premises. But the Admiralty had already made its decision in the conviction that economies could be made. Surgeon George Burn took charge of the building which Martin had found and, after agreement from the Portuguese government was obtained, the hospital opened at the beginning of October. 'It gives great satisfaction to the sick,' Martin assured the First Lord, 'as well as to all others who have visited it.'[34] Captain Frederick Warden of *Retribution*, who visited Lisbon in 1852, likewise remarked upon the transformation in medical provision. The hospital was clean and well conducted. As yet there were few patients, no books for them to read, the gardens might be put to better use by growing vegetables and it badly needed a clock. Its kitchen would also become stretched if more than 20 patients needed to be fed together. Yet all these deficiencies could be fixed for perhaps no more than £20. Under Burn's competent management 'the whole establishment is much cheaper to government (by nearly one third) than Dr. Mackenzie's sick quarters where, I have no hesitation in saying, it was a very doubtful benefit to send any patient'.[35]

Remote from London, foreign hospitals were never inspected by the Director-General. They mostly operated in uncomfortable conditions and according to the organizational competence and eccentricities of their Deputy-Inspectors or senior surgeons. Beyond naval duties, their medical officers were often called upon by communities nearby. Exposure to the elements could wreak havoc in ways which seemed almost comical when viewed from the safety of Somerset House. In the 1840s, for instance, the short-lived hospital at Port Essington was literally consumed by four species of Australian white ants. Thomas Huxley described it in 1848 as 'a low building with a white face and wide verandah'.[36] Unfortunately it had been built of eucalyptus, which proved to be a particular delicacy. Then there were the tropical storms, none more devastating than for the old building once a naval hospital on Barbados before its timely transfer to the army in 1816. The structure was demolished by a hurricane in 1834 along with its lodgings and other accommodation. Compared to hospitals at home, facilities overseas were basic, supplies and stores were more difficult to regulate and a reliable workforce was usually more difficult to find. Yet these establishments were vital for a navy whose reach spanned the globe. To the respite which they provided, many a sailor and marine owed his life when far from home in the nineteenth century.

CHAPTER 6

Minden on the China Coast

On 15 March 1842 a man-of-war slipped almost unnoticed out of Devonport. In sturdy condition and in full sail, there was no indication that she was different from any other vessel heading for the open sea. *Minden*, however, was an innovation. All but 20 of her guns had been stripped out and for three months she had been extensively refitted. The ship was commanded by Michael Quin and had a complement of 280 officers and seamen. But she also carried 27 other men and three women whose task was to care for sick and wounded sailors. *Minden* was the Royal Navy's first specifically equipped hospital ship. Her destination was the China coast.

Admittedly the navy had long used ships which held sick and wounded men, either moored in port or when transporting them ashore. Yet although such vessels had carried surgeons and dressers they never offered more medical attention than was available in most cockpits. *Minden*, by contrast, was a floating hospital. Part of her main deck and the whole of the lower and orlop decks were converted for medical purposes: the fore-magazine area was a storeroom for patients' effects and could be used for additional sick in emergencies. The space available was initially calculated as sufficient for up to 200 patients, though because most would be in oversized cradles the number was revised to 120. The iron bedsteads, bedding, furniture and utensils were those used at shore hospitals. Abundant sheets and bed-shirts were provided, water closets were fitted at convenient places and fixed and moveable baths were supplied. Appropriate books were selected for a small hospital library. Shifting, framed screens could isolate patients where desired, the ports had Venetian blinds and, to avoid spillage, mechanisms for suspending chamber pots alongside the cradles were used. The ward areas were well lighted by oil lamps while copious supplies of candles and candlesticks were carried for use during surgery. Cleanliness, both of the ship and the men, was given a high priority.

Impressive as all this alone would have been, *Minden* had two further revolutionary features. One was her hot water system whereby a labyrinth of tubes and stopcocks gave a constant supply to fixed baths, the wash-house and to general bathing and laundry areas. The boiler for this was located above those outlets; hot water simply flowed down the pipes as the cocks were opened. A generously proportioned cooking area with stoves for baking and boiling allowed food to be prepared for the sick. The other feature was the ventilation apparatus, installed at a cost of up to £400, which was designed to extract foul air and pump fresh air from outside to all parts of the hospital. The machinery was simple to maintain and the pressure of air flow could be adjusted in different places according to the area requiring ventilation. Although Quin commanded the ship, hospital functions were the responsibility of Inspector John Wilson. Wilson, author of the impressive and recently published *Statistical Report on the Health of the Navy 1830–36*, had overseen the fitting out since November 1841 and insisted that 'no such moveable hospital, in respect of magnitude, means of efficiency, and completeness, ever left an English port'.[1] The supplies of medicines, chemical preparations, comforts, nutrients and surgical equipment which *Minden* carried had likewise been left to his discretion.

Under Wilson were a surgeon, Alfred Tucker, and five assistants. There was one ward-master, equivalent to a matron, and 16 landsmen who served as nurses. The remainder of the hospital establishment comprised a clerk, a servant for the Inspector, a boy similarly assigned to the surgeon and the wives of three men on board who were employed as washers. Wilson recognized, however, that even with so many modern facilities at his disposal much would still depend on the quality of care and he worried about both the nursing staff and the food to be provided. One nurse could not attend more than ten patients and in the event of many serious cases an even more generous ratio would be needed. He also urged that better men would come forward as nurses if the rate of pay was advertised as being equivalent to that of able seamen. As for food, Wilson asked for either a professional cook or at least paying whoever was employed at the level of a superior naval rating. Sticking a landsman in the galley would not ensure properly cooked and nutritious food for sick and convalescent men.

Minden reached Hong Kong on 3 August 1842. From there she was sent up to the island of Chusan where she anchored two weeks later. *Minden* had been sent to support the Far Eastern squadron in the war which Britain had been conducting with China since the beginning of 1840. Provoked initially by the attempts of Chinese officials to stop the trade in opium at Canton by seizing the property of foreign merchants, the conflict continued intermittently, with both Britain and China conscious of national dignity and with neither amenable to diplomatic compromise. British forces had some successes to their credit. The navy had forced an entry to the Pearl River below Canton in 1840 and it had captured Chusan, six miles off the coast and close to the mouth of the Yangtse River. Early in 1841 the Bogue forts below Canton were reduced by naval bombardment and the town of Cheunpee was taken. British soldiers and marines captured the walls of Canton in March and in May a force of 2,500 men returned to force the city's surrender. All defensive positions in the Pearl River were also reduced in 1841. Yet none of this was sufficient to force any concessions from the Imperial government in Peking. Not only that, the war was proving costly both financially and in terms of manpower.[2]

With superior firepower, technology and military organization, both the army and navy had achieved their successes with few casualties against far greater numbers in battle. Losses from disease, however, proved to be another matter. This problem first appeared at Chusan between July and October 1840 where the initial military occupation comprising 3,500 men was within three months reduced to only 800 fit for duty. By the end of 1840 more than 450 of the force had died. The army was left in tents at waterlogged campsites, the climate was oppressive and the supply system broke down. Assistant surgeon Edward Cree, put ashore with soldiers from his troopship *Rattlesnake*, even had to drink from irrigation ditches filled with rotting vegetation, the water in which had run off nearby paddy fields. Poor command and disorganization were also to blame. The men on Chusan were increasingly packed into hopelessly inadequate field hospitals even as transport vessels lay empty just offshore and could have provided far healthier accommodation. In December 1840 the Governor-General of India ordered an enquiry into what had gone wrong at Chusan, and simi-larly into conditions in the Pearl River where men had been kept too long on cramped and unsanitary transports rather than landed at a secured site.[3]

Rattlesnake was in the Pearl River in May 1841 where again Cree witnessed a shambles unfolding. With the army ordered to take Canton, he observed that 'we have only 2600 men and a good many sick and wounded and the Chinese have 20,000 soldiers in the city'. Canton was captured despite the odds, but by the time the soldiers were back at the temporary base on Hong Kong in June 1841 many had died from fever and dysentery and more than 1,100 men were in makeshift hospitals. 'Half our ship's company laid up with fever,' Cree noted: 'many a gallant fellow who escaped in the field has succumbed to disease.'[4] Warships at anchor in the Pearl River and off Hong Kong had either skeleton crews or were judged unserviceable with interiors resembling hospital wards. Sickness and a want of adequate provision were reducing the British war effort to a state of disarray. With no supply base east of Singapore, supplying a fleet on the China coast inevitably posed problems although these had been expected. Indeed the First Lord of the Admiralty considered the naval force 'to have been very amply provided for'.[5] In the Pearl River things were not so bad since the crews of warships were able to trade for meat and vegetables rather than resort to salt provisions. Elsewhere, however, both the army and the navy were in trouble. Seamen in the Yangtse had to forage for fresh meat and vegetables and most ships were also running low on quinine and lime juice. In London, Burnett recognized in February 1841 that extra medical supplies were required in China and ordered four more number two chests and other necessaries to be sent out on the first available vessel: when a transport sailed in August Burnett had six tons of medical freight aboard.[6]

By mid-1841 the China squadron was also short of medical officers, and six newly recruited assistant surgeons were sent out. Burnett was now issuing medical chests intended to last two years instead of the normal 12 months. Treating its sick and wounded in China, however, the navy enjoyed one facility which made its care superior to that of the army. In June 1841, for an annual rent of £250, it had opened a temporary naval hospital in a large house at the Portuguese colony of Macao. The building had 20 rooms, nine of which were large enough to serve as wards, while the remainder provided ample storage space, accommodation for servants, bath-houses, privies, a cookhouse and a dispensary. A high wall beyond a small courtyard secured the hospital from intruders. James Allan, assistant surgeon from *Cruizer*, was put ashore to manage it – as he subsequently complained. The hospital could hold 100 patients and, though it never contained more than 76, Allan insisted that this was too many for one medic to cope with. His nosological return for the period June to September 1841 cited 92 cases of which only 40 were discharged cured. Twenty-three had to be invalided, 18 others died and the remainder were still receiving treatment. He hoped Burnett would bear in mind that he was sent only the worst cases, many of which had no hope of recovery.

Allan struggled on as best he could into the following year. Patient

numbers gradually diminished. The annual cost of maintaining the establishment was estimated at £2,400, with the medical officer's eight shillings
per diem being an additional charge. As the months passed, though, even
Allan came to see that life in Macao offered some advantages. The local
market afforded ample animal and vegetable produce and the meals of
patients on full diet were, in consequence, 'plentiful and nutritious'. Men
were given three meals daily. Breakfast at 8am consisted of soft bread, tea
and two eggs followed by a lunch at 1pm of 1lb of fresh beef, fowl or mutton
and a pint of broth with bread and vegetables. In the evening bread and tea
were again provided. Wine and beer were distributed at Allan's discretion
while those too ill for his full diet were issued a half or low diet instead.
Not only was the food good but he was able to hire Chinese cooks to make
rich and wholesome soups and animal jellies.[7]

Reports on the extent of sickness during the summer of 1841 made
depressing reading in London where Burnett reported the navy's growing
losses at the Admiralty. During the period 1 January to 31 October 1840
only 22 sailors had died from disease: a death rate of one in 129. In the
corresponding period since 1 November 1840, however, 39 had died from
total crews of 3,619 in the squadron: a death rate of one in 93. But it was
not the mortality rate which was degrading the navy's capacity. The sick-
lists during the period since 1 November 1840 totalled 2,247, most notable among which were 160 fever cases, 300 of dysentery, 215 diarrhoea and
521 with serious catarrh.[8] The Commander-in-Chief, Rear-Admiral Sir
William Parker, realized that he had to move his ships north in the hope
that cooler weather might restore the combined force, rejecting any suggestion of further operations in the vicinity of Canton. Parker captured Amoy
on 26 August, re-occupied Chusan on 1 September, took Chinhae on 10
September and Ningpo three days later. With his force now dispersed and
its state of health gradually improving during the winter, Parker devised
his own strategy for dealing the Chinese empire a decisive blow. With an
armada of men-of-war, transports, supply ships and surveying craft, 73
vessels in all, and with reinforcements which brought British land forces up
to 12,000 fighting men, his plan was to navigate the Yangtse as far as the
ancient capital of Nanking and to cut the artery on which Peking and the
north depended for its food supply – the Grand Canal.

Parker's 1842 campaign started well with the capture of Chapu in May.
Woosung was taken in June and Shanghai surrendered just three days
later. Now in the Yangtse, Parker believed that the problems of sickness

and supply, so evident in 1840 and 1841, had been overcome. Casualties, however, were heavier than before. Even when re-taking Chusan in October 1841 Cree had noticed stiffer resistance from Chinese soldiers and had to attend more wounded than usual. 'I had all the cots I could muster slung on the main deck,' he noted: 'quite a large hospital.'[9] But there was far worse to come in the Yangtse. In July 1842 the Chinese garrison at Chinkiang put up a stiff resistance when the British attacked and, in stifling temperatures, heatstroke accounted for yet more deaths and additions to the sick-list. Cree was unable to leave *Rattlesnake* on the day after the battle, having so many sick and wounded to attend. Moreover there was now sickness in all the ships with cholera aboard some vessels and fevers and diarrhoea becoming common. Parker struggled up to Nanking and blockaded the entrance to the Grand Canal. By the beginning of August, however, his force was reduced by illness to only 3,500 men fit for action. This might have been enough to take the city in an initial assault but, with no sign that the rate of sickness was declining, almost certainly not enough to hold it thereafter. Impressive as his flotilla looked moored in the river, Parker realized that his best chance lay in negotiations.

With fresh food again proving a problem for many warships in the Yangtse, Cree was certainly hoping that Parker's negotiations would soon end the war. On 22 August he went across to the flagship where he found Parker's surgeon 'up to his eyes in business' – as, he learned, was the case for those medical officers on other ships still well enough to perform their duties.[10] 'The sickness is considerable,' Parker confided.[11] Moreover whatever the outcome of the talks under way inside the city, Parker knew that getting his squadron back down the Yangtse would be more difficult than getting up to Nanking when the winds had generally been favourable. In the end Parker was spared the risk of an assault on Nanking. A treaty was signed on 31 August whereby the Chinese authorities ceded the base at Hong Kong to the British and opened five other ports to foreign trade. Surveying the state of the forces ashore at the time, one British army officer noticed how 'those buildings which we had appropriated for hospital purposes were crammed with patients'. 'The run upon the medicine, such as quinine and bark, so very efficacious in these diseases, was immense.'[12]

Making their way back to the sea, men-of-war and transports were so crowded with febrile soldiers and marines that sickness rates among the sailors soon soared. Some of the ships were so short of men who knew how to use sails that they simply drifted. One crew was described by a nervous soldier aboard as 'living skeletons' who were 'hardly able to crawl about the deck'.[13] *Belleisle* was among the first warships to reach the coast and her condition was not unrepresentative: only 75 among her complement of 250 sailors were able to work and the entire lower deck was an improvised hospital. As they straggled out of the river throughout September 1842, ships made their way to the anchorage at Chusan where, on 15 August, *Minden* had arrived. 'Better late than never,' Cree reflected.[14] *Minden*, however, was not immediately serviceable. Her decks were crowded with more than 70 tons of stores and until these were sorted and transferred to the army and other vessels no patients could be received. *Minden*, in fact, carried enough medical supplies for 5,000 naval patients over two years to the value of £2,855 and a further stock for 10,000 soldiers worth £3,566.[15] She was also encumbered with 700 bales of canvas and a large amount of cordage. With these cleared and with eight chests and other medical stores previously held elsewhere now brought aboard, *Minden* could be prepared as a hospital. To speed up this work, 18 Chinese carpenters were recruited to complete work on her decks.[16] Although the hospital was still not officially operational by 16 September, *Minden* began taking sick from other ships from that date.

With *Minden* at last functioning, Wilson took control of medical provision throughout the China squadron, thereby assuming charge of more than 80 surgeons and assistants. The ships at anchor at Chusan were mostly healthy but as those which had been in the Yangtse brought back their sick Wilson found his hospital in great demand. Most of the transfers to *Minden* were fever cases, though, as Wilson noticed, diarrhoea and bronchial complications often made treatment difficult. The hospital was soon admitting soldiers as well as sailors and marines: 50 febrile men from the 98th Regiment returning on *Belleisle* were taken aboard on 1 October. 'In all these cases there is exhaustion and emaciation, in many of them to an extreme degree,' Wilson noted. 'In a considerable number the powers of life are reduced to the lowest point compatible with existence.' Ulcers were sometimes so bad as to expose the bone while bed sores were becoming a problem. Yet *Minden* had only taken the worst cases off *Belleisle* and when Wilson visited the latter to inspect the rest of the regiment he was appalled by the general spectacle. 'The search for a healthy looking man is in vain,' he remarked. 'Everywhere, stretched helplessly on deck, suspended in cots and hammocks, or tottering unsteadily a few paces, are seen the subjects of wasting disease.'[17] The 98th Regiment had taken the worst losses of any unit in the Yangtse: its initial strength of over 800 men was reduced to only

70 who could perform even the lightest duty. Already 170 had died from disease and with more known to be ill on other transports that number was likely to rise.

As the days passed Wilson recorded a steady trickle of admissions. Undoubtedly the troop carriers suffered most but many warships carrying no soldiers still had a high proportion of their crews on the sick-list. In the week prior to 8 October *Minden* took in 82 patients, 14 of whom died soon after, while for the remainder there was little prospect of recovery. The intestinal tissue of many had been so destroyed, Wilson commented, that any attempt to cure them would have been pointless. Much of the hospital's work merely eased the suffering of the dying. Between 8 and 15 October Wilson recorded a further 11 fatalities, all but one from dysentery. The pressure on *Minden* increased on 22 October when a further 49 men from the 98th Regiment had to be taken. These were mostly long-standing cases of fevers and flux and, as with those arriving at the beginning of the month, many were simply brought to the hospital to die. The deplorable condition in which so many patients were transferred greatly distressed Wilson, not only because of the harrowing nature of hospital duty but because the resulting high incidence of fatality aboard would inevitably distort *Minden*'s real contribution to medical care in the fleet. The death rate among sailors admitted to the hospital was 25 per cent; among the soldiers admitted it was close to 50 per cent. He was able to report a modest improvement in the health of the ships assembled at Chusan by the end of October, although by mid-November, both on the warships and in the hospital, fevers and intestinal flux cases were on the rise again. By this time Parker was already making plans to leave China, to reduce the size of the squadron and to close the establishment at Macao. On account of the high levels of sickness and serious cases there, the Macao hospital, in fact, continued until early 1843. Wilson visited early in January 1843 and discovered only seven patients remaining. Allan had run the hospital well, he judged, and in 1841 it had undoubtedly proved its worth. The stores at Macao were all to be transferred to *Minden*.

By the end of 1842 Wilson and Burnett had both been able to analyse statistical returns for the summer months, 30 June to 1 October. Total sick-list entries from the China squadron amounted to 5,201, excluding soldiers. Eighty-eight seamen had died up to 1 October, 30 of them from cholera. Of the sick-list entries, 1,638 were for intermittent fever and 1,313 for intestinal flux, both diarrhoeal and dysenteric. On 1 October, 1,037 men remained on the squadron's combined sick-lists. Wilson noticed a low incidence of tuberculosis: it did not seem to be common in China. Nor, it seemed, were ulcers, serious as some cases undoubtedly were. Nevertheless, compared with annual average death rates throughout the navy in past years this statistical return for the third quarter in 1842 was dire. For the seven years preceding 1837 the mortality rate among serving seamen averaged 13.8 per thousand. On the China coast fatalities had been five times that level. Wilson derived no comfort from the navy's mortality rate being lower than that in the army.

Wilson added two warnings about interpreting these figures, however, given the trying circumstances in which they had been gathered. Firstly, diagnosis, especially on board ship, had often been difficult. On *Minden*, after careful examination, patients were sometimes found to be suffering from ailments different to those for which ships' surgeons had referred them. Secondly, it was not clear whether all the ships had their full complements on 1 July 1842; if not, then the ratios of death and sickness calculated against those assumed totals would be inaccurate and the rates of both even worse than previously given. As to what the next quarter's returns might reveal, Wilson had seen reports by several surgeons and by 19 November knew already of at least 13 deaths aboard other ships since 1 October and a further 29 on *Minden*. Taking all her admissions of sailors, marines and soldiers into account between 1 October and 19 November 1842, *Minden* had received a total of 223 men, of whom 73 had died.[18]

By the end of December only ten warships remained with *Minden* at Chusan; the rest had been dispersed either south to Hong Kong or else to collect invalids and to start their journeys home. There was also a dramatic improvement in health. Back in October the average sick-list for ships at the Chusan anchorage had been above 25 per cent of crews. Wilson calculated that the average sick-list now aboard the ten vessels left was about 5 per cent and that afflictions were mostly minor. This being so, *Minden*'s work in the north was essentially finished; the great wave of fever and dysentery produced by the Yangtse expedition had passed and regular ailments aboard warships did not require a hospital facility. At its peak *Minden* had housed 148 patients but by 6 January 1843 there were only 42, a number which remained steady until the end of February. Fatalities had effectively ceased by then. By mid-March *Minden* was receiving only occasional cases.

Minden was ordered south in April, first to Amoy and then to Hong Kong. To Wilson's intense annoyance, the ship was also ordered to transport

50 boxes of ammunition and other stores which he protested would impair its performance as a hospital. Quin made a similar representation to the senior officer at Chusan but the order was confirmed. Wilson therefore had to relinquish the orlop deck. Quin also pointed out that his ship had become short of crew by April 1843 and that he would have preferred to delay her departure. But *Minden* sailed on 8 May; Quin would have to pick up the necessary seamen at Hong Kong. Having observed *Minden* for more than six months at Chusan, however, the senior officer there reported to the Commander-in-Chief that it was a well-ordered vessel, her boats were always well turned out and 'the ship in many respects almost as efficient as if she were a regular man-of-war'. From a senior captain, this was praise indeed.[19]

Wilson's evaluation of his hospital ship, predictably, was by different criteria. Having reported all his statistics to London he reflected upon the context within which *Minden*'s services had to be set. The war with China had been unlike other campaigns: 'the force employed was at one time large; the ground occupied was so new as to be all but unknown,' he judged, 'and the diseases, though not new in essence, were also peculiar in many of their features.' At Amoy Wilson found time to indulge his scholarly inclinations, investigating common diseases among the Chinese, assessing traditional medical practices and describing sanitary conditions in coastal towns. Deformities and disfiguring diseases appeared common among Amoy's 300,000 population, with leprosy, eye and skin diseases and fever epidemics occurring regularly.[20]

At Hong Kong on 5 June 1843 Wilson discovered high levels of fever and flux aboard the ships at anchor. Hospital admissions resumed; by 7 August *Minden* held 92 patients. Nineteen had died during July. Such was the anxiety about the health of sailors and soldiers on the island that on 3 July Parker asked Wilson to join with Surgeon Daniel King from his flagship and John Reid, surgeon of *Agincourt*, to examine a number of sites close to where naval stores had been landed and soldiers encamped. Wilson concluded that these swampy areas with their decaying vegetation, along with the irrigation channels of terraced paddy fields, were the likely sources of disease at Hong Kong and he recommended draining the localities which affected shore installations. When dried, grass should be planted: the overall effect would be to break down the artificial barriers to natural drainage which traditional patterns of cultivation had encouraged and to allow a free flow of water towards the sea. Within a few weeks *Minden* was again admitting soldiers from the shore as well as sailors from the warships. 'From both sources, this hospital is full,' he noted on 27 September, 'and contains an immense proportion of bad, a large proportion of utterly hopeless cases.'[21] As in the Yangtse in the summer of 1842, it was once more the 98th Regiment that suffered most, with 25 per cent of a detachment dying from fever and flux during six months encamped on Hong Kong prior to October 1843. There was little excuse for this, Wilson asserted. In 1842 the 26th Regiment had suffered while ashore on the island, and earlier in 1843 the 55th Regiment's losses from fevers had likewise been severe. Hong Kong had potential as a trading centre, if the British government chose to retain it, but its development would depend on adopting extensive land improvements in order to make it habitable.

By October and November 1843 Wilson faced pressures comparable to those at the Chusan anchorage a year earlier. Eighty-four admissions in September alone brought the total sick aboard *Minden* at Hong Kong to 260 – way beyond the limit that could be accommodated in cradles below deck. Fluxes, complicated by fever, were the worst problem: 'most of them chronic and absolutely hopeless of cure', Wilson noted despondently. He painted a depressing picture of the routine in which he, Tucker and the assistants were engaged. Each day they 'go the same disheartening round, from bed to bed, hour after hour, seeing the sick men, who looked to them for relief, sinking slowly but surely'.[22] Even medical officers who had served in the West Indies declared that they had never seen men so debilitated by fevers or dysentery before. In October Wilson told the admiral at Hong Kong that he would be surprised if one in ten of his patients would ever be discharged back to their ships.[23] At the start of November he reported 99 in the hospital, with 44 deaths aboard in the past four weeks. As at Chusan in 1842 many men were being transferred *in extremis*. Even men discharged invalided were either not expected to survive the journey home or else would suffer for the remainder of their lives on account of the damage done to vital organs.

It remained the case until the New Year that, bad as the navy's losses were, the army on Hong Kong fared demonstrably worse. Half the 55th Regiment had died since April 1843 with only one-third remaining serviceable. *Minden* lost 16 per cent of patients admitted in December 1843 – 17 men in all, of whom 13 were soldiers. The overall figure for the hospital would almost certainly have been worse, Wilson confided to Burnett, had he not managed to transfer a further 18 soldiers to an army installation ashore. Not only that, the old problem of supplies had surfaced again owing to the large run on many medicines and comforts. Tucker became aware of this in his daily running of the wards and wrote officially to Wilson in the knowledge that the hospital's plight would thereby be forwarded to London. Breakages of bottles and other glass containers as chests and crates were banged around on transport vessels, and even in the storage areas on *Minden*, made matters worse: fortified wines, which Tucker administered to men too weak to eat properly, suffered in this way and he had been reduced to buying inferior stocks from merchants and others on Hong Kong at greatly inflated prices. Aside from the magnesia, sulphate of zinc, chalk, camomile flowers, citric acid, quinine, carbonate of ammonia, castor oil, various powders and tinctures and the other aromatic substances which he listed, Tucker also needed sago, rice and barley as staples for his sick-diet. The last shipment of barley had decomposed *en route* to China; the solution, he suggested, was to purchase these foodstuffs locally since, unlike the wines and medical ingredients, they were abundant at Hong Kong and money could be saved. Burnett approved of that. Overall, though, Somerset House did not take kindly to any complaint from *Minden* and judged the supply system to have worked well. *Minden* had gone out with 12 months' supplies for full hospital operation and those had lasted a year from the summer of 1842. A further six months' supply had been sent on a troop ship which had arrived as planned and would last at least until April 1844. Parker confirmed that *Minden* 'has admirably answered the purpose contemplated by their Lordships and has proved a great comfort'.[24] Burnett would therefore hear of nothing which called into question such approval for his department.

Overwhelmed though *Minden* had been in the autumns of both 1842 and 1843, with her chaotically crowded decks and despite Tucker's anxieties about essential supplies reaching her in time, few who had served on the China coast would have disagreed with Parker's evaluation. At both Chusan and Hong Kong there was a broad conviction that holding the sick afloat was a great deal better than landing men to suffer an unhealthy environment. After Hong Kong was occupied, rumours abounded that a military hospital would soon be erected and that, at least for the soldiers, more familiar surroundings might become available. But as one army surgeon, Chilley Pine, explained as early as March 1841, although it was invariably more convenient to work at a land establishment than in the cramped conditions of a ship, 'unless <u>good</u> hospitals are provided I think it would be better to leave the sick in the hospital ships'.[25] Once Hong Kong became British, however, building a shore hospital became a matter of debate for both services. Rear-Admiral Sir Thomas Cochrane, in charge there in September 1842, stressed that naval surgeons had more than sufficient work among their crews and in future would not be able to give assistance to Chinese workmen injured ashore, at the gaol or to the increasing number of merchant vessels calling. The island would need its own surgeon and assist-ant, the costs for which might be borne by a small tonnage duty levied on ships entering the port.[26]

Early in 1843 Hong Kong was surveyed by the surgeon of *Nimrod* with a view to discovering a suitable site where a shore establishment might be sheltered in winter and enjoy the cooler effects of sea breezes in the heat of summer. But finding a site and building a hospital were two different things. Parker told Burnett in September 1843 that there were no skilled craftsmen, no overseers or clerks of works, and not even any Royal Engineers who could design and organize construction. All materials and fittings would have to be shipped out from Britain and the expense would be consider-able. Where labour was available locally the quality of work to date had been very poor. Merchants had commissioned Chinese builders to put up houses but the structures had been located on sandy ground and without foundations. Inevitably most had been undermined during heavy rain. The army would doubtless establish a field hospital for the diminishing number of troops kept at Hong Kong but, for the navy, a shore hospital seemed a remote prospect and *Minden* should therefore remain moored close by. Cochrane was against building ashore on principle, believing Hong Kong to be too unhealthy a location. Throughout the war, men afloat had recov-ered more quickly from illness than men ashore; Cochrane therefore, advo-cated leaving *Minden* in the Far East until she became unfit for use. Given the options, the Admiralty requested Burnett's opinion on what should be done with its only hospital ship.

Whatever plans Burnett may have harboured for *Minden* after service in China, the opinions of both admirals in the Far Eastern squadron left little scope for argument. In any case, Burnett had no alternative suggestion for naval hospital provision at Hong Kong. Seamen in south China were exposed annually to the dangers of remittent and intermittent fevers which, he explained to the Board, arose from the malarial and marsh miasma of the general neighbourhood. There was no point, therefore, constructing a land hospital in a place inherently unhealthy. Until such time as Wilson's sweeping public-health recommendations about drainage and changes in agricultural practices were implemented, the problem of medical accommodation was most readily and least expensively solved by towing *Minden* to a safe place, dismantling her masts and rigging, paying off her crew and using her solely as a fixed floating hospital with only medical staff and a handful of sailors for maintenance purposes aboard. In February 1844 Parker was informed by the Admiralty that since the government had decided to reduce the number of ships on the Far Eastern station, and would probably do so again in 1845, the whole question of building ashore had been shelved. Potential hospital sites would be made over to the navy and retained but *Minden* would stay at Hong Kong with Tucker as surgeon in charge.[27]

With the arrival of cooler weather in December 1843 the state of the squadron gradually improved. Parker noted that the crews generally were healthy, though at Hong Kong the rate of improvement was stubbornly slow. Not until 1 March 1844 did Wilson feel confident that the maladies of autumn 1843 were finally over. Most ships had fewer than 3 per cent of their seamen on the sick-lists and the ailments reported were no longer of a serious nature. There were ulcers, bronchial infections, venereal complaints and shipboard accidents to tend to, along with 'abuse of what the ancients called non-naturals and other forms of misconduct'.[28] As for *Minden*, only 13 patients remained aboard in March 1844 although the number rose to 40 in August. In April 1844 Parker received instructions from London finally to hand over his command to Cochrane and to reduce its size to just 15 warships for all service east of India.

With his duties now light and with Tucker running the hospital, Wilson again had time for the scientific pursuits he most valued. He resumed his research into the nature of contagious disease – why some ships fell prey to it more easily and why, even within those, different men similarly employed either evinced resilience or quickly succumbed. He looked back too on the efficacy of the treatments he had employed when trying to contain the various epidemics of fevers, flux and dysentery in 1842 and 1843. He had tried bleeding, leeches, blistering, the application of heat, calomel, quinine, saline draughts and opium as deemed appropriate, and although he could detect no pattern whereby treatment had proved successful nevertheless his meticulous notes gave an insight into his medical philosophy. Admittedly his successes had been modest in number, though that did not imply that his efforts had been either inefficient or unskilful. A practitioner's ability was not measurable in crude statistics and rates of mortality: 'it may be more difficult to save one life in one degree of disease than twenty in another, though both pass under the same name'.[29] Reporting failures could be as instructive as bragging of successes. A good surgeon was always ready to learn, even if no more than to avoid making the same mistake again.

Wilson's experience with men returning prostrate from the Yangtse in September 1842 confirmed another of his medical opinions: the inutility and even harm in using calomel for tropical diseases. Properly administered and in small doses a mercurial treatment might have value, as many of his colleagues who had served in the tropics insisted, but, given indiscriminately and under the erroneous conviction that if it was not working then the dosage simply needed to be increased, Wilson came to the conclusion that it actually destroyed life. 'Routinism, the besetting sin and bane of medicine, is apt to be indulged in treating tropical diseases,' he reflected, 'and in nothing is the tendency more displayed than in the use of mercury.' But here was the doctor's dilemma: did medical practice abandon long-standing treatments which still attracted much professional support just because something new was proposed? 'Exaggerated commendation of new medicines, or of new or rare applications of them, has proved a great hindrance to the advance of therapeutical knowledge,' Wilson judged.[30] Expectations were raised to unreasonable levels and then, when the limitations of a new therapy were discovered, the disillusion which followed led to its abandonment, notwithstanding that in the right cases a proper application had brought benefit. The slovenly way in which medicines and substances were used also hindered medical progress. Poultices, for instance, were frequently improperly applied. It was not sufficient to give directions and then retire, especially in the navy where those who helped in sick-bays or hospital wards were often poorly motivated and lacked even rudimentary training. A surgeon, by frequent inspection, must assure himself that what had been prescribed was fully carried out.

The relative quiet on *Minden* for much of 1844 also gave Wilson a chance to extend his observation of Chinese practice and the incidence of particular afflictions. There had been some first-hand opportunity to do this at Chusan in 1842 when local people had approached *Minden* either to have wounds dressed or diseases examined. One severe case of elephantiasis was treated on board and some improvement recorded. Whether on the hospital ship or ashore at Amoy and Hong Kong, Wilson's ability to investigate traditional medicine was, as he admitted, largely limited to what he could see with his own eyes: fevers, digestive disorders and respiratory diseases were, he concluded, as common among the native population as among foreigners, though probably less likely to prove fatal. Cholera cases were reported, although Chinese doctors appeared to be in denial that so devastating a malady could exist or be propagated on their own soil, describing it, admittedly plausibly, to be a foreign import. Wilson was horrified by foot-binding. Furthermore the more he saw of China's population the more he judged that ophthalmia must be widespread after passing so many who were either partially or totally blind. His conclusions regarding ancient arts of healing in China were generally unfavourable and the standard of provision for most people was abysmally low. Soap and water, he opined, would work miracles for large sections of society.

Nothing better illustrated the tranquillity which Wilson was enjoying than his nosological returns for the six months from May to October 1844. He had forecast well in advance that sickness rates would decline steeply from their 1843 levels and he took great satisfaction in being proved correct. At Hong Kong men were healthier than those elsewhere on the Far Eastern station and fatalities in 1844 were only a quarter of those experienced in 1843. Sick-lists on the ships varied between 4 and 8 per cent of their crews: in 1843 several ships had up to 20 per cent of their men out of action. The figure for invaliding was also much lower, as was that for fatalities on the hospital ship where only 13 per cent of patients had died between May and October 1844 compared to more than 33 per cent over the same six months in 1843. Things did begin to get worse in November 1844 when 20 soldiers from the 98th Regiment were brought aboard, followed by 20 more in December, but Burnett's recommendation to the Board at the end of the year remained that the squadron was well provided for and, given its reduction, no longer required the supervision of an Inspector. His other recommendation, which the Admiralty implemented in August 1845, was that *Minden* should be officially designated a foreign naval hospital.

Now almost three years in the tropics, Wilson's health was beginning to deteriorate. In March 1845 he was invalided and forced to return to England. Even though weakened and towards the end of his time in the Far East, Wilson still had sufficient concern for the health of the squadron to report on the unhygienic state in which the crews of the various ships slept. With the help of three surgeons still at Hong Kong, Wilson investigated the state of bedding and blankets aboard naval vessels, finding them depressingly filthy and a potential source of disease. Cochrane conceded that in his experience these items were rarely washed, even on ships otherwise kept clean, and ordered captains to ensure that all blankets be washed with soap and aired at least once each summer and the bedding material and hair beaten, teased and dried.[31] Once Wilson had departed Tucker moved into his quarters aboard *Minden*. The hospital had only 16 patients in early April 1845 and none of them was serious. Furthermore numbers were likely to remain low in light of the shore facility for the few soldiers left on Hong Kong which the army was constructing. Yet Tucker had only a brief opportunity to run a naval establishment. His letters to Burnett spoke of his own suffering from remittent fever from July onwards and though he struggled on surveying stores and preparing medical returns it was clear that he was seriously ill. Tucker died on *Minden* in November 1845. Responsibility for the hospital was now entrusted to Robert Bankier.

Bankier had served on *Herald* during the war although his ship had not been in the Yangtse. Distinguished by having won the Blane Medal while still an assistant surgeon, Bankier was conscious of his own abilities and inclined to treat other medical officers rather haughtily. Most colleagues believed that Bankier had seen his move to *Minden* as a step to Deputy-Inspector or to a prestigious hospital posting, hence his irritability as the years passed and nothing was forthcoming. Bankier inherited 31 patients in November 1845, some of them seriously ill. The hospital, nevertheless, was reducing its establishment; in January 1846 the nurses and servants who had sailed with *Minden* in 1842 were discharged for their passage home. Nursing and washing were henceforth performed by eight staff, seven of whom were locally recruited Chinese. The hospital was almost empty for the first half of 1846 until four warships returning from the coast of Borneo in August required 38 admissions, mostly fever and dysentery cases but a few with spear wounds. Bankier lost five men from the 38 admitted. That was depressing enough, given that it was his first real test in charge. By then, however, anxiety was also caused by the decision to move the hospital to *Alligator* and to leave *Minden* as a store-ship for medical and other supplies.

The naval hospital at Hong Kong was transferred to *Alligator* on 9 September 1846. Most medical staff at Hong Kong believed that this was a mistake. *Alligator* could not hold so many patients, although with the station now reduced to only a handful of ships which were at different times away from Hong Kong that was not the real problem. *Alligator* was, as one of its assistant surgeons, Alexander Mackay, who joined in 1849 complained, 'a miserable jackass frigate, which had seen a good deal of work'. Unfit for further service as a man-of-war, she was first turned into a troopship and then dismantled for hospital service. Her cabins were cramped, the cradles were unavoidably level with the ports and insufficient boats for junior medical staff were available. 'I have little hesitation in saying that many a valuable life was lost by the ill-judged economy which placed more value upon old ships' stores than upon the lives of men,' Mackay confided.[32] Unsuitable as *Alligator* was, Bankier had 44 sailors to tend by the end of October 1846, mostly suffering from chronic dysentery. Mercifully his load was down to only seven by March 1847.

The hospital carried on uneventfully for the remainder of 1847 and into 1848. Bankier's principal problems were with dysentery cases, although those were not necessarily local but were men brought to him by warships arriving at Hong Kong. The island itself seemed healthier than in previous years: indeed, when Cree left in 1846 he remarked on the changes which had taken place since his arrival in 1841 and how a handsome town was developing. *Alligator* had 24 sick on board in April 1848; with three assistant surgeons still on the establishment, however, this did not create much pressure. Patient numbers were much the same a year later, though Bankier, briefly with 66 in his care in March 1849, refused more cases from ten warships arriving at Hong Kong which he did not consider sufficiently urgent. *Alligator* could not hold any more, he wrote in justification; he regretted refusing any sailor for whom hospital care might be better than that available on a ship, yet his decision was unavoidable because *Alligator* 'is not fully adapted for the purposes of an hospital'.[33] Not only was she short of space and facilities but the men admitted appeared to recover very slowly.

Alligator functioned so long as her numbers never rose much above 30, although even with manageable numbers the complaints never stopped. Ventilation, especially in summer, was bad. Noise and odours were insupportable at times and her lower deck was overrun with vermin. Burnett felt that he had to persuade the Board to transfer the hospital back to *Minden*. The latter would, of course, require restoration after years of neglect and Burnett did not refrain from expressing his regret that his only hospital ship had been downgraded to a storage vessel. The matter was made more urgent when there was no seasonal falling off in demand in November 1849 and Bankier once more had to refuse further admissions. But the most the Board would permit were extensive cleaning, platform additions for increased storage and repairs to *Alligator*, which provided only two months of respite elsewhere while the work was being done. In the course of 1850 conditions gradually deteriorated. With her expanded capacity *Alligator* had 78 patients in June, mostly from *Serpent*, half of whose crew had contracted fever, bronchial afflictions or gastric irritation while on shore leave. Even so, to ease the overcrowding Bankier had sent some patients to space available on *Minden* with the obvious disadvantage that the hospital's medical and other staff were now dispersed.

Only when the Commander-in-Chief, Far East, Rear-Admiral Charles Austen, joined the debate about hospital provision did the Admiralty seem to attach any importance to Bankier's predicament. Austen insisted that *Alligator* was too small for the navy's requirements and that the minimum hospital capacity at Hong Kong should be for five officers and 80 men. The surgeon's cabin and pantry were adequate but there was only a tiny mess place for the two assistant surgeons still on the medical establishment. The two cabins designated for officers were not in use, which was just as well since one of them had to double up as an office. The modest improvements made to *Alligator* at the beginning of 1850 were the most that could be done: no more beds could be squeezed in, building more cabins on the main deck would obstruct the already poor ventilation, while if cabins were constructed on the quarterdeck they would cut the walk required for convalescing patients. Austen advised fitting up a larger warship for hospital use – in particular one which would allow well-proportioned mess and sleeping places for the assistants whose duties, for much of the year, he described as arduous. Yet although he had joined with Bankier in condemning the current arrangements, Austen's recommendation differed from what Bankier wanted insofar as Bankier favoured a shore establishment rather than a floating hospital. Being on the island might be less healthy, but Bankier argued that this would be counterbalanced by the extra space available and the ease with which treatments could be administered. Isolating patients with different diseases would be simpler too, and exercise for convalescents would obviously be facilitated. His views were not accepted. Although the navy still had a 12-acre site at Hong Kong, building a hospital on it remained out of the question. A decision was finally made early in 1851 for which Austen expressed his appreciation to the First Lord: 'The arrangement for converting the *Minden* to an hospital ship and the *Alligator* to a coal depot is exactly what I could have wished.'[34] Medical staff thus looked forward to returning to *Minden* and the implicit recognition thereby that the five years spent in such adverse conditions on *Alligator* had been a mistake.

Minden re-opened as the Hong Kong naval hospital on 22 April 1852. For the remainder of the year the ships in harbour were healthy and the hospital often had no more than ten patients. Bankier reflected that he had spent 14 years in the Far East. The oppressive climate had weakened him and he advised Burnett in May 1853 that he was having difficulty recovering from an illness which had developed when recently visiting Shanghai. It was, though, nothing which a change of air and 15 months' well-earned leave in England would not cure. But the illness was hepatitis and Mackay, who watched Bankier struggle back aboard *Minden*, recognized immediately that his case was hopeless. After Bankier died in June 1853 Thomas Keown was transferred from the flagship to be hospital surgeon and storekeeper. Keown, however, was not impressed with the way in which *Minden* had been restored and, with much more sickness to contend with than Bankier had experienced in 1852, soon made his views known. *Minden* had 106 patients on 26 December 1853, diminishing only slightly to 82 a month later. The manner in which *Minden* had been knocked about in recent years greatly impaired her functions. She also had to accommodate the second master and a clerk sent over from *Alligator*; even worse, Keown penned furiously, 'our ships are allowed to make and mend sails on board; this in addition to her being a store ship and, by a late order, a receiving ship also.'[35] Burnett took up Keown's case in London. When ill or injured, he urged the Board, sailors needed quietude which was not available in a hospital used for so many other purposes. Not only was *Minden* used for sail making but men were sent aboard from other ships for cannon and small-arms practice. Keown meanwhile continued to have a steady flow of admissions, taking in 33 sailors from the French warship *Sibylle* in March 1855 which swelled his list to 65 at a time when he had only one assistant surgeon. His job was made more difficult by preparations to move the hospital and its stores to *Hercules* for a few weeks while the sides of *Minden* were repaired. When *Minden* was returned to him he hoped that she would revert solely to her original function. Hong Kong had become a more important naval base in recent years. In November 1855 the station comprised 3,200 seamen.

Keown's complaints about facilities at Hong Kong were shared by all medics who had been there. Mackay certainly left a vivid summary of his experience. 'Did not sleep over well during the night,' he jotted in May 1854. 'Had the nightmare which took the shape of an order to proceed at once to Hong Kong, quite enough to frighten one out of sleep.'[36] Under no circumstances, he later added, would he try for the position of surgeon and storekeeper in charge of *Minden* if the opportunity arose. The chance, however, was never likely to arise. When repair work began in 1855 the bottom of *Minden* was discovered to be rotten and she had to be towed into dock. The hospital remained on *Hercules* where Keown had to find space for about 50 patients throughout July and August, taking in men from *Rattler* and six from an American frigate, all of whom had been wounded during clashes with pirates. There were 100 men aboard *Hercules* by the end of October and still Keown had only one assistant. The problems were mostly ulcers, rheumatism, bronchitis, dysentery, remittent fever and syphilis; his number was still 64 at the end of November when news arrived from the dock-yard that *Minden* had been condemned, her timbers being so extensively rotted that she could no longer be rendered serviceable. Stranded for the foreseeable future on *Hercules*, Keown resurrected the question of a hospital ashore, not because all previous objections to an establishment on Hong Kong had been overcome but simply because it was impossible to run any facility which was constantly being moved from one ship to another.

Minden was not replaced with a shore establishment. In 1856 and with above 50 sailors constantly requiring hospital accommodation, the navy assigned *Melville* to be moored in the harbour and fitted out for a maxi-mum capacity of ten officers and 110 seamen. With this increased size the hospital would henceforth be allowed permanently one surgeon and two assistants. Keown was consulted on how the vessel might best be adapted and, replying to the Commander-in-Chief, referred to some of the features which had made *Minden* so advanced in her design. Proper rooms for nurses and other staff would be needed, as would water closets, washrooms, bathing facilities, spaces where patients could be taken when confined to cots, and dry storerooms for hospital supplies. Unfortunately the conversion proved to be a protracted process. In March 1857, with the navy engaged again in war with China, the hospital still had not moved from *Hercules*. The Medical Department understandably protested when it discovered that *Hercules* was also being used as a powder magazine. Abandoned prior to being eventually sold off in 1861, *Minden* remained the model for a hospital ship 15 years after her original fitting. Her contribution on the China coast after August 1842 had been considerable, both during war service and later in the harbour at Hong Kong. Successful as *Minden* proved to be, though, the Royal Navy fitted out no further hospital ship until 1854 when *Belleisle* was despatched to join the Baltic fleet.

CHAPTER 7

Baltic and Crimea

Burnett's medical service faced its sternest trial in a European war after the summer of 1854. A political crisis, originating with Russia's claim to be protector of the Greek Church in the Ottoman Empire, had unfolded during the preceding year and then intensified when the Russian army occupied Turkey's Danubian principalities. As at the time of the Mehemet Ali crisis in 1840, the British government resolved to preserve Turkish power in the Balkans and Near East; this would act as a restraint on the expansion of Russian influence. This time, significantly, it would do so in conjunction with France. The Mediterranean fleet, under Vice-Admiral Sir James Dundas, was reinforced and held six miles south of the Dardanelles in Besika Bay. The Turks insisted that Russia withdraw from the principalities and on the day before their ultimatum expired in October 1853 the British and French governments ordered warships to anchor off Constantinople as a gesture of support. War was not yet felt to be inevitable but moving men-of-war through the Dardanelles was an obvious signal to the Russians.

Besika Bay was an unhealthy anchorage and sickness became a problem as early as August 1853 when fever spread among the 16,000 seamen aboard British warships. Wind blew foul air from nearby swamps along with the stench from rotting offal strewn across the beach outside a French slaughterhouse. Having requested a medical opinion, the Commander-in-Chief subsequently ignored advice to move at least some of his squadron. Moored close by off the island of Tenedos, George Mackay, surgeon on *Bellerophon*, was faring no better. He had 58 fever cases by 25 August and since not all could be fitted into his sick-bay had resorted to stringing up hammocks on the main deck. Furthermore the admiral refused Mackay's request that drills and gun exercises might be suspended because of the disturbance to his patients. It was becoming clear that extra supplies were needed. These went out from London in September; for the moment, that particular problem was containable.

Even from this early date there was a problem collecting and coordinating data from many different vessels. Burnett first learnt of this from John Stewart at the Malta hospital who advised that a supervising medical officer would provide 'something like uniformity of management and centralise the information for you'.[1] But it was not just information which needed centralization. A clear medical authority was required in the Mediterranean fleet in order to prevent disputes about judgements and seniority. Mackay, in fact, was already embroiled in one dispute about rank regarding the fever aboard *Bellerophon*. Dundas had ordered the captain and surgeon of his flagship, *Britannia*, to visit *Bellerophon* and, with the surgeon from *Rodney*, to find out why Mackay had so many cases. Mackay was livid at being investigated by surgeons his junior. His own captain supported Mackay's protest but the admiral's orders were plain enough. 'I stated that I could not look upon Mr. Rees, the surgeon of the flagship, as my senior officer, or in any way entitled to enquire into my treatment or practice,' Mackay wrote indignantly to Burnett.[2] It was an embarrassing occasion for all three surgeons, with the whole show acted out in the presence of Mackay's assistants. Nothing untoward was found. Safely back on *Britannia*, surgeon John Rees explained almost apologetically to Burnett how he had been ordered to visit other ships before and how he always tried to proceed with tact and caution. Fever in the fleet was, mercifully, both mild and manageable, he reported early in September, but had it been more severe then the lack of a senior medical officer with clear authority might have been more keenly felt. Rees did not ask for the job, though from his correspondence he clearly saw himself as the obvious candidate.

Still smarting aboard *Bellerophon*, Mackay realized that this issue could never be resolved among competing surgeons. Furthermore, without a medical officer holding the rank of Inspector to advise him the Commander-in-Chief had been making his own medical judgements; it was Dundas, for instance, not Rees, who had moved *Bellerophon* from Besika Bay to Tenedos and placed unnecessary quarantine restrictions on the ship. Tenedos was just as unhealthy as Besika Bay; Dundas had merely succeeded in raising fears about an epidemic among *Bellerophon*'s crew. It was essential to get a doctor on to the flagship whom the admiral might consult 'without appearing to descend from his dignified position'. An Inspector would thereby 'uphold the respectability and independent character of the medical officers of the naval service'.[3] Being ineligible for such an appointment himself,

Mackay's recommendations were received in London as a genuine expression of service requirements. By the autumn of 1853 there were 14 men-of-war in the eastern Mediterranean. An Inspector's task, however, would be more than just to visit, to coordinate medical provision among a large number of vessels and to exercise authority over all their surgeons. Mackay also envisaged a research role. An Inspector would visit towns and coast-lines in the vicinity of any anchorage in order to anticipate health problems; topography, climate and local circumstances would all be studied and the Commander-in-Chief advised accordingly. Bathing and exercise routines for seamen would also come within his remit.

Rees watched the build-up of the fleet in the Bosphorus during the winter. Public opinion in both Britain and France was hardening in favour of war, particularly after Russian warships destroyed much of the Turkish navy while anchored at Sinope on 30 November. But even if war came, Rees assured Burnett, the fleet would not be engaged before next spring. In the meantime all was well: crews were generally healthy and ships were well supplied and in a good winter anchorage about nine miles from Constantinople and six miles from the entrance to the Black Sea. Rees declared that he was preparing for 'those greater responsibilities which in the event of war will devolve on myself as surgeon of the flagship'.[4] Shore-leave for more than 6,000 men in the course of the winter posed the usual medical problems, especially with an abundance of cheap spirits available. The Royal Navy entered the Black Sea in January 1854. It was accompanied by French men-of-war and escorted Turkish troopships conveying soldiers to the frontier. Soon the British had 22 warships and ten smaller vessels beyond the Bosphorus. Four per cent of crews were on the sick-lists. Rees remained well satisfied. He was, needless to say, even more so a few weeks later when promoted to Deputy-Inspector.

In February 1854 the British and French governments presented an ulti-matum for Russian troops to withdraw from the Danubian principalities. This being rejected, war against Russia was declared on 27 March.[5] Rees meanwhile continued with his preparations, confident that the Russian navy would never come out from its base at Sebastopol to risk a battle. Equally, however, he anticipated no immediate naval action against Sebastopol, since the narrow channel into the port could easily become blocked if just three attacking ships were sunk by its defensive batteries. Sebastopol was undoubtedly the prize. It would, however, require a combined operation with the army and would doubtless cost many lives. To allow for naval casualties, arrangements were under way for a forward hospital on the Bosphorus, north of Constantinople at Therapia which could hold more than 100 beds and which would save otherwise having to transport serious cases back to Malta. In April 1854 Rees urged that ideally 200 beds would be available at Therapia and that appropriate equipment should be shipped from Malta without delay. Men wounded during naval bombardments against Russian shore guns could thereby be accommodated in comfortable surroundings within 36 hours of any engagement. This would give the Royal Navy better medical support than its French counterpart which currently provided 70 hospital places for its ten warships in the allied fleet.

Odessa was the first scene of naval action in the Black Sea. On 22 April 1854 five British and three French warships attacked the port's defences and its merchant vessels.[6] Rees watched excitedly from *Britannia* how the steamers paddled to and fro to make it hard for Russian guns to find their range; the engagement silenced the Russian batteries and inflicted considerable damage on the harbour and its craft while sparing the town and civilian property as far as possible. Admittedly it was a small affair: the British lost one man with only nine others wounded. But seeing the ships in action was a wondrous sight, Rees reported to Burnett. Crews were cool under fire and junior medical officers pushed themselves forward to do duty. A few more medics would be welcome, but the majority of those on the station were men of superior calibre and all medical arrangements were working well. This was a reflection on the improvements to the service instigated by Burnett since the 1820s, Rees added sycophantically: the availability of more surgical texts, regulations for battle preparation, the introduction of chloroform and the use of cotton wadding all marked significant advances since the Napoleonic Wars. Alas for Rees, despite having made no secret of his own ambitions, he was not appointed to take charge of the fleet, being sent instead to run the Bermuda hospital. David Deas arrived in the Black Sea as Deputy-Inspector in August 1854.

Between the action at Odessa and his departure for Bermuda, Rees became largely occupied with the deteriorating health among the crews of many ships. *Britannia*, off Sebastopol in mid-May 1854, had fever aboard. Rees managed this with a liberal use of quinine though he was not sure that other surgeons had done so well. Scurvy was another problem, brought on because so many men had been confined to the lower decks during cold weather and fed too much on salt provisions. But the greatest danger proved to be cholera which was spreading rapidly by early August. *Trafalgar* had 33 deaths between 9 and 13 August. *Furious* had 19 deaths by 21 August. Her surgeon collapsed, having exhausted himself caring for his dying assistant, and by the time another assistant surgeon arrived to take charge the entire crew was seized with panic. Aboard *Albion*, 39 men were dead by 19 August. It was, however, Rees's *Britannia* that suffered most. Between 9 and 19 August she lost 112 sailors and marines, producing chaotic scenes 'perhaps without parallel in the history of our service'.[7] Men simply fell down all over the ship and were carried in a stream towards the sick-bay. This was soon overflowing, requiring the sick and dying to be laid out on both sides of the middle deck. It was impossible even to keep a register of cases: on one day alone 50 seamen succumbed. By 24 August fatalities on *Britannia* had risen to 132, with two-thirds of her crew affected. By that date the ship had mostly been evacuated for fumigation. The final toll was 139. Within just five days 229 men on *Britannia* had been diagnosed with cholera with a further 400 suffering from diarrhoea among her complement of 920 men.[8] Most of the fleet in the Black Sea was now anchored at Baljick where Deas joined *Queen*. It was a depressing spectacle and a far cry from the encouraging tone in which Rees had written to Burnett four months earlier.

Before joining *Queen* Deas had visited the small division of the fleet to the south at Varna where more than 60,000 British and French troops were camped in readiness for the expedition to the Crimea. Conditions there were bad too, for both soldiers and sailors. The army lost about 1,260 men to disease on the Bulgarian coast in the summer of 1854; cholera accounted for almost three-quarters of these. Naval captains and surgeons off Varna urged Deas to retrieve their missing assistant surgeons, many of whom Dundas had ordered to Baljick. Given the obvious shortage of young medics on the ships, Deas willingly agreed. Reaching Baljick, however, he realized why the assistants had been moved: the shortage there was even more acute and the extent of sickness greater. Men-of-war close by *Queen* all had cholera aboard and several had medical officers who were too ill to work. *Queen* had a complement of 1,000 men, no assistant surgeon, and Deas soon found himself helping out in the sick-bay instead of tending to his own duties. By 24 August, 301 seamen had died from cholera in the Black Sea fleet and many new cases were still being diagnosed. The epidemic eventually claimed more than 400 lives. Having experienced at first hand the strain placed upon the obviously insufficient number of doctors, Deas reported how medical staff were 'overworked and exhausted'.[9]

Unfortunately the situation was about to get worse. On 20 September 1854, having landed in the Crimea just two weeks before, the army fought its first battle at the River Alma.

Shortages of medical officers in the navy were exposed, however, even before cholera made its appearance in the Black Sea. Towards the end of 1853 Burnett had required all surgeons on half pay to declare their availability. The shortage, as usual, was among assistant surgeons, for which there were 21 vacancies in April 1854. The Medical Department meanwhile had only five applicants to be examined for entry. Seven full surgeons were still performing the duties of assistants, while three druggists had recently been employed to compound medicines where no assistants were available. In July the Admiralty ordered another trawl of the half-pay list to try to discover whether any surgeons or assistants recently certified as unfit were making a timely recovery. A string of enquiries arrived at Somerset House from over-aged practitioners or those otherwise unqualified, but Burnett would make no concessions on that account. His view, stated for the House of Commons on 31 July 1854, was that the Black Sea fleet was short of neither surgeons nor assistants. Technically that was so. It was not, however, the whole truth. The reason why there were only 21 vacancies for assistant surgeons in the navy was because of a change of regulations in 1851 whereby three-deck vessels, which formerly carried three assistants, now bore only two, while frigates, which formerly carried two assistants, now bore only one. Only an admiral's flagship was now staffed with more than two assistant surgeons. Levels of medical provision by 1854, thereby, had arguably ceased to take account of the possibility of war.[10]

The Royal Navy operated in a second theatre of war, the Baltic, where Vice-Admiral Sir Charles Napier commanded. Napier's purpose was to implement blockades and harass enemy shipping, to engage the Russian navy if possible and to reduce Russian shore installations and fortifications. By April 1854, upwards of 25 ships with crews of over 17,700 men had assembled in the Baltic. On paper, this was an impressive fleet; the ships, however, were undermanned and their crews too often a mixture of the aged and inexperienced. As for medical staff, Burnett conceded in July that four vessels sent to the Baltic were each missing an assistant surgeon. Against that, though, the Baltic squadron had one benefit – a hospital ship. This owed nothing to the First Lord of the Admiralty, Sir James Graham, who clung to the view that rolling seas always made a ship a bad hospital.[11] Overcoming this inertia, nevertheless, *Belleisle* was converted at Devonport between March and May 1854. Stripped down to six guns, she carried a complement of 240. Within that total were its medical staff, comprising an Inspector, Alexander McKechnie, a surgeon in charge, Robert Beith, an additional surgeon and two assistants. To support the hospital she carried a clerk, 14 male nurses and the wives of three of them as laundry staff. As refitted, *Belleisle* held 155 iron beds of the sort used in home hospitals, 118 of which were on her lower deck, 30 on the orlop deck, two in an operating ward and five in main-deck cabins reserved for officers.[12] *Belleisle* joined Napier at Baro Sound on the southern coast of Finland on 5 June. Days passed unloading provisions brought out from England and then preparing to receive patients. As *Belleisle* arrived warships were moving to attack Helsingfors and to probe the defences of the fortress at Sveaborg, in respect of which McKechnie anticipated casualties almost immediately. But there was no significant fighting and only five wounded were admitted. Although by the end of June the hospital had taken 57 cases, of whom eight had died and six been invalided, the problem for the fleet, as in the Black Sea, lay with disease and the availability of medical officers rather than with action against the enemy.

Those difficulties had, in fact, surfaced even before the hospital ship arrived. James Salmon, surgeon aboard *Neptune*, found that he had an epidemic on his hands in May 1854. Unfortunately he had misdiagnosed seven sickly sailors and not taken isolation measures. It proved to be smallpox and he soon had more than 80 cases. The middle deck of *Neptune* had then been given over as an extended sick-bay. Salmon received the help he needed from his captain when enforcing quarantine and detailing nurses but was refused a small steamer to be set alongside to hold infected men. Cots, screens, bedding, clothing, utensils, buckets and pans were all disinfected with a solution of zinc chloride in an attempt to contain the outbreak. It was only on 1 July, however, that McKechnie felt confident enough to write home that the smallpox on *Neptune*, and also that aboard *Cumberland*, was under control. But at least Salmon had sufficient hands available on *Neptune* to do his bidding. By contrast, Walter Dickson, surgeon on *Archer*, protested that he had been left without the assistant surgeon promised before leaving England two months previously. Dickson had more than 100 seamen on his sick-list, several of them dangerously ill and needing constant care. He lacked not only a qualified assistant but even a reliable sick-berth attendant. If *Archer* went into action matters would become even worse, he predicted. Then he would need to perform surgery rapidly, administer chloroform and secure arteries, and 'such help as could be got from ignorant and inexperienced bystanders could hardly fail to accelerate rather than retard a fatal issue'.[13] Dickson reverted to the familiar surgeon's plea for properly trained and permanently attached sick-berth staff, especially on larger vessels.

Smallpox and a shortage of medical attendance were not the only short-comings which greeted *Belleisle* on arrival. McKechnie was also struck by problems of supply. Meat and vegetables, mostly purchased in Stockholm, were restricted and of poor quality. Most crews had been on salt provisions for some time and lime juice would soon need to be issued. On investigation, however, the squadron had only small supplies of juice; the general health of crews would soon deteriorate in these circumstances. By the beginning of July 1854 the larger part of the Baltic fleet had moved to threaten Kronstadt. Other ships, both British and French, were in the Gulf of Bothnia while *Belleisle* remained with about a dozen warships off Sveaborg. McKechnie, therefore, found it hard to collect information though knew that several ships already had cholera aboard. Cruising at sea and using zinc chloride were the answers to this, he later advised Napier. But the disease, as in the Black Sea, proved difficult to contain and with the warships back at Baro Sound again on 9 July the extent of the outbreak became clear. There had been 152 cases: 45 fatalities, 11 men sent to the hospital ship and 59 still under treatment on different vessels. *Belleisle* had 40 sick and wounded aboard, though only four were cholera cases. By 16 July, 74 men were under treatment for cholera in the Baltic fleet; on 24 July McKechnie reported that the death toll had risen to 64. The problem, he concluded, lay with the anchorage.

Baro Sound contained too much decaying vegetation, and the land which enclosed it resembled a bog. The squadron, therefore, should be moved. Napier responded vaguely. 'He is always very kind to me,' McKechnie recorded after a meeting; the gist of the Commander-in-Chief's reply, however, was that whatever might be wrong with Baro Sound it was not as rocky or unsafe as other places visited. Napier confided that he intended to take ships up to Kronstadt again and so cholera might be dealt with by that means. Meanwhile it was slowly dawning on McKechnie that there was no clear idea about what the navy might achieve in the Baltic. To date there had been only unopposed actions to burn Russian dockyards and storehouses at Brahestad, Uleaborg and Tornea in the Gulf of Bothnia, followed by an unsuccessful raid by boats on the port of Gamla Carelby on

7 June. None of the officers to whom McKechnie had spoken seemed to expect much fighting. Russian warships would obviously never come out for a battle; equally, though, the strength of Russian shore fortifications meant that British naval losses, and those among accompanying French soldiers, might be considerable if serious attacks were attempted. Yet doing nothing, while the health of the fleet suffered, was also unsatisfactory. So much medicine had been expended on various ships that their surgeons were turning to *Belleisle* for emergency supplies – 'which I cannot comply with', McKechnie observed.[14] The one spare medical chest which he had brought out from England had long ago been given to a man-of-war badly afflicted with cholera.

While Napier considered what to do next and McKechnie continued to monitor the incidence of cholera, John Gallagher, surgeon on *Arrogant*, raised a more specific issue on behalf of the sick and wounded. Since most of the vessels in the Baltic were steamers, enemy fire would no longer be directed at masts and rigging, as in the age of sail, but would be aimed at the hull, as close as possible to the waterline. Keeping the wounded in the lowest part of the ship was therefore no longer so safe. Gallagher proposed that prior to any engagement the storerooms used by carpenters and boatswains immediately below the lower deck, but above the gunners' storerooms, should be emptied and allocated as sick-bay accommodation. In London the question was referred to the surveyor of the navy who, while acknowledging Gallagher's concern, concluded that the idea was impractical since it would be nigh impossible, with the ship on battle stations, to find anywhere else to put the carpenter's stores. But Gallagher's observations about the changing nature of naval warfare were not confined to this. In recent years, with chloroform becoming widely used in surgery, the old cockpits no longer sufficed because of the fumes. Wherever medical staff worked, pipes from outside the vessel would in future need to be led into the operating area so that fresh air might circulate.

The only major engagement in 1854 came when the Aaland Islands forts at Bomarsund were reduced by naval bombardment and captured by French soldiers between 8 and 16 August. More than 2,200 Russian prisoners were taken. Napier had warned McKechnie of this attack a few days in advance, advising him to restrict admissions to *Belleisle* so that those severely wounded might be brought aboard. *Belleisle* had 59 patients on 7 August and McKechnie noticed that the hospital was already running out of several medicines and was anxiously awaiting fresh supplies. By 21

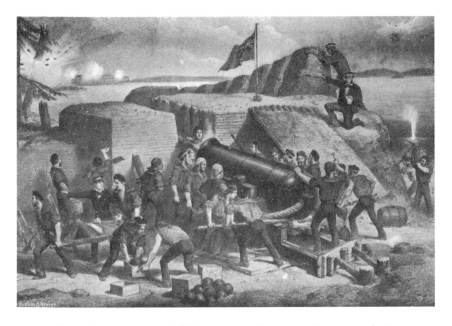

5. Removing the wounded from a naval battery at Bomarsund: 1854.

August, after Bomarsund, *Belleisle* had 85 patients. There would, however, be no further campaigning in the Baltic that year. The French soldiers, who had also suffered much from cholera after the assault at Bomarsund, sailed home for the winter in September while *Belleisle* was ordered back to England conveying 75 wounded or invalided men. Napier faced public criticism for indecision when he returned to Portsmouth in December and was relieved of his command. In the course of the 1854 Baltic campaign only 15 seamen had been killed by enemy action.

Before *Belleisle* left the Baltic, McKechnie was visited by Edward Cree, surgeon from *Odin*, who took the chance to look over the hospital. Twelve years earlier Cree had been able to investigate *Minden* in just the same way when an assistant on the China coast. 'Everything very nice and clean, but pretty full of our sick and wounded, beside the worst of the Russian wounded,' he recorded.[15] With McKechnie gone, Frederick Le Grande, surgeon on Napier's flagship, *Duke of Wellington*, took charge in the Baltic. *Belleisle* reached Plymouth on 13 October where 45 patients need-ing residential care were moved to the East Stonehouse hospital. Thereafter McKechnie wrote up his statistical report. Though not all were men-of-war, there had been about 50 British ships in the Baltic with combined crews

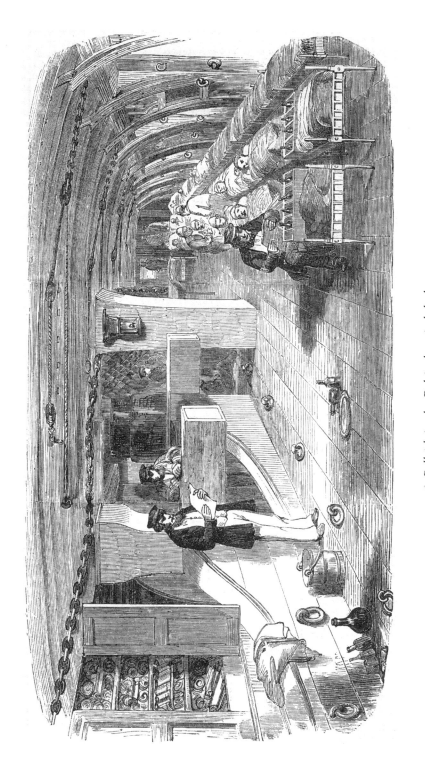

6. *Belleisle* in the Baltic: hospital deck.

of over 20,000 seamen. He divided the 1854 campaign into two parts. For the three months 1 April to 30 June there were 8,531 cases on the combined sick-lists. Eighty-one men had died, 60 from disease and 21 from accidents. For the two months 1 July to 31 August the sick-lists amounted to 4,418 with 72 fatalities. Deaths therefore totalled 153 from among 12,949 sick and wounded. Cholera was by far the largest killer. Throughout June, July and August, McKechnie calculated 285 cases in different ships of which 107 died and 178 recovered. Comparatively few of those cases came to *Belleisle*. The efforts of the hospital ship, however, were reported in great detail. She admitted a total of 234 patients while in the Baltic. Ninety-five were discharged cured, 57 were invalided and 31 had died; others were sent to home hospitals. Six major operations of surgery were performed aboard. Back at Somerset House Burnett pored over the costs of such provision. *Belleisle* had been equipped with medicines and stores to the value of £2,259 when she left England in May 1854.[16] The hospital had never been stretched to capacity but it had done its job well and been an asset to the fleet.

Keeping track of supplies to both the Baltic and Black Sea fleets and providing for the hospital ship were additional pressures on the Medical Department brought about by the war. Ensuring sufficient hospital space for casualties returning was another. At Haslar, plans for more furniture, water closets and stores were drawn up in February 1854. The washhouse also needed enlargement. Plans, however, were one thing, builders another. In November Richardson, as Inspector, while assuring the Admiralty that a number of wards were ready to receive invalids, had to admit that over-all progress had not been as rapid as anticipated. Haslar suffered from 'the slowness of the workmen who are paid by the day and are not insensi-ble to the comfort of under-employment under cover'.[17] Meanwhile East Stonehouse reported that, like Haslar, it was ready to take up to 50 army casualties if necessary. But beyond this capacity at the two largest home hospitals Burnett considered that two further establishments should be created. Firstly, the old facility at Deal with 200 beds was re-opened in March 1854. Its total accommodation expanded to almost 300 in August. Secondly, the building at Yarmouth, long used by the army to house lunatics, was restored to Admiralty authority and refitted as a hospital. Yarmouth was set aside for army casualties in November, by which time sufficient supplies had been shipped from Deptford to allow up to 350 cases in an emergency. At Somerset House the administrative burden for all these arrangements was borne largely on the shoulders of William King Fossett, since those senior had proved not up to the task.

While home hospital provision was necessary for the seriously sick and wounded, that could only be of value to those able to undertake the voyage to England. The front line in hospital provision clearly had to be closer to the fighting, which, in the case of the Black Sea theatre, meant Malta and the temporary naval hospital taking shape at Therapia. Being the main supply base for the Mediterranean fleet, the Malta hospital was overwhelmed with demands for medical necessities almost as soon as war was declared. On 6 May 1854 Stewart confessed that his dispensary arrangements had fallen apart. Seeing the urgency, Burnett appointed a dispensary assistant for the hospital to be paid five shillings per day plus rations. As for capacity at Malta, Stewart assured the Admiralty that, since the hospital was stocked to hold 300 patients, about 250 could readily be accommodated, although if more space were needed then storerooms, passages, corridors, the duty room and a building currently used by convalescents would have to be converted. That would provide room for about 450 cases. Beyond that, in an emergency, total capacity might be raised to 520 in the summer months by using four verandahs. With extra provisions, Malta could doubtless cope. Indeed by September 1854 the First Lord seemed sufficiently impressed to observe that 'measures have been taken to render the hospital establishment at Malta more effective'.[18]

Progress at Therapia, by contrast, appeared to be painfully slow. Although a large three-storey house close to the beach had been procured from the Turkish authorities and stores brought up from Malta, many improvements were necessary before patients could be admitted in the numbers anticipated. Burnett had reservations about the accounting system for supplies which Dundas had authorized: Burnett wanted the establishment victualled like a sick-mess aboard ship whereby the savings on men's normal rations were credited to cover the costs of sick-diets and medication, rather than have money change hands on the spot. This was an economical system. It was how *Minden* had operated at Hong Kong, it was how the temporary hospital at Lisbon was victualled and it was the procedure recently adopted with much success at Ascension Island. However, converting and fitting up the property, its stables, sheds and hay-loft were a more pressing concern, although, as Rees explained, this need not be costly if done by naval carpenters. In February 1854 surgeon John Davidson arrived to supervise the work required at Therapia. Neither Rees nor Dundas was pleased to see him.

'My coming out has not been acceptable to the authorities,' Davidson reported back to London. Rees proved 'very forward in offering me assistance', while the Commander-in-Chief dug in his heels and refused to consider any changes to the victualling procedures which he had stipulated in December 1853. Furthermore no one seemed to have mentioned how intolerable the hospital would become in winter. The old house was a wooden structure, full of windows, and although Rees had managed to get it into a state of modest repair it would require many stoves to keep it warm. There might be a problem with storage too, Davidson observed: 'the upper floor is so frail as to render it dangerous to put any considerable weight upon it'. As for staff, Dundas had left him with one assistant surgeon, which would obviously not be enough if capacity rose to 100 beds. He needed a dispensary man to compound medicines; that would at least leave his assistant free for medical duties. He also needed nurses: at present some volunteers from the fleet were ashore, but these were inadequate and when spoken to in anything other than complimentary terms immediately expressed a wish to return to their ships. These obstacles notwithstanding, Davidson managed to find himself another assistant, a clerk, a steward, a cook and a marine who acted as a washer. He had a marine corporal and three privates as guards and five nurses. It was a start. More men might become available as needs arose. As war was declared Davidson already had 45 patients under his care, most of whom had been victims of fever. Even at this early stage the strain was beginning to tell. Davidson warned Burnett in April 1854 that 'my mind is so <u>unhinged</u> that I find difficulty in discharging the hospital duties'.[19] Burnett was not interested. With Davidson now confirmed as surgeon in charge at Therapia, Burnett had no intention of bringing him home.

Little changed at Therapia in the course of the summer. In April Davidson asked for clear instructions about where he should draw future supplies; on that, Burnett ruled that only orders for equipment and stores unattainable at Malta should be forwarded to London. Yet even assuming that the hospital could get all that it needed, Davidson still had the problem of storage: not only had he insufficient space but the only rooms available were insecure and thefts could not be prevented. His own health improved in May although he was still anxious about the way in which the hospital was audited, which he knew to be inconsistent with the Admiralty's Foreign Hospital Instructions which Burnett required him to enforce. 'I have only charge of the medicines and medical necessaries,' he pointed out to Burnett. Under Dundas's arrangements, with which Rees had too readily acquiesced, it was uncertain who was responsible for other stores, patient lists were forwarded to the Commander-in-Chief and records of sickness were returned to the ships from which the men had come rather than to Somerset House. Davidson derived considerable comfort, however, watching the fleet leave the Bosphorus for Odessa, which meant 'less interference with hospital affairs' from either Rees or the admiral.[20] Rees did not return to Therapia until June 1854 when, now Deputy-Inspector, he took it upon himself to visit and report on the state of the hospital. It was a tense occasion.

Rees had no criticism of the hospital; on 10 June its 37 patients were being properly cared for in clean and well-ventilated conditions. But he was critical of Davidson for having done nothing about the accounting system other than to complain. Rees accepted that the arrangements which he had made with Dundas were not to Burnett's liking. The problem, however, was that the victualling system which Burnett wanted could only be administered via a ship's paymaster, who would account for patients as supernumerary sailors borne on the flagship. How could this operate when there was no ship permanently anchored close by? Davidson had known this weeks before; in fact, Rees had pointed out that Burnett's instructions were impracticable when Rees had handed over authority. 'I advised him to study the subject <u>at once</u> and submit to you his opinion,' Rees informed the Director-General. 'I regret much that he did not <u>then</u> follow my advice.'[21] But whether Davidson was at fault for either ignoring the issue or failing to keep Burnett fully informed mattered little: without a ship's paymaster in the vicinity the hospital had to continue to buy meat, bread and vegetables locally. Davidson tried to keep a record of expenditure as best he could. No wonder staff at Somerset House despaired.

When Deas took charge in the Mediterranean after August 1854 the burden of responsibility was largely lifted from Davidson's shoulders. Deas told him to buy what he needed until a reliable supply system from Malta was in place. Meanwhile at Malta Stewart had engaged six nurses at 2/1d per day plus rations to work at Therapia, although since none appeared able to write his name there was clearly some question of how useful they might be. Cholera brought Davidson a few more patients: he recorded 52 at the start of September. But he had now lost his clerk, which would prove to be an even greater problem if the navy went ahead with a plan to set up a store for the service afloat at the hospital. Stewart again obliged, sending someone from Malta. Davidson did not wish to seem ungrateful but regretted that the man's English was rather limited. Amid this ramshackle organization, a marine sergeant in the guard doubled up as hospital steward for an extra shilling per diem, while the privates chipped in as nurses, washers and cook, pending the arrival of staff recruited at Malta. Davidson knew that he was disliked among senior naval commanders for his constant complaining; indeed he suspected that some took delight in his frustration, so much so that in November 1854 he informed Burnett that he was on the point of resigning. This had to be prevented, Burnett pleaded at the Admiralty: surely some way could be found for naval commanders in the Bosphorus to make better provision for the hospital? He commended Davidson as a surgeon of the highest character who had shown great professional commitment since taking charge at Therapia. 'Were he to be driven out of the service of the hospital, I know not where to look for a competent successor, not already employed, which would be very disastrous for the service.'[22]

Confronted again with the hospital's difficulties, Dundas ordered Deas to conduct another inspection. On 25 November Deas thereby drew Dundas's attention to the continuing confusion with the accounting system and the language deficiency of the Maltese clerk, both of which meant that Davidson was spending too much time away from medical duties. Deas discovered that the clerk of *Viper* had volunteered to assist at the hospital and urged Dundas to give authorization. The building work was also behind schedule and, with winter approaching, patients were already suffering the damp. Worst of all, however, were the nurses. Those found by Stewart at Malta had proved to be useless: they did little more than eat their food and take their money and had all been dismissed. Men had again been drawn from the fleet, though given the quality of those sent for this work additional misery was thereby frequently inflicted on the sick and wounded. Therapia needed one nurse for every three patients. That meant 14 at least and then further reliable men to act as cooks and general labourers. And competent men, once found, should be allowed to remain. Finally Davidson should be given disciplinary authority over seamen assigned to hospital duties; this currently rested with the captain of the nearest man-of-war. With so much cheap alcohol obtainable in the vicinity, keeping order in the hospital was proving difficult, yet when no ship was close at hand Davidson had no recourse to punishment in cases of drunkenness, neglect or insubordination. Having Deas with the fleet was certainly making a difference. He had managed to speed up the building work and, much to everyone's delight at the hospital, had obtained a second house from the Turkish government to be used as accommodation for medical staff. The latter he achieved by fostering good relations with the British embassy at Constantinople.

Even so, there was a limit on how much time Deas could devote to the Therapia hospital. It could at least tend the sick and wounded, which was more than could be said for the steamers sent to collect casualties from the beaches after the battle of Alma. Filthy and overcrowded vessels with the barest medical assistance struggled to convey diseased and wounded soldiers from Balaclava to the military hospital in the Bosphorus at Scutari. The navy sent medical staff ashore to help army surgeons overwhelmed with work, yet men died as they waited, as they were brought aboard and in appalling conditions on the journey. Edward Pearce and Harrison Smith, both assistant surgeons from *Britannia*, suddenly found themselves in charge on one troop ship ferrying the wounded to Scutari. It was, they reported to Deas, an upsetting experience. No naval officers were aboard to prevent helpless men being robbed by others or to superintend the messing. They had no nurses or orderlies to empty bed pans; between decks about 200 men were laid out on hay or on bare wood with little prospect of worthwhile medical attention. Among the 52 who died aboard many had also contracted cholera.[23] William Reynolds was another assistant surgeon despatched for duty among wounded soldiers on the transports. Medical cover was hopelessly inadequate, he recounted. There was a string of amputations to perform; meanwhile 'from want of dressing and exposure on the field, maggots of a very large size formed in some of the wounds'. Deas's initial estimate of 1,400 dead and wounded was initially disparaged as extravagant. 'Alas, they were far under the truth,' he assured Burnett on 27 September.[24]

On 17 October 1854 a squadron comprising more than 50 allied warships, led by *Agamemnon*, made an unsuccessful attempt to reduce the Russian forts protecting Sebastopol. Almost all the attacking vessels were damaged, some badly so, while 44 British seamen were killed and 266 wounded. George Mackay described his cockpit on *Agamemnon* in the midst of the action. The ship was hit many times by Russian shore guns, in consequence of which the wounded were carried down or lowered in chairs while Mackay and his assistants worked at the table to amputate and dress horrific wounds caused in the main by exploding shells. Gunners stayed below to comfort their friends, which might have impaired the ship's fighting capacity, Mackay jested, but for the fact that the smoke of battle above was so thick that it was impossible to take aim at anything. Smoke from the guns, from the cockpit's lamps and from the candles used at the operating table made the use of chloroform impossible: only when the engagement had ended was it used for his last two cases.

James Donovan, surgeon of *Sanspareil*, worked in similar conditions. *Sanspareil* had 11 killed and 60 wounded at Sebastopol. Donovan had to perform limb amputations with only one inexperienced assistant aboard and had to watch a sailor die when forced to abandon a thigh operation because he had insufficient space among the broken bodies all around him and could scarcely see what he was doing for the suffocating smoke.[25] Naval casualties were also mounting among the brigades of sailors and marines which had been formed to support the army ashore at the siege of Sebastopol. Deas reported 15 killed and 85 wounded there up to 30 October. Davidson would have to do the best he could at Therapia, given the demands on Deas elsewhere. Deas believed that there was more scurvy at Therapia than anyone was prepared to admit; nevertheless the hospital's fundamental problem was that the Admiralty was not making sufficient provision for the force now employed in the Black Sea.

Uncertainties about supply were to be expected given the long line of communication from London to Malta, the Bosphorus and the navy's principal unloading station in the Black Sea – Balaclava. A flotilla of over 40 transport craft brought stores and equipment into the port at Constantinople where too often they were just abandoned. Medical provisions were sent to the wrong destinations or else simply disappeared. In May 1854 Captain Peter Christie, the chief agent of transports in the Black Sea, longed for changes to the way in which the movements of men, horses and supplies were handled at Constantinople and looked to Rear-Admiral Edward Boxer, who assumed control there, to make improvements. But as the military build-up continued, conditions deteriorated. On 10 June Christie confided that Boxer's arrival had only increased his workload because Boxer lacked method in much of what he did, while obliging Christie to keep him constantly informed of all that was happening. 'Most naval men know nothing of the difficulties of the transport service,' Christie protested at the end of September 1854.[26] Howard Banks, surgeon on *Terrible*, echoed that sentiment. The transports bore no medical staff and no one knew or seemed to care about their crews. Diarrhoea, fevers and dysentery were widespread among these vessels and cholera certainly existed too. That was hardly surprising, Banks concluded when called out from *Terrible* to tend some of the sick, since the holds were full of liquid draining from the horses' stalls.[27] On 19 December Boxer calculated that he had 145 transport craft under his orders. For the few medics on warships still held in the Bosphorus the transports were becoming a vexing duty.

When Deas arrived in August 1854 he was presented with transport problems straight away. 'Seldom a day passes in which complaints of medicine chests not having arrived at their destination to or from Malta are not made,' he informed Somerset House. It subsequently transpired that several chests had been discovered in the holds of transports. Jars and canisters regularly went missing after arriving at Constantinople, receipts were not collected and neither Deas nor anyone else had time properly to investigate what was going wrong. 'I could not have taken more trouble,' Deas assured Burnett, 'had they belonged to myself and been filled with gold.'[28] Even when barrels and casks did arrive, the quantities in which they had been packed and despatched made effective use well nigh impossible. There was no one available to divide their contents, shipped in bulk, into smaller amounts for distribution among the many vessels and shore locations. In the Black Sea everything suddenly became even worse on 14 November when a violent storm sank over 30 vessels, damaged a number of other transports with many of their stores and temporarily closed the harbour at Balaclava. As winter advanced the appalling conditions among soldiers in the trenches before Sebastopol were becoming obvious. Deas now feared for the sailors and marines, both those serving alongside the army and those still on their ships. He wanted the stores and supplies which John Churcher, acting as agent for the Therapia hospital, had brought out from England early in December 1854 to be shipped straight to Balaclava. But Deas could not persuade Boxer to act promptly. It was also hard to find beds and several medical comforts. It had become impossible to acquire more blankets to supplement the inadequate numbers initially issued. Surgical instruments were also in short supply: by the end of 1854 those of many surgeons had become worn out, spoilt by the weather, or, in the confusion of war, either lost or stolen. Although stocks of medicines would last a while longer, other stores were running low and the lack of fresh food was increasing the incidence of scurvy. Furthermore, with over 3,000 sailors and marines now serving in brigades, Deas found that much of his time was spent making arrangements ashore rather than being able to concentrate on the needs of the fleet.

It was clear by September 1854 that, since there would be no major engagement for the fleet in the Black Sea, guns, marines and sailors could safely be landed to fight alongside the army. More than 400 marines had initially gone ashore to cover the army's landing at Eupatoria; they fought off a Russian attack in October and defended the town until relieved by Turkish troops in December. A larger marine contingent of over 1,000 men, formed at the end of September, was sent to guard the heights above Balaclava. A separate naval brigade was likewise created and, with its ships' guns, howitzers and rockets, moved up to assist outside Sebastopol. By the time of the bombardment on 17 October the navy had on shore 1,786 officers and sailors, 1,530 officers and men of the Royal Marines and the 400 men still holding Eupatoria. Deas assigned a surgeon and two assistants to the naval brigade, choosing another surgeon and assistant to go with the marines. Not only were medical officers required to accompany these brigades, increasingly so as the size of the force ashore grew, but hospital arrangements were also needed for them at Balaclava, the supplies for which would not be available from men-of-war.

Well before the end of October the Medical Department recognized that with so many sailors and marines doing duty alongside the army, three extra surgeons and three more assistants should be sent out to the Crimea at once and a further one of each rank sent to help Davidson at Therapia. When with the brigades, medical officers should be issued with sets of field instruments and portable medical chests. They would also need bedding suitable for wounded men kept under canvas and bearers detached from warships to carry stores and equipment. Needless to say, these extra supplies required from home imposed a further strain on Somerset House. 'We are still all bustle here,' Burnett wrote wearily on 31 October, 'but I shall get off the medical stores today.'[29] By November 1854 most of the sailors and marines landed were at Sebastopol but the extra medical officers required were nowhere to be seen. Up to 1 November, 25 men had been killed in action with 61 sick and wounded moved to a makeshift hospital established aboard *Diamond* in the harbour at Balaclava. The naval brigade was camped in tents, each containing 14 men, about two miles east of Sebastopol. Initially this had been a good location but once storms made the ground waterlogged the brigade had to be moved to the south, a greater distance from their gun positions. By 20 November more than 65 sailors had been killed or wounded at the batteries. Sickness provided a further 781 cases, of which 223 were either on *Diamond* or returned to their

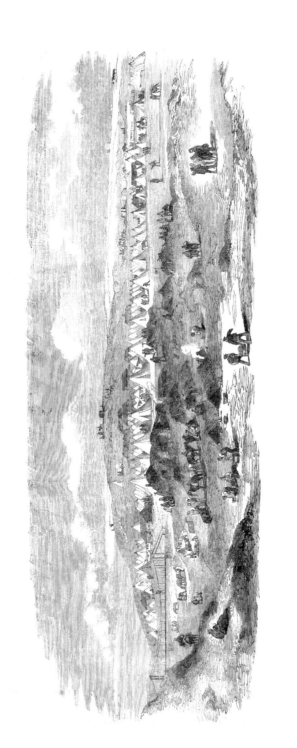

7. Naval brigade camp before Sebastopol.

own ships for treatment. Diet was now a major problem as fresh meat and vegetables were desperately short. The sick were also being kept too long in camp because the state of the roads made conveyance back to the ships impossible; this made diarrhoea and cholera in the camp more difficult to contain. The marine division, which fought at the battle of Inkerman on 5 November 1854 and was thereafter supplied by the army in forward positions at Sebastopol, was in an even worse condition than the naval brigade. 'My orders were not to supply the marines,' Deas later reflected. However, despite being forbidden to help them, his instructions were 'never to prevent either of the marine medical officers <u>stealing</u> what they required'. With over one-third of the marines sent up to the foremost trenches either dead, sick or in hospital, no wonder Deas despaired that 'I have today got an occupation which so far as I see is quite beyond me.'[30]

Facing a disintegration of naval medical provision in the Black Sea in January 1855, Burnett was obliged to report that he had no more medical officers for active service. He could immediately place 30 or 40 assistant surgeons, if available, and by the spring, with further warships likely to be in commission, the shortage would be closer to 100. Painful as it was to concede the point, Burnett informed the Board that emergency, albeit temporary admissions to the service would have to be made. This would have been easier to do a year earlier, he acknowledged, since many young men, otherwise lacking the statutory qualifications, 'have been swept up by the army department, the East India service, and by the mercantile steam vessels carrying surgeons'. The Royal Navy would therefore have to invite up to 40 medical students aged between 18 and 22 to join for six or seven months until the end of October 1855. These recruits would serve either in home waters or with the Baltic squadron thereby releasing qualified assistant surgeons for duty in the Black Sea. The students would need good testimonials and to have attended six-month lecture courses in anatomy, surgery, medical theory and practice, and either chemistry or *materia medica*. They should have six months' practical experience at a hospital, poor house or public dispensary and spent six months compounding medicines. If these criteria could be met then they would be interviewed in London for positions as dressers to help naval surgeons. Pay would be six shillings a day. Students chosen would be subordinate to assistant surgeons and would mess with midshipmen. Come October they would all be discharged to return to winter studies at their medical schools. How would all this be received in the universities, Burnett speculated? 'Professors and teachers in the country and in Scotland are inimical to the medical service of the navy,' he reminded the Board. Nevertheless by extending these generous terms of employment to students 'they might be probably disarmed and converted into friends'. It was a desperate scheme; indeed, Burnett confided, 'nothing but the most pressing necessity could have induced me to moot it'.[31]

Hard pressed as the navy was, Burnett would still consider no concessions towards older men who had either once been in the service or who offered themselves for home appointments. He was sure that his offer to medical students would give enough eager young men a chance to do their patriotic duty. When forwarding the statistics required for parliamentary questions in February 1855 he acknowledged that the navy was now short of 72 assistant surgeons. Twenty-eight full surgeons were performing the duties of assistants, which left 44 vacancies on ships and in hospitals unfilled. There were currently only three candidates for entry examination. By 21 May, however, Burnett was pleased to note that 73 student-dressers had been engaged. Such information was welcomed by members of the government increasingly criticized for their handling of the war and it offered some reassurance to an anxious public. It provided no immediate relief, though, for the sailors and marines still suffering in the Black Sea.

Michael Cowan, assistant surgeon on *Agamemnon*, saw some of these shortcomings when escorting sick and invalided men to Therapia in March 1855. Little, it seemed, had changed from the chaotic scenes witnessed aboard transports at the Alma six months earlier or throughout December and January when a total of 7,941 diseased and wounded soldiers had been embarked at Balaclava for military hospitals in the Bosphorus. 'I found that not a single thing was provided for the men; no medicines, no nothing,' he wrote home. He went to complain to the admiral's secretary and managed to get some supplies of medicine. Beyond that, though, '[I] had to battle it out the best way I could as to provisioning the men and getting utensils for their use'.[32] There was no executive officer to look after the men's papers or to sort out the constant confusion. The transport vessel was not fit for purpose and Cowan spent most of the voyage just trying to keep the patients comfortable.

Once at Therapia, however, Cowan could have felt less cause for criticism. When inspected by members of the British government's Sanitary Commission, sent out to investigate the health of the armed forces in the East, in March 1855 the hospital was judged to be satisfactory, despite the fact that the old buildings which housed it imposed severe constraints on

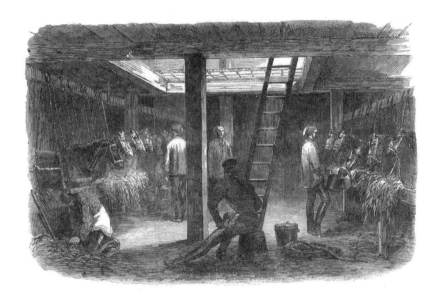

8. Horses on transports bound for Balaclava.

what could be done. It now had a permanent agent, William Penfold, who arrived in December 1854 and who took over after Churcher was moved to take charge of the naval depot at Balaclava, and a clerk, Edward Carter, who was appointed in February 1855. They took charge of the stores and accounts. Moreover, after the disastrous experiments with nursing staff recruited in Malta and the poor quality of the men detached from ships to replace them, a group of eight women under Eliza MacKenzie arrived from England in January 1855. Throughout December and January Davidson had been admitting men diseased, frost-bitten and malnourished from the siege of Sebastopol: on 20 January, 74 marines were brought in, giving him suddenly 160 patients to care for in the main house and aboard an old transport, *Cornwall*, sent by Boxer, which was moored offshore and served as accommodation for convalescents. Relations with Boxer had remained strained for much of the winter. *Cornwall* was 'an old leaky ship', Davidson moaned.[33] She was unfurnished and her master refused to cooperate. All the men whom Boxer had sent to her as nurses had been either useless or dishonest and when Davidson asked for a warship to be stationed nearby, on the grounds that it would be more use to him than doing nothing in the Black Sea, Boxer took great offence that a surgeon should offer an opinion on naval deployment and reprimanded him accordingly. Then Boxer took exception to a reference in one of Davidson's private letters to the manner in which some smallpox cases had been transferred to the hospital. This was an implicit criticism of a senior officer. Boxer therefore referred the matter to the new Commander-in-Chief, Mediterranean, Rear-Admiral Sir Edmund Lyons, who had replaced Dundas on 31 December 1854.

Davidson was also rebuked over stories of hospital indiscipline which had come to Boxer's attention. 'I think him unfit to have charge of the hospital in a military point of view,' Boxer advised the Admiralty.[34] It was a great relief for Davidson, therefore, when Boxer was moved from Constantinople to take charge of the shipping at Balaclava in January 1855. Boxer's transfer came after accounts reached London of delays in disembarking wounded men destined for the military hospital at Scutari and of the poor arrangements in place at Constantinople for unloading, storing and forwarding provisions. Boxer had 'caused much confusion and no system' at Constantinople, a member of the Board of Admiralty confided.[35] Davidson had the further satisfaction of being raised to Deputy-Inspector shortly after. At the start of February 1855 there were 159 sailors and marines at Therapia. This was down to 80 by 1 March. Men were still coming in with dysentery, bronchitis and pneumonia, Davidson observed, yet 'they are no longer the deplorable looking objects who were received in January'.[36] Those arriving from Balaclava now were generally better fed and better clothed. Supplies were clearly getting through to marines in the trenches before Sebastopol while sailors in the naval brigade had become adept at scrounging fresh meat and other delicacies around their camp site. The long Crimean winter was finally over.

Many of Davidson's patients, being from the naval brigade and marine division, were forwarded from *Diamond* at Balaclava. *Diamond*'s surgeon was William Smart. He had one assistant, Edward Pearce. By common consent, Smart was both an able medic and an excellent organizer. Deas nevertheless observed in December 1854 that *Diamond* was far from being a hospital ship. Deas had trouble getting sufficient beds and mattresses even for her, let alone for her overspill vessel, *Pride of the Ocean*; indeed his modest success was achieved only by cadging equipment from men-of-war and transports. *Diamond* was, in fact, the picket ship at Balaclava, moored in such a way that her remaining guns swept a valley and thereby forestalled any Russian assault on the British lines. As wounded, diseased, crippled or half-starved men could be brought down from forward positions during the winter, so Smart had the unenviable task of saving who he could. Fever, diarrhoea, dysentery and scurvy accounted for most of Smart's 47 cases at the end of 1854. But at least most supply problems ended at Balaclava when Churcher arrived, bringing with him a sufficient quantity of medical provisions. These, once unloaded, would last a while, Deas reflected; it depended, of course, for how long seamen were to be kept fighting ashore. The brigade had 1,250 sailors camped at their gun batteries with a further 440 kept aboard *Sanspareil* to move stores. This transport duty was proving to be as perilous as working the guns and, as far as Deas could tell, was reserved for sailors who had dared to complain about their lot. Roads were icy, explosives were dangerous and many men, often intoxicated on the journey back to *Sanspareil*, fell into deep mud and froze to death. By the end of January 1855 Smart had upwards of 120 seamen in his care.

Deas feared that the state of health among the marines was probably much worse than among the sailors. Unfortunately he could not discover the truth, he informed Burnett on 29 January, since the road between Balaclava and the marines' trenches had become impassable. Undeterred, Deas secured a mule and 30 men from the naval brigade and, laden with medical comforts, set off to find the marines. His party eventually got through with medicines, fortified wine 'as well as some oranges and lemons', he recalled with evident pride. Given the roads and with so many sailors physically weakened by the effects of cold and hunger, supplies had to be packed in weights not exceeding 30lbs, otherwise they were too heavy to be carried. With such pressing matters to hand on which the lives of many seamen depended, Deas was not impressed when rebuked that statistics concerning men ashore were not being forwarded to London quickly enough. 'I must say that it is frequently no easy matter to write in a tent,' he observed pointedly, 'and there are frequently difficulties in getting the letters conveyed after they are written.'[37] Burnett did not raise the issue again.

On top of their immediate difficulties at Balaclava, Deas and Smart also knew that it was an unhealthy location for any hospital or receiving vessel. As winter ended the port was being extensively developed to provide a long wharf frontage, a railway line and cranes to lift heavy equipment from the ships. All this was necessary because Balaclava was small and not easily accessible for the large number of craft coming in and out, which had contributed to the problem of supplying the army since landing in September 1854. Thousands of troops, horses, fodder and military stores were being unloaded in a crowded harbour usually containing up to 200 craft and a floating population of several thousand people. This produced a vast amount of rotting debris and decomposing cattle carcasses, despite Boxer's efforts to keep the water clean. The solution to this problem for the navy's medical facility at Balaclava was to construct huts and to transfer everything from *Diamond* on to dry land.[38]

Hut construction, however, advanced slowly. Even though the building materials were being landed in January, Christie observed that 'they get them away very slowly' on account of the shortage of horses and bad roads leading up from the port.[39] Still no huts were erected to take the sudden flow of casualties from the naval brigade in the second week of April 1855 when 16 men were killed and about 70 wounded. Deas, now promoted to Inspector, made a hurried visit to Balaclava but discovered that Smart had everything under control. The marines fared better. Their wounded were housed in huts already erected on a well-chosen site, to which Boxer wished to send all the sick sailors from *Diamond* until Deas managed to persuade him that the accommodation there would not be able to cope and that the naval brigade needed its own huts. Boxer resisted this suggestion until the end of April when finally building began nearby in Cossack Bay, which Deas assured the Admiralty was an excellent location. Huts made it much easier to separate the sick from the wounded. This became more urgent after cholera was diagnosed in the brigade camp and cases were being brought aboard *Diamond* which could not be isolated from the 35 sailors wounded at the batteries whom Smart admitted between 1 April and 1 May. Everything on *Diamond*, however, seemed to meet with widespread approval. Deas had reported favourably on all that Smart had done since October 1854, while Davidson wrote in glowing terms of the condition in which *Diamond*'s sick and wounded continued to arrive at Therapia. In May the huts for both the marine division and naval brigade were inspected by the Sanitary Commission. Deas reported their findings enthusiastically to London: 'we have put it quite out of their power to offer even one suggestion of an improvement'.[40]

❧

As improvements were acknowledged at Therapia and in the Black Sea during the spring and early summer of 1855, so preparations were under way for another naval campaign in the Baltic. The new Commander-in-Chief was Rear-Admiral Sir Richard Dundas, from whom a more adventurous strategy was expected. In anticipation, *Belleisle* spent the winter refitting at

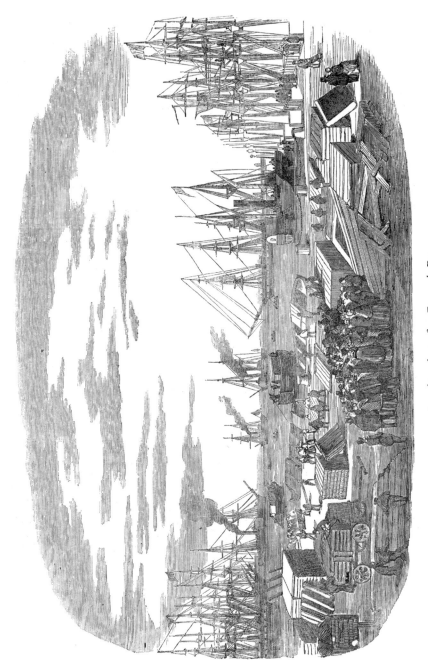

9. Loading huts for Cossack Bay.

Devonport in order to expand her hospital facility and to eliminate some of the shortcomings which had been identified in 1854. The noisy capstan, which had so distressed sick officers on the main deck, was relocated above, while the 'small, wretched dog-holes, called cabins' set aside for their use were converted into two good-sized officers' wards. The lower deck was also cleared of cabins and, opened up as a ward, could take an extra six beds. Hospital accommodation was thereby increased to a total of 167. Its staffing level was raised too. Robert Beith remained in charge, with the newly created rank of staff surgeon, with two other surgeons, James Martin and Samuel Wells. Thomas Breen and William Stephens were the two assistants, helped in their duties by five extra nurses and five student-dressers. By 1855 *Belleisle* was also equipped with a 'highly serviceable washing machine'. This had the great advantage, Beith later recalled, of enabling the hospital 'to dispense with the uncertain and capricious services of some troublesome washerwomen'.[41] But operational improvements could not be achieved solely by alterations aboard, Burnett advised the Admiralty early in February. *Belleisle* could not be in many places at once; she therefore needed a couple of small steamers attached as ambulances to carry patients from different vessels and locations and to ferry the sick and wounded back to Yarmouth as required. McKechnie, who was preparing to go out again as Inspector for the Baltic fleet, also had suggestions. In 1854 there had been insufficient nursing staff for nightwatch duties and he was not convinced that this issue had been adequately addressed. Nurses should be not only numerous enough but have the pay and rating of able seamen. He wanted better food for the hospital too, in light of the difficulty of obtaining soft bread during the previous summer. McKechnie therefore asked that a baker be engaged for the hospital, to hold the rating of second-class petty officer. Equipped even more lavishly than a year earlier, *Belleisle* returned to the Baltic in May 1855.

The Baltic fleet in 1855 contained above 18,000 men. Unlike 1854 its warships now comprised exclusively steam vessels. Yet as in 1854 sickness showed itself right at the start of the campaign. The flagship, *Duke of Wellington*, experienced an outbreak of smallpox before *Belleisle* arrived, which obliged her surgeon to cordon off one side of the middle deck for infected sailors and to make urgent enquiries among the whole crew regarding previous vaccination. Nor was this the only problem which came to light in May. Three sailors had died of exposure on *Colossus* in circumstances which, her surgeon asserted, revealed the navy's indifference

towards ordinary seamen. *Colossus* had been at Jamaica until December
1854 where, given generous shore leave, many of her crew had squandered
their money. Back in Plymouth in March 1855 the men had sold their clothing to cover further shore expenses. The surgeon, John Carruthers, watched
the crew re-embarking unequipped for the Baltic and urged the captain to
ask for extra clothing. Since the paymaster would not advance money to
profligate men who already owed much from credit extended in the past,
Carruthers settled for an assurance that enough frocks and coats would be
collected at Spithead before finally leaving England. *En route* for Kronstadt,
however, it became clear that neither clothing nor sufficient blankets had
been brought on board. There was some cloth on the ship, but since most
men were unable to sew this was of limited value and the suffering, mostly
from lung infections, continued until emergency provisions could be transferred from the flagship on arrival. Carruthers's concern for the crew was
not appreciated: he was advised not to write critically again unless such
letters had first been approved by his commanding officer.[42]

Smallpox soon became a more widespread worry. By mid-May it was
obvious that a temporary hospital would have to be set up where isolation
could be guaranteed. Nargen, at the entrance to the Gulf of Finland, was
rejected as being too close to the enemy coastline. This left Faro Island,
back towards the Swedish coast, as the most suitable location. There would
be no problem equipping such an establishment: 100 hospital beds and
other furniture were all in store at Deptford ready to go out whenever
needed. *Duke of Wellington* had 41 smallpox cases by mid-May. There had
been 46 others aboard *Arrogant*, 24 of which had already been landed on
Faro along with six attendants, one student-dresser and such medicines,
comforts and cooking utensils as the surgeon in charge, John Gallagher,
had requested. A few cases of measles were likewise moved to Faro. Once
his smallpox cases had been put ashore, the surgeon on *Duke of Wellington*
set about cleansing the vessel with disinfectant, scrubbing everything in the
sick-bay and persuading the captain to allow a whole day for the crew to
wash and air their clothing and bedding. *Belleisle* arrived at Faro on 24 May
in the midst of this activity and McKechnie went ashore immediately to
inspect the arrangements. He found 61 men under Gallagher's care in two
wooden buildings which had been quickly converted for naval use. There
was no means of heating, yet McKechnie reported that all the patients felt
comfortable and appreciated the care bestowed.

With *Belleisle* operational, stores and provisions for Faro were placed under the control of the hospital ship and Gallagher returned to *Arrogant* on 2 June. McKechnie sent Breen ashore from *Belleisle* to take charge, with three nurses, two seamen as cooks, a corporal and four marines. Gallagher had kept all the accounts prior to his departure, assuring the Medical Department that he had exercised due economy in victualling men at 1/10d per day for a total cost of £146. His medical chests were made over to Breen for use ashore or for transfer to *Belleisle*. But the disease had not been stamped out on *Duke of Wellington*, which reported eight further cases on 4 June. Five men had died on Faro by this time and although many had recovered and returned to their ships it was impossible yet to close the establishment. Indeed *Belleisle* still had sailors digging a well there two weeks later. The last six patients were discharged cured only on 4 July. For any future emergency, a lease was taken for the nearby small island of Bungaör where huts and a cookhouse were erected. However, no staff were detached for service on Bungaör and the stores landed were eventually collected by *Belleisle* in October 1855 prior to her return to Plymouth.

With limited action in the Baltic, McKechnie's duties were minimal compared to the worries faced by Deas in the Mediterranean. *Belleisle*, indeed, had been sent to the wrong place: that, at least, was the opinion of surgeon John Sabben when helping aboard transports between Balaclava and the Bosphorus in January 1855. Men lay helpless and dying on bare decks exposed to the cold, Sabben reported in horror: 'Again I beg to suggest,' he implored Burnett, 'had there been such accommodation as a vessel similar to the *Belleisle* could have afforded, these men would have been transferred to Scutari hospital in 30 hours instead of 14 days.'[43] As it was, *Belleisle* had admitted only 12 patients from the Baltic fleet by 6 June and in conditions which would have been regarded as luxurious in the Crimea. Daily supplies of milk, eggs, bread and poultry came aboard and any other articles of diet required, including fresh beef, were readily obtainable. By 30 June the hospital ship had still treated only 34 men in total: 'a fact which either speaks well for the sanitary condition of the fleet,' Beith contemplated, 'or ill for the arrangements which have been made for the transmission of the sick'.[44] It was, in fact, the former. At Faro, throughout most of June and July 1855, the medical staff, nurses and student-dressers had little to do. Even the engagement at the Sveaborg forts, where the Russian arsenal and magazines were destroyed on 9 and 10 August, resulted in only four casualties – all the result of accidents.[45] On 15 August Beith reported 66 seamen registered in the hospital, though many, rather than undergoing treatment, were invalids waiting to be taken home.

Apart from accompanying men-of-war to Sveaborg after 6 August the greatest excitement aboard *Belleisle* was when sent to collect 101 invalids stranded on the Gottland coast where the transport *Cottingham, en route* for England, ran aground on 7 August. The incident was embarrassing for the navy but brought great credit to the medical service when the role played by the accompanying surgeon, Robert Wallace, became clear. Confronted with many men fearful of going down with the ship yet too weak to save themselves, Wallace had both the knowledge and presence of mind to explain that, being built in compartments and the rear ones being undamaged, the vessel could not sink, however low in the water. He had the patients moved to a safe deck while constantly reassuring them that with the sea calm and the night so clear there was no immediate danger. Wallace appeared almost to take command of the stricken ship. 'I gave orders then to have the boats lowered and kept alongside,' he later reported to Somerset House. 'At about 7am I had all the people landed.' [46] Having one of the student-dressers with him, Wallace gave instructions about care for men while transported in the boats and then joined the last boat off *Cottingham* in heroic fashion. Everything he had planned was efficiently performed and without any injuries. On landing, he observed the men cooking from the supplies of rice, barley, sago, tea, sugar, wine and preserved potatoes which he had asked the captain to put ashore, along with a galley cooker and a stock of coals. Once landed, he found carts to move men who could not walk and he organized a building large enough to provide shelter. Tins, plates and hammocks were also removed from *Cottingham. Belleisle* picked up all the men on 17 August where they remained until sent on to England ten days later.

Belleisle left Faro Sound on 17 October 1855. Having accommodated 60 patients for most of August and September she was loaded with other sick and 11 invalids before sailing home. On arrival at Deal, 79 of her 94 patients were sent to the hospital. McKechnie, however, went on to Portsmouth where he compiled his report. Between 1 April and 17 October 1855, he calculated, there had been only 109 deaths among the 22,000 men whom he estimated had served in the Baltic. Thirty-three of those were from falls, drownings or in action; 76 were due to disease. This compared favourably with a corresponding total of 339 fatalities in 1854, 107 of whom had died in the outbreak of cholera. Cholera claimed only two lives in the Baltic in 1855. Smallpox had been more of a problem in 1855 but generally the ships had been healthy and their crews well fed with ample meat and vegetables.

Along with smallpox, fevers and pulmonary disease accounted for most deaths. *Belleisle* had never been full. Her hospital had admitted 217 patients between 24 May and 17 October 1855; of these, 87 were discharged cured, 22 were invalided, nine had died, 18 were sent to England in another vessel and the rest sailed home aboard. While in the Baltic during 1854 *Belleisle* had received 172 patients, with 72 discharged cured, 22 deaths, 68 taken home and others sent away. *Belleisle* made a final, uneventful voyage before the end of the war, returning with 108 patients from the Baltic on 30 April 1856. She was decommissioned a week later.

Not only had the navy made ample medical provision for the Baltic theatre: it also made more than adequate arrangements for receiving the sick and wounded in hospitals at home. Arrangements in 1854 had included accommodation for the army: 100 soldiers were to go to East Stonehouse, 100 to Haslar, 150 to Deal and 300 to Yarmouth. 'It appears, however, that not a man has been sent to Haslar, Plymouth or Deal where three or four hundred beds have been provided for,' Burnett pointed out in February 1855.[47] Not only that, the army had possession of what was until 1814 the old naval hospital at Gibraltar which could house more than 300 patients. Deplorable as conditions at Scutari and at other military hospitals in the Bosphorus were, the army, overall, did not lack hospital accommodation and the navy certainly had not been reluctant to help. The Medical Department was informed that it was unlikely that the army would need so many beds reserved at Yarmouth beyond May 1855; reserving 200 for soldiers would now be quite sufficient. Yarmouth, in fact, remained available for use by both services throughout the war. After Burnett's retirement Liddell managed to repel a request from the mayor of Yarmouth to use the building as a barracks for the East Norfolk militia, which he did by reminding the Admiralty how much it had invested there. Letting healthy men use it as a barracks would degrade the facility and soon make it unfit to serve as a hospital for either soldiers or sailors. 'All our medical preparations during the war have been conducted on these principles of not meeting existing emergencies but making the necessary deliberate preparation for them prior to their occurrence,' Liddell reminded the Board with an air of self-congratulation.[48] That was not how things had appeared a year earlier. Yarmouth, though, was an example of prudent planning. It was finally closed as a temporary naval hospital in September 1856.

Deal was also maintained until the war ended, closing in October 1856. When sick from the Baltic were sent there late in 1855 Liddell decided that he had better conduct an inspection. *Belleisle* had landed 96 cases at Deal, mostly with chronic conditions, he subsequently reported. The establishment was a credit to its Deputy-Inspector, James Wingate-Johnston, who ran it in a clean and well-ordered fashion. It benefited from reliable nursing staff: the same five women who had been engaged when the hospital opened in February 1854 were still there. Provisions at Deal were particularly noteworthy. The food was well cooked, with the diet 'adapted to the taste of the most fastidious patients'. Liddell was impressed with the dispensary and with the range of comforts available. Indeed the visit was a great success until he strayed beyond the areas which Wingate-Johnston had wished him to see. Other parts of the building, long disused, were decayed by leaking water pipes. The boiler was so corroded that it flooded its surroundings and could not heat water quickly enough when baths were required. The lighting was dim and gas fittings were needed. More defects might have been discovered, Liddell speculated, but for 'a smokey chimney that drove me out of the place'.[49]

John Drummond, Deputy-Inspector at Chatham, was more fortunate when he received an unscheduled inspection on 19 June 1855. Returning from a well-publicized visit to the army hospital at Brompton, Queen Victoria, glancing from her carriage, noticed invalids at the gate of the Melville and decided to go in. Drummond had taken some precautions, just in case. Each man from the Crimea had his name, ship, cause and place of invaliding by his bed in order that they might be asked about their recovery and experiences. The royal party moved through the kitchens, operating theatre and three of the wards, of one of which, Prince Albert was unmistakably told: 'now this is just the thing as it ought to be'. Fever cases and wards with infectious diseases were avoided, but in other particulars Drummond was asked occasionally uncomfortable questions about numbers per ward, nursing requirements, gas and water supplies, washing facilities and how the hospital was managed. No prior preparations had taken place, Drummond begged to explain: the Queen saw how patients were always treated. The occasion was a spectacular triumph, Drummond hastened to assure the Lords of the Admiralty. More gratifying still, 'it appeared evident from the remarks of everyone that this establishment contrasted most favourably with those of the army department'.[50]

Both the Melville and the Marine Infirmary at Woolwich were, in fact, full with patients from the Baltic and Black Sea by June 1855 and Liddell thereafter advised that any further consignments of men for hospital care should be sent to Yarmouth. East Stonehouse also had many more admissions than usual even though the army was slow to take up the accommodation allocated there. By 21 February 1855 there were 356 patients on its victualling list and arrangements were being made to receive a further 50 or more cases. The level of stores held at East Stonehouse was thus raised from that sufficient for 400 men to that required for 800. The hospital was also short of medical staff – a problem temporarily solved when Thomas Breen was removed from *Belleisle* during her winter refit at Devonport. Haslar was also requesting additional medical officers as the numbers of sick and wounded coming off ships at Portsmouth increased steadily throughout February and March 1855. Haslar had 391 patients on 24 February; by 31 March the number was 608.

To make matters worse, Haslar faced another epidemic in the spring and early summer of 1855 when, as in 1853 and 1854, scarlatina broke out among the fleet at Portsmouth. *Excellent*, which acted as the training vessel for recruits, was the warship most affected: her surgeon, James Salmon, found it impossible to contain the disease without redistributing both newly raised men and her own crew in port. From Haslar, Richardson warned Burnett that a sudden influx of scarlatina cases would jeopardize his preparations for accepting war casualties: he had 30 patients in isolation on 7 March and had no alternative but to open two more wards, with a combined capacity of 110 beds, to take the increased numbers anticipated. This, he reflected, was on top of the two wards already filled with 24 smallpox patients and another ward for measles. Two days later Haslar had 60 scarlatina victims and there was no assurance that transfers from *Excellent* had ceased. Salmon had cleared *Excellent* of its marine cadets and about 200 boys, all of whom were hurriedly given leave. With only 400 men aboard at least the problem of transmission caused by crowding was diminished.

But in April the disease came back and referrals to Haslar resumed. Syphilitics were also requiring treatment in greater numbers than usual: 151 were in Haslar's surgical department by late March. This made it difficult to assess how many men returning from the Crimea could be taken. As things stood, 354 of the 581 beds in the Inspector's division at Haslar were occupied, as were 237 of the 352 in the Deputy-Inspector's surgical wards. The hospital did not have a staff allocation to cope with these numbers, Burnett reported to the Board. Not only were its three surgeons currently doing the work of assistant surgeons, since there were only four of the latter, but more senior staff were required for the most serious cases. One additional

Inspector and a further Deputy-Inspector should therefore be appointed at once. Men referred to Haslar from other institutions or from ships where even competent surgeons could not cope merited 'the undivided skill and attention of our most talented practitioners'.[51] He had every confidence in the rising generation within the service; there was, nevertheless, no substitute for experience.

By May 1855 Salmon was desperate to bring the epidemic on *Excellent* under control. Men and boys ready for service with other ships had already been transferred to the hulk *Melville* in order to reduce the number remaining aboard; on *Melville* they were inspected twice daily by a medical officer. No sailors were to be moved from either *Excellent* or *Melville* to any other warships until 14 days had elapsed since the last scarlatina case was confirmed. But fresh cases continued to appear on both vessels; 51 scarlatina sufferers were in Haslar by 9 May. Nine more had to be sent during the next couple of days, at which point Salmon had to admit defeat and advised the captain to abandon ship. Worse still, almost half the men coming back from Haslar relapsed soon after. *Excellent* needed to be purified and a separate hulk provided for convalescents. But no second hulk was forthcoming at Portsmouth. Salmon then went over to Haslar and had an equally disappointing meeting with the hospital's Deputy-Inspector, Peter Leonard, who refused to readmit all the men who had previously had the disease or to hold all future cases sent to him until such time as Salmon believed the danger aboard the ships at anchor had passed. It was a hospital's job to cure and then discharge patients, Leonard pointed out abruptly. Haslar had already set aside a much needed ward for convalescent scarlatina cases. What more could the hospital be expected to do?

With *Excellent* evacuated for thorough cleaning, 220 of the regular ship's company were put on to another nearby vessel, *Camperdown*, while all her 210 new recruits and boys were kept aboard *Melville*. But still one or two scarlatina cases were going ashore to Haslar every day. Then the disease died down and sailors moved back from *Camperdown* to *Excellent* on 6 June. But within a week it reappeared and the trickle of patients sent to the hospital resumed. Within days it had become a flood, with 13 admitted at Haslar on 13 June, 36 on the following day and 26 more on the day after. At this point Salmon concluded that the problem was not exclusively medical: men who knew that they were infected had not been coming forward and were thereby mixing with healthy messmates for far too long. He went onto *Excellent* and *Camperdown* twice daily in order to inspect everyone personally, he assured Liddell, and was becoming expert in picking out premonitory symptoms: 'the tone of voice – a huskiness or hoarseness, often indicates the disease when the patients are desirous of concealing its existence', he advised.[52] The staff at Haslar would certainly have been grateful for Salmon's belated insight. By 15 June 1855 he had sent 179 scarlatina cases to the hospital since the epidemic started.

Whether Salmon had identified the real reason for the persistence of the epidemic or whether the disease had simply run its course by July 1855 was impossible to determine. Inspecting *Camperdown* below decks in mid-June, however, might have given pause for thought. Admittedly the vessel was better than any hulk he had ever been on: it was well ventilated and, after copious application of disinfectant, it smelt clean enough. 'I must say the ship is however infested with rats,' he confided.[53] That being so, it was difficult to know just how much difference cleaning out the holds, moving the stores and whitewashing and painting the decks would make in the long run. Salmon kept a strict eye on the movement of sailors. No one returning from leave was to be allowed any contact with the company of *Excellent* until Salmon had conducted a personal examination and, once aboard, no one should be allowed off any of the holding vessels until 14 days after the last diagnosis. Haslar had now agreed to hold scarlatina patients for as long as the pressure on its accommodation would allow. With the men and boys from *Excellent* dispersed and with measures in place to seek out the disease before it could spread, Salmon felt confident that he had at last stamped it out. Not until early July, though, had there been no fresh case for more than a fortnight, at which point Salmon decided that *Excellent*'s seamen could be released from the hospital and from his other quarantine restrictions. It was fortunate that neither the navy nor the army in 1855 had made a greater call on Haslar's resources.

As in 1854 it was not only medical staff whose stamina was tested by the war. At Haslar an increased administrative burden fell on John Russell's shoulders, who, not unnaturally, asked for a review of his agent's salary of £400 per annum. Burnett advised the Board in April 1855 that this was justified: Russell was as correct and zealous as any government employee and there was no doubting his value to the hospital. This problem of overburdened administrative staff continued within Somerset House where Liddell soon realized that the department was unable to keep pace with the volume of work generated in the past two years. He needed two extra clerks, in the same way that the other civil departments of the navy had been granted additional staff since the war began. The evidence produced to justify this request was certainly impressive. In the past year, he wrote in July 1855, the number of letters received, recorded and requiring reply had risen by 2,247. In 1852–53 the department had to meet 711 demands for medicines and stores: in 1854–55 corresponding demands totalled 1,040. Comparing the same periods, the number of medical appointments had risen from 269 to 373. The size of the navy was also much greater: there had been 160 ships in commission in 1852 whereas there were 260 in 1855. On top of all that, the creation of temporary hospitals at Therapia, Yarmouth, Deal and the holding centres for Russian prisoners of war at Lewes and Millbay had required an enormous amount of administration. So too had all the arrangements necessary for fitting, equipping and staffing *Belleisle*. Perhaps the impact of war on the Medical Department had been more gradually felt than in other branches of naval service, Liddell added tactfully, and it had therefore been possible to defer decisions about its size. By the summer of 1855, however, the pressures were obvious and the department was falling into arrears with much of its routine work.[54]

While processing data reaching London was admittedly a growing problem, gathering it and then finding time to write up what was demanded was a more immediate concern for those serving in the Black Sea. Deas commonly excused incomplete reports on the grounds that the day was simply not long enough. On 14 February 1855 he informed Burnett that he kept no copies of letters sent to London to which he could subsequently refer. He was always on the move from Balaclava to Therapia, to the flagship in the Bosphorus and among the ships off Sebastopol, and, since it was impossible to take a clerk with him, transcribing correspondence was out of the question. His health was also suffering under the strain, which left him only the option of never writing or, as time allowed, sending the Director-General his 'crude but honest professional opinions as they are formed'. The Commander-in-Chief, he understood, had complained that duplicates of Deas's despatches were not forwarded to him, which, if construed as an indication that the Inspector was no longer fit to perform his duties, would allow Burnett to ask the Admiralty to supersede him. Alarmed at the prospect, Burnett discreetly directed that Deas's letter was 'to be returned'.[55] The hospital at Malta was also coming under pressure by the early months of 1855 as more cases were being landed either from the fleet or sent by Davidson from Therapia.

Malta had 201 patients on 7 March, having at one time been down to its last nine beds. The hospital had ample supplies of medicines and comforts: the problem was, and would remain, finding nurses to care for men shattered by exposure and malnutrition. By 7 May the patient list was down to 98, a level at which it broadly remained until Stewart's departure on 17 August. Stewart was replaced as Deputy-Inspector by James Salmon, newly promoted after his struggle with the scarlatina epidemic at Portsmouth. Salmon found the staff at Malta eager and well ordered; there was no suggestion, therefore, that the hospital could not handle an increased load. On arrival, however, Salmon felt that Malta had acquired a bad reputation. Too many seamen believed that Malta was merely a collecting point for invalids and that referral there meant their war was over and that a trip home to England was guaranteed. As far as Salmon was concerned, cure and discharge to regular duties was the order of the day; patients otherwise became depressed, often believing that they were in a worse condition than was really so, which frustrated efforts to cure them. But who could blame an ordinary sailor or marine for wanting home if this attitude was to be found even among medical officers? In December 1855 Salmon was obliged to report on Seth Sam, assistant surgeon from *Harpy*, whom Davidson had sent as a patient from Therapia. 'His case was his own production,' Salmon concluded. 'During the period of his remaining under my care I never could satisfy myself he laboured under any disease.'[56] On being discharged from hospital by order of the Commander-in-Chief, Sam resigned from the naval service.

With the army's siege of Sebastopol the focus for the war, the navy's contribution, other than a bombardment prior to the capture of most of the city on 9 September 1855, was largely confined to the marines and naval brigade ashore, to a raid on Kertch on 24 May, to operations in the Sea of Azov during the summer of 1855 and the destruction of Russian forts and batteries at Kinburn between 15 and 17 October.[57] While these actions all posed their own problems of supplying the ships and treating the wounded, Deas was also confronted with a continuing shortage of assistant surgeons and in June 1855 by a serious outbreak of cholera, especially among the transport vessels, at Balaclava. Towards the end of March 1855 Boxer had estimated 135 vessels of all descriptions jostling for space in its overcrowded harbour. By mid-May cholera had appeared and Deas worried that if it spread there would not be adequate medical cover. 'Perhaps the brigades are sufficiently supplied,' he reflected, 'but they are so to a great extent at the expense of the ships.' During bombardments the surgeons of many warships were already greatly overworked. They could probably cope, he concluded; 'But what is to become of the <u>thousands</u> of men who have no medical attendance in the transports and merchant ships?' Even in normal times conditions aboard these craft were bad and when cholera had struck in 1854 their crews undoubtedly suffered far worse than those aboard men-of-war. Furthermore when a medic was sent to tend to disease on a transport it could only be at the expense of sailors or marines elsewhere. 'I again and again saw our own men partially neglected, and our medical officers completely knocked up from the incessant calls made by the transports for relief,' Deas reminded Liddell. If cholera really took hold in the harbour 'I know not where to put my hand upon either surgeon or assistant.'[58]

Liddell agreed to send three further medical officers out to Balaclava. Unfortunately it was too late. By the start of June cholera was diagnosed at the naval brigade camp and was evident among the transports. On 1 June Boxer's nephew, who acted as his clerk, died of the disease at Balaclava. On 5 June the admiral himself succumbed, despite having both Deas and Smart in attendance. Rear-Admiral Charles Fremantle was now appointed superintendent at Balaclava, at which point it became clear that Boxer had not been a great deal more successful trying to instil order there than he had been previously at Constantinople. It was not Boxer's fault that the harbour was so small, yet it seemed to Fremantle that not much had been done to provide adequate storage houses in anticipation of another winter in the Crimea. By the summer of 1855, 90,000 men and 20,000 horses were being supplied through Balaclava. Congestion and logistics aside, there were also disciplinary difficulties with many of the merchant seamen over whom, officially, the Royal Navy had little control. This did not stop Fremantle from trying to end quarrels between merchantmen and having troublemakers among their crews thrown in irons, put on diets of bread and water and flogged if necessary.[59] Amid all this, surgeon Thomas Costello did what he could as the cholera spread.

Costello had been assigned to the transports and merchant craft at Balaclava; in effect, he acted as the harbour's sanitary officer. Without any assistant he moved among the vessels, advising on hygiene, treating the sick and compounding medicines. This he did between October 1854 and August 1856, treating on average 100 patients a day – a task made more arduous by many craft being moored at a distance from the harbour and their crews, being of many nationalities, often unable to communicate in English. Many of the crews were malnourished, drank excessively and, given the damp and dirty accommodation aboard their vessels, were prone to infection. When cholera arrived they had no defence and as Costello knew from his experience in 1854 there were no cures, only sanitary precautions. At the peak of the epidemic he was tending 35 cases simultaneously aboard different transports and private vessels. The harbour still contained floating debris and dead animals while powerful odours emanated from several points on the beach and quays. Deas continued to report cholera on British warships well into July 1855 and sporadic cases among transport vessels entering the Bosphorus as late as December. It ebbed and then returned without warning, Deas observed wearily, having just lost one of his oldest friends in the service to the disease. For Costello, the worst was over before then. By the time he left Balaclava, exhausted, in August 1856 he had attended 2,329 patients for all ailments in the harbour during the previous 20 months. Half of them had been suffering from fevers or bowel complaints of one sort or another.[60]

Bad though conditions were in the port at Balaclava during the summer of 1855, the naval brigade ashore was already benefiting from the huts in Cossack Bay. These and others for the marine division were mostly completed by May. Up to 180 sick seamen could now be tended ashore rather than on *Diamond* and its auxiliary vessel. By late April casualties could be brought down from the marine camp by railway. As for the sailors, their camp was moved to higher ground in May after cholera claimed the lives of a handful of men. The naval brigade, however, made comparatively little demand on its medical officers until 6 June when its batteries recommenced their bombardment of Sebastopol. Within a week it had 90 wounded, with as many again in the week which followed. It was a heavy list, Deas observed, although sailors who could be moved were soon made comfortable in Cossack Bay. Smart took 40 wounded into the huts in June 1855. They were all 'in admirable condition', Deas discovered when he visited on 2 July.[61] Those kept at the brigade camp were also doing well. By the end of July only 39 of the naval brigade's 1,295 men were on the sick-list, 16 still registered as wounded.[62] The marine hospital establishment, with capacity for 80 patients, was rather fuller; in the trenches before Sebastopol, Deas concluded, the marines were more prone to fevers and bowel disorders brought on by fatiguing duties. Back in the Bosphorus Davidson was finding his duties a good deal less stressful than they had been six months earlier. Having been given use of a second house and an extensive garden for convalescents, many of the problems caused by overcrowding at Therapia were eased by April 1855. The hospital could now accommodate 380 men. Given its size, in July Liddell persuaded the Board to place Therapia on the same footing regarding its staffing and victualling arrangements as the navy's permanent overseas hospitals.

Until his retirement Burnett worried about the costs incurred at Therapia. They were high, Davidson conceded in May 1855, particularly costs charged as servants' wages. But that was because of the accounting system whereby large working parties of sailors sent ashore to equip the buildings had to be victualled through the hospital, there being no other category for them. Supply problems also continued to push up the hospital's expenses. Stores long on order from England failed to arrive regularly, which meant that provisions and extras needed for his worst cases had to be acquired in Constantinople where prices and labour rates were high. Then there was the additional burden imposed on the hospital by admitting sick from the transport service. Having seen the state of the transport and merchant vessels at Balaclava for himself, Deas had authorized sending the worst fever cases down to the Bosphorus. Burnett could not disapprove the Inspector's compassion, though in reporting this departure from the rules to the Board he stressed that Therapia had only been created to receive sick and wounded from the fleet. If fever was introduced into the hospital by patients from the transports this might jeopardize the lives of seamen already there. It was a legitimate concern, although given Davidson's current list it could scarcely be argued that the hospital was unable to cope. Therapia had 60 patients on 1 June; only 43 had been brought in during the whole of May. The health of the fleet was generally good, Davidson observed. Furthermore there had been a significant improvement regarding nursing since Eliza Mackenzie had arrived. When two of her nurses had to return home due to ill health in May 1855 Davidson realized just how much his hospital had come to depend on them. He urged Liddell to find replacements immediately.[63]

Davidson's only real concern by the summer of 1855 was how best to prepare his establishment for another winter. For one thing, the ramshackle heating arrangements from 1854 had to be improved. Until now, ships' stoves installed in the building, and long tubes running from them, had been the only means of warming the hospital. The stoves could only burn wood, which was often so wet when brought in that water ran across the floors. These stoves also gave off so much dirt that it was impossible to keep the wards clean. The most costly remedy would be to install proper pipes to circulate hot water and hot air. For half the cost, however, four chimney stacks could be erected and hearths for open fires put in wherever needed. Eleven grates and a kitchen range designed to improve the cooking were duly ordered from Deptford although as late as mid-August those were still awaiting shipment. This need not have been a serious delay: with the cold weather still several weeks away there was ample time. A month later, however, Davidson no longer felt so optimistic.

In the course of August the hospital had started to fill again. It admitted 137 cases, mostly of dysentery, diarrhoea, fevers and rheumatism during the month. By 1 October Davidson had a list of 108. Much of this new influx came from the marines outside Sebastopol. Many of them had been in the Crimea for ten months, Davidson discovered, and their constitutions were broken down by chronic infections. Yet he had the means to cope with that. By far his most persistent problem was the builders engaged to erect new chimneys. The initial contractor had offered to put up the stacks required for about £400 but had since disappeared claiming pressure of other work. His replacement quoted £830 for the job but could not complete until the middle of November. Davidson had been compelled to approve the latter, thus adding to overall costs. Moreover, since the stacks would need to be built in pairs in order to meet the deadline there would be far greater inconvenience to the hospital than he had anticipated.

When Deas visited again in mid-October 1855 he witnessed the disruption and the inevitable reduction in accommodation. Yet this would only be temporary: the benefits from fires and cleaner air would soon make such inconvenience worthwhile. Already, Deas observed, the plumbing was much better, with cisterns and proper water closets fitted inside the building in addition to facilities outside. Not only did Davidson at last have the prospect of accommodation fit for purpose: along with the two surgeons and two assistants on the establishment he was now able to concentrate on medical duties free from the burden of hospital management. Penfold, as agent, with the support of a clerk and a steward, with his assistant, took care of the administration. They had between them four labourers who served as boatmen, gravediggers, manglers in the laundry or in other work as required. In addition to its medical staff, Therapia had 16 competent male nurses who worked alongside MacKenzie and her two lady and six paid nurses. Four seamen were detailed to do the cooking, the food provided was good and the laundry was well organized with a drying house available. Therapia was a credit to the navy, Deas concluded, and could withstand whatever the winter might bring.[64] In fact, it brought very little. The fall of Sebastopol just three weeks earlier had meant the end of any large-scale hostilities. The hospital's list was merely 38 by 1 February. By then there were already fewer warships in the Black Sea; indeed by early 1856 it was hard to see where more admissions would come from.

Pressures on the Therapia hospital had been decreasing since the early summer of 1855 in proportion to Smart's success creating his own estab-lishment at Cossack Bay. Both the naval brigade and the marine division were inspected by Deas on 18 August, who judged that the men, casual-ties from the fighting aside, were in reasonable shape. The former had 41 men sick while the latter returned 177. Unfortunately several of the medi-cal staff ashore were among those unfit for duty, which meant that Smart's experienced assistant had to be released from Cossack Bay to work at the front during the final assault on Sebastopol. The marines, however, were approaching the end of their tether, Deas wrote to London: the men 'looked worn and shattered, like used up, to use a vulgar, but expressive phrase'.[65] The young of the division were faltering under the hardships of work and exposure while the older men were increasingly succumbing to disease. All of Sebastopol was in allied hands by 11 September 1855, follow-ing which it was naturally assumed that the naval and marine brigades would be disbanded. Deas was at once beseeched by the medical officers attached to try to find out what was to become of them. But if the prospect of an immediate journey home lay behind their enquiries then several were destined to be disappointed: most were ordered either back to their ships or to remain with Smart at Cossack Bay. The greatest prize had been captured but the war was not over.

Prior to the order to break up the naval brigade camp on 15 September there were 47 sailors ashore listed as wounded and a further 33 undergoing treatments for disease. Those unable to return to their ships were sent to the huts at Cossack Bay. The marine brigade, meanwhile, had a sick-list of 145. Yet the marine camp was greatly improved from the dreadful condi-tions in which the men had been living six months earlier. The army had improved its supply system and, since the marines were treated as soldiers, they had acquired access to medicines and comforts of all descriptions. If the marines were to remain in camp their only requirement would be some good-quality huts, which might be easily met by transferring those soon to be dismantled at Cossack Bay. The stores accumulated by Churcher at Balaclava were available to be dispersed between the marines, the hospital

at Therapia and ships of the fleet. On 30 September both Churcher's victualling establishment and the Cossack Bay hospital facility were closed, the
latter following a final inspection by Deas. By then Smart had only 12 of the
naval brigade remaining, one of whom died within hours of the Inspector's
visit, while the others were all fit enough to be shipped to Therapia. Smart
returned to *Diamond* to await further orders. He had been with the naval
brigade since it first landed, Deas reminded Liddell, and had been a pillar
of strength in the Crimea: 'I have no words to express the degree of admira-
tion and gratitude I feel.'[66]

While Smart's year with the naval brigade launched him to prominence, the Crimean campaign was a tragic end for his counterpart with the
marine division, Edward Derriman. Derriman had been senior surgeon in
charge of the shore hospital for marines until taken ill with peritonitis early
in September 1855. He died on 5 October, leaving behind, Deas reflected,
'an establishment which would have done credit to the oldest Inspector of
hospitals we have'. For Deas, the loss of Derriman epitomized the sufferings of the marines throughout the siege of Sebastopol. Even when that
battle was won they were not released to their ships, as were the sailors,
but sent, still as a division, as part of the attack against Kinburn. Surely
the marine brigade was no longer needed, Deas appealed to Liddell after it
returned from Kinburn at the start of November? 'The majority are <u>shaky</u>,'
he confirmed;[67] it would be better to send them home and then bring them
back, if needed, next year rather than disembark them to survive another
Crimean winter. Deas expressed relief when news eventually arrived that
the marine brigade was to be disbanded. By the end of November 1855 the
Royal Navy was effectively out of the Crimea and all sailors and marines
had been re-embarked. From a total of 4,469 sailors and marines landed to
serve in brigades ashore the navy lost 100 killed and 475 wounded in enemy
action.[68]

Davidson carried on until the Therapia hospital was closed on 25
July 1856. By September 1855, however, most of his work was done. After
succeeding Burnett, Liddell compiled a clear record of the hospital's contribution to the war, drawing together all the returns made between 1 January
and 1 July 1855. Therapia had admitted 647 cases during those six months,
73 of whom had died, 51 were invalided and 463 were either discharged
cured or sent as convalescents to Malta. In fact on 1 July 1855 Davidson had
320 vacant beds – evidence indeed that the navy was well prepared for all
eventualities.[69] Admittedly Davidson had never been a great accountant, but

even that criticism subsequently appeared unmerited when Penfold, as full-time agent after December 1854, begged to be excused for similar failings in February 1856. There were losses from stores and in the accounts which Penfold simply could not explain. Carelessness under the pressure of work, unreliable staff, unruly sailors sent as nurses and thefts from intruders had made it impossible to safeguard public property as he would have wished. Davidson's otherwise tranquil life at Therapia in 1856 was disturbed only by having to keep MacKenzie's nurses occupied now that there were so few patients to look after. He certainly failed with Louisa Drake who was found intoxicated in the wards on 6 January and who had to be suspended and sent home. The arrival of Elizabeth Dunn from England to serve as ward matron in March 1856 was intended to solve that problem. Dunn would mess with the female nurses, Davidson ruled, 'and thus be a check upon their conduct'.[70] As it was, Dunn had little to do. The hospital had about 30 patients for most of the time after March 1856; on 15 June Davidson reported only three admissions during the previous week, none connected with the war, and that most of his stores, furniture and bedding were being transported to Malta. Staff and remaining patients followed ten days later. The keys to the building were handed to the embassy in Constantinople for return to the Turkish authorities on 28 July. Davidson arrived in England with Deas on 15 August.

Davidson's success at Therapia, like that of Smart at Balaclava, went far to ensure that the naval medical service in the Black Sea was spared the criticism heaped upon the army.[71] Pressed as the Therapia hospital was in January 1855, the conditions encountered by MacKenzie on arrival bore no comparison with the desperate accommodation and shortages of every description which had greeted Florence Nightingale and her nurses at Scutari just weeks before. Of course, the navy did less fighting, had longer to prepare and, the marine brigade aside, its men were not exposed to the appalling conditions suffered by the army before Sebastopol in the winter of 1854. The navy's medical failures were largely confined to hopeless inadequacy when conveying the wounded from Balaclava to the Bosphorus and among the merchant craft and transports in the harbour at Balaclava both before and during outbreaks of epidemic disease. The army lost over 18,000 men in the war. About 1,800 were killed as a result of enemy combat; the remainder died from disease. The navy lost 2,029 men from the Baltic and Black Sea fleets. Of those, 227 were killed or died from wounds in action and 228 died in accidents or drownings. Deaths from illness totalled 1,574, of which 861 were from bowel disease, mostly cholera, 217 from respiratory infections, 172 from fevers and 29 from smallpox. The navy also invalided more than 3,700 men between 1 April 1854 and 1 April 1856.[72]

Supplying the Mediterranean station had not been without problems in the early stages of the war but, for the most part, neither ships nor hospitals were ever seriously deficient. By the summer of 1855 there was an embarrassment of stores in the Mediterranean, as Deas indicated in August when explaining his arrangements for warships recently sent into the Sea of Azov. Medicated wine was abundant; indeed, 'they have quinine enough to poison half their numbers'.[73] There was, though, a difference between quantity and quality. James Jenkins, a surgeon with the naval brigade throughout 1855, reminded Liddell of this when assessing the efficacy of chloroform during amputations. He had difficulty both inducing and maintaining unconsciousness: the stuff was effectively useless. Liddell wanted to know whether Jenkins had been using naval stores or been dependent on issue from the army. In either case, quality was not just a function of manufacture but of careful handling. Had it been kept cool and stored in dark places or 'knocked about in half-full bottles?' It was a delicate substance, Liddell continued, which would decompose quickly if those precautions were ignored. 'I am anxious to know whether it has failed in other hands in the Crimea.'[74] Given the constant problem of transporting, tracking and storing anything in the navy, it was perhaps remarkable that such complaints about the quality of medical supplies were not more common.

While Deas, Davidson and Smart in the Mediterranean theatre, and McKechnie and Beith in the Baltic, took much of the credit for the navy's favourable showing when it came to medical organization, they in turn depended heavily on the surgeons and assistants who worked under and alongside them. Often tireless in their medical duties, when not stretched to their limits many were absorbed in military matters, had opinions about their naval commanders and were eager to be amongst the action. Michael Cowan's frustration aboard *Agamemnon* as the siege of Sebastopol reached its climax in 1855 typified the enthusiasm of most of the navy's young medics. 'Eternally the same day after day, hankering after Sebastopol,' he wrote impatiently. 'We must do something soon or the winter is on us.' Cowan went with the squadron to Kinburn and Odessa in October 1855 where, after being lost in thick fog for a while, he had the opportunity to see the Commander-in-Chief come aboard to inspect the ship. 'Old Lyons is such a queer fellow that one requires to be made aware of all his eccentricities,' he confided to his mother.[75] The good news, however, was that in the forthcoming attack against the Russian defences at Kinburn *Agamemnon* would have place of honour, with the fire from two mud batteries and another fort to contend with. Whether his mother shared this eagerness for action was not recorded.

Where the navy was criticized for shortcomings, insufficient assistant surgeons was usually the response – either as being the problem or to excuse deficiencies elsewhere. Deaths and sickness among medical officers in the Black Sea soon exposed inadequate staff levels there while the Baltic fleet maintained its numbers by recruiting dressers from the universities. In both theatres, experienced surgeons were short of qualified support and had to perform duties stipulated for their juniors. This problem was never overcome and once the naval and marine brigades ashore had to be provided for it was inevitable that many ships would have reduced cover. Even after Sebastopol fell and the brigades re-embarked, Deas still insisted that he could not find sufficient doctors for vessels going into action. He had already distributed several medical officers exhausted from shore service around the fleet when they should really have been sent home to recover. This had not proved to be enough, however: 'To supply four vacant ships I know of but one assistant,' he confessed.[76] It always came back to the old argument about recruitment – but not only of sufficient numbers. Although so many young practitioners had proved a credit to their profession, Deas maintained that colleagues with the desired skills and academic accomplishments remained too few. Only by making the navy a more attractive career could Burnett's dream of a service at the leading edge of medical science ever be realized. But in war, qualities other than intellectual refinement had a vital part to play. George Mackay watched in September 1854 as sailors and marines rushed ashore from *Agamemnon* to help casualties brought down from the Alma. Laden with cots and stretchers, seamen saved the lives of many men that day. On the beaches, Mackay observed, 'the energies and skill of the medical officers of the fleets were called into requisition'; as the wounded arrived at collection points 'medical men of all grades vied with each other in their efforts to assist and alleviate the sufferings of our gallant soldiers'.[77] As long as the commitment was sufficient, who in such circumstances was to say what qualities mattered most in a naval surgeon?

CHAPTER 8

Modernization and 1914

William Burnett's retirement marked the end of an era. Having presided over the department since 1832 and been previously influential on the old Victualling Board, he had shaped the navy's medical service and by 1855 either admitted or promoted every man working aboard ships or in hospitals, infirmaries and dockyards around the world. At the age of 76 he was among the last survivors of the age of Nelson. A meticulous organizer of men and resources, Burnett was widely respected for having done much to raise the status of surgeons. Throughout his time Burnett had shown firmness when confronted with indiscipline or negligence, yet, as those who wished him well in old age often revealed, a kindness too towards assistants starting their careers or struggling with adversity through no fault of their own. Alexander Mackay, on *Fantome* in Australia, reflected that he had ever found his chief energetic and thorough, despite the advancing years. Mackay, like many, regretted Burnett's departure: 'it will be a difficult matter to find an equally able man to fill his vacancy'.[1]

The background to Burnett's decades at Somerset House had all too often been budget economies or drives for administrative efficiency. After 1815 that was understandable, though with Britain's commerce and empire gradually expanding the annual naval estimates were always politically contentious. The estimates for 1835 were a paltry £4.5 million. From that low point expenditure slowly rose again as worries about Russian, American and French naval activity increased fears at home that Britain had become ill prepared for any challenge at sea. In 1845 the budget was above £7 million, with 40,000 sailors and marines allowed. But money remained tight. Although between 1848 and 1853 the annual estimates were consistently above £6.5 million, at its hospitals and afloat Burnett always felt vulnerable to cutbacks in relation to departments which had more clout at the Board of Admiralty.

In Burnett's time a clear progression of rank between assistant surgeon and Inspector became evident and the service acquired public recognition for its contribution to scientific enquiry and public health. But he was seldom free for long from the problem of recruitment; an establishment large on paper always contained many unfit, half-pay surgeons and, all too frequently, insufficient young assistants upon whom, in practice, so much of the tedium devolved. Improving its image in university medical schools seemed a forlorn task. Pay and prospects were invariably regarded as better in the army while, even among those who heard the call of the sea, disillusionment with naval realities, combined with invaliding and deaths in tropical climates, produced a wastage rate which only added to Burnett's difficulties. When Burnett called up eight new candidates in March 1848 he was obliged to warn the Admiralty that they were the last on the list. Things became no better. There were 309 assistant surgeons in 1846; in 1850 the total was 294 and 261 by 1852.

Surveying the service in 1853, Burnett advised the First Lord that this problem was being made worse by the promotion of so many assistant surgeons, 38 of whom had been raised to surgeon since 1851. All had been deserved and, of course, promotions were essential for morale. Nevertheless in consequence the navy had 15 surgeons who had not worked since being upgraded, whereas most of the 38 vacancies automatically created at the lower level remained unfilled. The timing of war against Russia, therefore, could scarcely have been worse. The estimates jumped from £7.2 million to over £15 million, ships were suddenly commissioned and the number of seamen and marines rose from 45,500 in 1853 to 63,500 in 1854. 'We are indeed deplorably in want of assistant surgeons, and the same will soon be the case with surgeons,' Burnett confessed in October 1854.[2] Taking student-dressers for the Baltic in 1855 was a bitter pill to swallow: the navy's appeal to patriotic duty had only managed to raise the number of assistant surgeons from 267 in January 1854 to 288 in January 1855. The number of surgeons fit for work remained at 320. The service's poor reputation and its chronic inability to recruit even for the needs of war hung as a cloud over Burnett's final year in office.

Yet the war also revealed something of the improved professional standing, certainly for senior surgeons, within the navy. Some had always had occasion to acknowledge the help of a commanding officer, but in an earlier age few would have dared present their captain with the demands issued by John Sabben on *Sphinx* at Sebastopol in October 1854. Prior to going into action, Sabben stipulated exactly where the cockpit should be located, his needs for lighting, tables, swabs, chairs for the wounded, buckets, water, drinking vessels, restorative wine and spirits and enough kindly men assigned as attendants. Above all, the most intelligent seamen were to be given instruction in ambulance and on the use of tourniquets. The captain agreed without hesitation.[3] Surgeon Edward Heath also took an assertive line after a gun on the main deck of *Dauntless* exploded in April 1855. Four men were injured; it would have been much worse had not other guns and men been moved away beforehand. By the time *Dauntless* went in for the attack on Kinburn in October 1855 Heath had the captain's consent for every precaution. He had moved out of his original cockpit and had a storage area fitted up for receiving the wounded. Ropes were strung above the upper deck to catch falling spars and rigging while splinter nets were spread inside the ship to limit the amount of wood scattered if hit. Heath and his assistant also undertook an educational function. Gun crews and all petty officers were instructed in the use of tourniquets 'in addition to such points of surgical haemostatics as we thought might prove useful'. Tourniquets were widely distributed and reserve supplies placed in several convenient locations.[4] Commendable as such harmony during action between surgeons and captains was, it did not address wider grievances still felt within the medical service in the late nineteenth century.

The Therapia hospital, Smart's work on *Diamond* and in the Cossack Bay huts, and Deas's tireless efforts to ensure that supplies and men were properly located drew accolades from within and outside the service. The naval brigade and marine divisions ashore, though their medical cover was sorely stretched at times, were also kept in fair condition, while back at Malta the large hospital coped with cases arriving from the Bosphorus. In light of their accomplishments, many medical officers expected rapid promotions and were quick to express disappointment when left off the lists. Deas, Davidson and Stewart at Malta were all promoted in 1855. Smart, however, had to petition in January 1856, reminding the Director-General that he had taken 740 cases onto *Diamond* from camps ashore, dealing thereby with fevers, dysentery, cholera and upwards of 200 gunshot wounds. He was not raised to Deputy-Inspector until 1858. While the work of a few senior medical officers and several others attached to the soon famous naval brigade was recognized, medics who had served throughout the war with marines in the trenches before Sebastopol or at gun batteries generally felt passed over. Yet in all weathers and frequently exhausted, it was they who had to rush to where the wounded lay. 'In doing so,' assistant surgeon John Cotton on *London* wrote indignantly, 'we had ample proof that neither shot nor shell discriminates between the surgeon and his patient.'[5]

Deas drew attention to assistant surgeons who had impressed him in the Black Sea as best he could. William Baird, he felt, was a particular omission from the promotion list. Although Baird had only entered the navy, aged 21, in 1852 and had not yet passed the examination for surgeon, Deas reminded Liddell in July 1856 how throughout the war Baird had been 'tossed from ship of war to ship of war, and from transport to transport, in a manner that must have been very distressing'. Yet to Baird's great credit, 'no such ill usage ever caused the least abatement of the most ardent zeal'. After Baird was ordered back to his own ship in an emergency, Deas was obliged to move him once again, this time to act as Smart's assistant at Cossack Bay. Smart, despite feeling insulted by the meagre 2/6d per diem offered him for his additional duties at Balaclava, found time to support his erstwhile young colleague. 'Pass without delay, and make a push at the Admiralty for your promotion,' he urged Baird.[6] Yet medics did not just feel neglected by their masters at the Admiralty: the senior service as a whole never seemed to get the recognition it deserved. Deas was annoyed that Sir John Hall, Inspector-General of army hospitals in the East, had received a higher order of decoration from Napoleon III when they went to Paris in 1856. For himself he did not care, but advised the Board to watch that the navy was not so slighted in future. That was easier said than done. Almost half a century later, James Porter, senior surgeon with the naval brigade in South Africa, voiced frustration that the navy always lost out when honours were distributed.

Porter joined as assistant surgeon in 1877. By then the Royal Navy was fast changing and in some respects was unrecognizable from the era of Trafalgar. In the second half of the nineteenth century iron replaced wood, steam became universal and gun turrets superseded the broadside of the old three-decker man-of-war carrying a thousand crew.[7] Taxpayers generally accepted that ruling the waves did not come cheap: the annual naval estimates rose from under £12 million in 1860 to nearly £19 million by 1895. But the number of vessels declined slightly after the Crimean War. From a peacetime peak of 266 ships in commission in 1847 the number dropped to 250 in 1860 and to no more than 200 in 1871. Manpower was also reduced. The wartime vote of 70,000 sailors and marines in 1855 was pared to under 60,000 by the late 1870s, leaving many executive officers on half pay with scant prospect of employment. Unchallenged on the high seas, the navy was increasingly expected to fight on land. Naval brigades were ashore during the 1857 Indian mutiny, in both China and Burma in 1858, in New Zealand between 1860 and 1864, during the Ashanti War in 1873–74, and in South Africa at the time of the Kaffir War in 1877–78, the Zulu War of 1878–79 and the first Boer War of 1880–81. The medical service won its solitary Victoria Cross amid fighting on Crete in 1898, Porter's naval brigade served with distinction during the second Boer War, while another was formed in China to combat the Boxer Rebellion of 1900.[8] Increasingly, service with sailors and marines ashore became the opportunity for medical officers to make their mark.

But it was not just the technology and operational requirements of the navy that were transformed in the late nineteenth century. Its character was also changing. Writing in 1871, one informed commentator observed the emergence of a different class of seaman. Gone were the days when riotous sailors, paid off with £50 in their pockets, would be fleeced or squander it all in a couple of nights in the backstreets of Portsmouth, Plymouth or Chatham.[9] The navy was becoming an increasingly professional service, comprising volunteers trained to handle sophisticated weaponry and equipment. Porter echoed this after 22 years of service in 1899: discipline was now maintained without brutality and men 'fit to go anywhere and do anything!'[10] Life on the lower deck was noticeably better than for previous generations – as statistics proved. Deaths from all causes in the Royal Navy were 22 per 1,000 in 1857, 11.5 in 1867, 8.3 in 1887, 5.2 in 1897 and only 3.3 per 1,000 by 1907 – a level maintained until the First World War. Deaths from disease alone dropped from 12.1 per 1,000 in 1856 to 6.5 in 1868 and 4.8 in 1887. The trend continued: the ratio was down to 1.4 per 1,000 by 1936.[11]

To some extent this could be explained by advances in medicine and surgical procedures. The fevers which so ravaged crews off the coasts of Africa and in the West Indies in the early nineteenth century were gradually tamed by the widespread use of quinine from the 1840s onwards. Burnett included the use of its precursor, Peruvian bark, in his guidance for the health of crews during the 1841 Niger expedition, alongside the need for cleanliness, dryness and ventilation on all vessels, superior victualling, regular meals, limited exposure to the sun, dry clothes and no overnight boat duty. The problem, even six years later though, was that 'it is hard to get officers or men to take this invaluable medicine as a powder even when mixed with wine'.[12] Trials showed that mixing grains in bottles with

Tenerife wine both prevented decomposition and made it palatable. After 1848 it was an obligatory daily issue by surgeons on the West Africa station for men going ashore, in boats or otherwise exposed to a dangerous environment. By 1851 reluctance to take quinine wine had disappeared. Robert Bernard in the Mozambique channel recorded how 'at first the men shewed a great dislike to it but after a short time took it willingly and latterly called for it if it was omitted to be given'.[13] The preparation used was 'devised with our chemist', Burnett reported to the Board. Manufactured in casks at Deptford, the navy's quinine was the best available. 'It has never been in any pharmacopoeia and is a suggestion entirely of our own.'[14]

As quinine transformed the treatment of fevers, so chloroform and more effective disinfectants were extending the possibilities for surgery. To reflect this, in 1852 Burnett revised the list of medicines to be issued, which required some minor changes to the layout of medical chests. The change was not radical enough for William Graham, surgeon aboard *Vengeance* in the Mediterranean in 1853. Admittedly zinc chloride had achieved much as a disinfecting agent throughout the fleet and in naval hospitals, while introducing new medicines was to the credit of the Medical Department. But where was cod liver oil in the updated schedule? This was 'a medicine of such great notoriety in the present day', he remarked, and exceptionally helpful in cases of phthisis and all diseases connected with the lungs.[15] By the time of the 1882 Egyptian campaign, rapid relief for those fallen provided a further innovation. This was not so obvious at Tel-el-Kebir where Eveyln Pollard, dodging the bullets, moved among the wounded applying dressings and providing comfort in the time-honoured manner of surgeons in the field. Earlier, while surgeon with marines in a small action at Mallaha junction on 5 August, however, Pollard recorded how medicine had changed since 'the hypodermic injection of morphia was used freely to all who suffered pain'.[16] At the end of 1899 Porter felt confident that advances in medicine and hygiene would render British losses in South Africa fewer than in wars conducted previously in pestilential climates. Pinned to the ground under Boer fire as a patient was killed beside him, such confidence must have seemed misplaced. As his brigade gradually advanced, however, Porter was able to resume his dressings while 'serving out morphia, brandy and water etc.'[17]

There was, of course, far more to preserving the health of seamen in the late nineteenth century than better medicine and greater comfort when patching up their wounds. As senior naval officers were well aware, even in the 1840s, the fitness of men started with recruitment. In 1846 the Admiralty informed Admiral Charles Ogle at Portsmouth that too many unfit boys had been accepted.[18] In the Mediterranean three years later Vice-Admiral Parker reflected that 'stunted, undersized men should not be entered'.[19] From the 1860s onwards the navy took a greater interest in the regimes aboard training vessels and at the Greenwich naval school, where exercise, diet and cooking were repeatedly reviewed and the growth of boys monitored.[20]

The navy became a more benign environment as the century wore on. Aboard ship, the savage discipline of Nelson's day, still evident on some vessels in the 1830s, was progressively eased following the 1835 Royal Commission on naval punishments. Solitary confinement tended to replace the lash. In 1839, 2,007 men were flogged; by 1847 the number was down to 860, though captains retained considerable discretion. After 1846 naval punishment returns were required by parliament and were regularly submitted after 1853. The navy suspended peacetime flogging in 1871. It disappeared entirely in 1879.[21] Punishments aside, the lower deck was also a healthier place – as Captain Adolphus Slade wrote to his friend, Captain Charles Eden, at the Admiralty in 1852. Mortality on his ship was down more than half from the levels of the 1840s. Slade attributed this to the comforts available below, principally the superior deck-ports and the stoves lighted day and night for warmth and to avoid dampness.[22] Men were increasingly instructed in personal hygiene and sanitation: bathing, regulation uniforms and the regular washing of clothes became part of the responsibilities of every captain and medical officer. This was far removed from what Burnett had witnessed when first inspecting Britain's naval hospitals in the 1820s: he had been horrified how 'the clothing brought from the ships by the patients generally came in a very dirty state, and, on the individuals being discharged, the clothing was returned to them to carry on board of ship in the same filthy condition'.[23] By the 1890s Porter rejoiced at the arrival of electric lighting on many naval vessels. Refrigerators and freezers were another luxury, he wrote home in 1898. His new machine could make a hundredweight of ice a day: 'Splendid affair for sick in hot weather.'[24]

Yet for many medics and executive officers these advances paled in significance when compared to the benefits of limiting alcohol consumption. That problem had always been acknowledged: controlling the habits of men for whom excess was often their only relief from the rigours of life at sea was, however, difficult in practice and bound to breed resentment.

Nevertheless by the 1840s the issue had to be tackled. Thomas Dunn, surgeon on *Fisgard*, calculated that half of all accidents and diseases and nearly 90 per cent of crime in the Royal Navy, both at sea and in harbour, were alcohol related. The Admiralty was concerned to make punishments more humane, he observed in 1847; why not, therefore, strike at the real root of the problem? Rear-Admiral Dundas confided to the First Lord in 1849 that drunkenness on ships was breaking down discipline and that flogging men for drinking was not working.[25] Halving the grog allowance in 1850 was therefore widely welcomed, although it had always been known that the willingness of many sailors to sell their issue caused as much trouble as the initial distribution. Robert Bernard sensed in 1851 that drunkenness was already less common: surprisingly, the men 'appear to have become quickly reconciled to the change'.[26] The problem never disappeared, although in his 1862 report Milroy contrasted the service favourably with that of 40 years previously when every day a half-pint of spirits had been doled out to every man and youth. Thereafter a maximum strength for naval rum was fixed in 1866. In 1881 the issue of spirits to officers and men under 20 years of age was stopped.

While acknowledging a number of improvements by the 1860s Milroy nonetheless concluded that better hygiene and care of seamen could still reduce sick-lists by 10 per cent. His opinions thereafter influenced changes in the naval medical service and the closer attention paid by executive officers to the health of crews. 'The more that the medical officers of our ships are regarded in the light of preservers of health and not merely of healers of disease,' Milroy advised the First Lord.[27] According to some medics, stamping out smoking was a further step which should be taken. John Nihill, assistant surgeon aboard *Cockatrice* in 1852, conceded that although the public cherished the image of a sailor puffing happily at his pipe in a moment of relaxation, 'few can imagine that the excess to which it is carried contributes to lay the foundation of much permanent debility and disease'.[28] Even if regular sailors could not realistically be restrained, surely it was possible to dissuade boys and new recruits from taking up the habit? The Admiralty had, in fact, issued a circular letter regarding tobacco in 1846 which another campaigner, Vice-Admiral Parker, welcomed as giving him authority to restrict smoking throughout his Mediterranean command. He had forbidden it for everyone below 19 years of age and in 'any enclosed berth'.[29] No officer aboard his flagship smoked, which would set an example throughout the fleet. Parker was probably deluded, though no doubt tobacco was never seen in his presence.

The limits of medical knowledge made two common scourges of sailors and marines difficult to control before the twentieth century. The first was venereal disease. Lock hospitals to provide secure retreats for women on the streets of Portsmouth and Plymouth were proposed and some experiments conducted in the 1850s, although the navy recognized that it could only treat a fraction of those infected. At overseas ports even fewer checks were available. Malta did its best. John Dunlop, surgeon on *Superb* in 1852, was impressed with the small number of infections picked up there, which he ascribed to the system for inspecting prostitutes. Yet, as with smoking, only so much could be done. Malta's precautions were commendable but, as Dunlop recognized, 'the greater number and the worst cases were contracted after the ship returned to England'.[30] In any case, venereal disease was as much a moral as a medical problem and was frequently regarded as a consequence of excessive alcohol: if the navy dealt with that fundamental evil then immorality, like crime, would diminish naturally. John Drummond, Deputy-Inspector at the Melville in 1853, was among those advocating lock hospitals for women in the naval towns: syphilis was neither sufficiently acknowledged nor taken seriously enough. It was not an issue which society wished to hear about, yet it was 'a source of loss to the country to such an extent that it cannot well be estimated'.[31] It was destroying the navy's best men. The East Stonehouse hospital, after consulting with local police, reported that there were likely upwards of 3,000 prostitutes in the Plymouth area in 1853. Between 1851 and 1853 the hospital had admitted 570 syphilis cases – almost 30 per cent of its entire intake. Haslar meanwhile had about 70 syphilitics at any time, with a further 30 men on average undergoing treatment at marine headquarters. The cost of all this to Haslar was £2,767 per annum. In 1856 the Director-General estimated that whether due to hospital expenses, care in marine barracks or treatment aboard ships, syphilis at Plymouth cost the Royal Navy about £8,000 per annum, excluding further losses via invaliding and pensions.[32]

With estimates of 2,000 prostitutes in Portsmouth in 1863 and a further 1,000 distributed between Chatham and Woolwich the scale of the problem in the late nineteenth century remained apparent. Indeed data collected for 1862 indicated that of the 88,611 men admitted to naval hospitals at home and overseas, 7,367 were classed as venereal, with the overwhelming majority syphilitic. In different locations the army was similarly affected. A parliamentary committee was set up to investigate ways of reducing infection rates in 1864 at the same time as the Contagious Diseases Act introduced compulsory medical inspections in designated towns for women reported as prostitutes. Needless to say, Portsmouth, Plymouth and Chatham were on the list – as were Woolwich and Sheerness. More legislation, in light of the 1864 committee's findings, followed in 1866 and 1869. To a degree, the blunt instrument of these Contagious Diseases Acts did produce a measurable success. From the high levels of 168 cases per 1,000 men in 1856, 125 in 1862 and 104 in 1863, the rates of men afflicted with venereal complaints declined sharply to 53 per 1,000 in 1868 and 48 per 1,000 in 1874. But the Acts were unpopular and after their repeal levels rose again in the 1880s. Decreases resumed in the decade before 1914, largely explained by statistical distinctions now drawn between primary and secondary syphilis and the eventual discovery of more effective treatments than mercury. Into the early twentieth century, however, syphilis remained the most frequent affliction on naval sick-lists.[33]

The second disease prevalent in the navy which medical science could do little to remedy was tuberculosis. It was naturally associated with the conditions in which seamen lived, though in the 1850s was also considered by some medical officers to be accelerated by drink and debauchery – a judgement apparently confirmed by the incidence always being higher among ordinary seamen than among officers. Tuberculosis seemed to increase as scurvy declined, although no connection between those trends could ever be established. It was established, however, that the problem grew worse after steam power became widespread, thereby reinforcing opinions about foul air and poor ventilation being a root cause. The idea that germs in sputum might spread the disease was not widely accepted until the causal bacillus was isolated in 1882. But as with so many diseases in the nineteenth and early twentieth centuries, identification and cure were different things. In the three years 1856 to 1858 deaths from tuberculosis ran at 2.6 per 1,000 men with a further 3.9 per 1,000 invalided. As late as 1901–5 the mortality rate in the navy was still more than twice the level in civil society; thereafter the incidence of tuberculosis in Britain generally halved between 1921 and 1936 whereas in the Royal Navy it remained unchanged. Considering why sailors suffered so much, a parliamentary committee in 1911 returned to the old problem of recruitment: were many men brought up amid poor housing conditions, bringing the disease into the service with them, albeit at a stage too early to be detected? As so often in the past, naval medics were enjoined to conduct stricter examinations for those enlisting.[34]

❧

Although seamen could not be protected from all ailments they might encounter, better food and clothing and the benefit of smallpox vaccination at an earlier age did make them increasingly resilient. Compared to the merchant navy, those who served on HM ships enjoyed far higher standards of comfort and provision. Between 1857 and 1867, for instance, the overall death rate in the Royal Navy was 15 per 1,000 men; in the merchant navy it was 24 per 1,000.[35] But the navy did not just keep men healthier at sea. When accident or illness befell them they also received better nursing by the late nineteenth century. Aboard ship, poor nursing had long featured among complaints by surgeons. Robert Grigor, for one, raised the issue directly with Burnett just weeks before the latter retired. Grigor was profuse in his praise for all that Burnett had done to improve medical treatments, to make living quarters aboard ship healthier and to build up a corps of medical staff which was second to none in public service. But help for surgeons in the sick-bay was no better than during the Napoleonic Wars. Instructions to captains issued in 1833 required them to make provision for sick-berth attendance but in practice this represented little advance on the old loblolly boys. A steady man 'very naturally becomes discontented and wishes to get away as soon as possible'.[36] The only solution, Grigor urged, was to persuade the Admiralty to attach first-class petty officer rank to this vital employment. In truth, for 30 years Burnett had expressed sympathy for those who toiled in this way for so little reward throughout the fleet and in the navy's famous institutions and he had recommended deserving individuals for specific advancements and pensions. But he had arguably done almost nothing to alter the ad hoc and increasingly inefficient structures under which they worked.

As Director-General between 1855 and 1864, Liddell cared about nursing. He was, however, more interested in the quality provided at naval hospitals. Indeed in 1861 Alexander Mackay recognized that nothing had altered afloat and was preparing to reiterate Grigor's point about upgrading sick-berth stewards on large vessels. But nursing was not the only deficiency and Deas, drawing on his experience in the Black Sea and having consulted with fellow senior medical officers, advised as early as March 1855 that the service had to change in other ways. The old system whereby surgeons returned so many purely professional documents, such as the ship's basic nosological statistics, through the captain was at best cumbersome for commanding officers and at worst an insult to experienced doctors. A greater range of medicines, surgical appliances and comforts were also needed: the contents of a number one chest no longer reflected modern medicine, while the list of additional equipment needed was extensive. Pillows, cushions, better-stuffed beds, more blankets for the sick-bay, oiled cloth, waterproof sheeting and superior splints were all in demand. Larger issues of calico, lint and sponges were required, as were better surgical instruments to take out on boat service. Food had to be improved too: preserved potatoes, vegetables, chocolate, milk and beef essence should be available in all ships rather than found sporadically throughout the fleet.[37] No Director-General was ever likely to disagree. The problem at Somerset House was, as always, where was the money to come from?

The Crimean War brought the issue of day-to-day costs to the fore: the old sick-mess fund, which paid for the victualling of those on naval sick-lists, had essentially failed under the pressure of soaring demand. The fund had been in surplus to the sum of £5,015 in 1846 and, confident that the fund could bear further charges, Burnett had persuaded the Admiralty to transfer to it the cost of providing medical necessities. However, during the three years 1853 to 1856 a total of £5,676 had been charged to the sick-mess fund for care aboard ships against a figure of only £1,060 received. The surplus could have absorbed this imbalance had the costs stopped with naval vessels. But charges for hospital comforts at Lisbon, Ascension and the expensive establishment at Therapia had also been diverted to the sick-mess fund and by January 1857 there was a deficit of £409. Liddell had now to devise a way of salvaging the whole system whereby sick and hospital diets were funded. Closing Therapia in 1856 and halting other hospital costs against the fund stopped the problem getting worse. Liddell concluded nevertheless that more would be necessary in order to balance the books. He persuaded the Board that Burnett's 1846 funding transfer would need to be unscrambled, thereby restoring the sick-mess fund to its original function 'to provide hospital diet for the sick of H.M. fleets'.[38] To place the fund back on a sound financial basis many of the costs incurred, including those at Lisbon, Ascension and Therapia, would need to be recovered from a separate Admiralty vote. But with his rescue measures in place, Liddell still had to convince the Board that the difficulty would not arise again, for which purpose it was necessary to reveal where money in the past had gone. To the Medical Department's embarrassment, research unearthed two glaring accounting discrepancies.

The first of these related to the unusually large quantities of preserved meat issued to naval crews on surgeons' recommendations during the war. Surgeons had treated this supply as part of naval rations, nominally charged the same as fresh meat at 4d per pound, so long as quantities remained within the Admiralty's approved scale of victualling. Yet whereas 4d per pound was a realistic cost price for fresh meat, the cost price for preserved meat was upwards of 11d per pound. The difference had been charged by paymasters to the sick-mess fund. Liddell soon slammed the door on that loophole. In future, he informed the Board, preserved meat would not be allowed as an article of diet: it would be issued only to the sick when fresh meat was unavailable. The second discrepancy that came to light concerned unauthorized payments to attendants and cooks. Such men had frequently received £1 per month out of the sick-mess fund in order to keep up their spirits when tending the sick and wounded, or, in the case of a cook, to procure a reliable man who knew how to prepare the special diet dishes ordered in the sick-bay. Since these underhand payments were condoned by most ships officers as the only way to get competent men to volunteer, Liddell recognized that there was no realistic scope for economy here. The Board confirmed that irregular sick-berth attendants and diet cooks could receive 'the usual gratuity', although in light of a recent pay increase no further sums were to be given them.[39] By August 1857, however, Liddell had found one other area for tightening. Having clawed back on preserved meat, he managed to extend restrictions on the purchase of medicines beyond the Admiralty scale. Only special needs could justify such provision.

When urging measures to overhaul the service in 1855, Deas touched upon the plight of surgeons whose work was hindered by unwilling or incompetent helpers in the sick-bay. Like Grigor and Mackay, his solution was to introduce a first-class petty officer rating for experienced attendants in large ships, while in smaller vessels to ensure that men who volunteered were excused other duties. But Liddell's priority remained hospital provision, mindful as he was of the shortcomings exposed by Davidson's difficulties with nursing staff at Therapia and of the deterioration in nursing care commonly perceived in the home hospitals. Nevertheless the contribution of some excellent men who had either left their ships or come out from establishments in England to work in the unglamorous environment of temporary naval hospitals was acknowledged. Henry Meadows was one. He had volunteered for duty at Therapia in June 1854 when dispensary assistant at Haslar and he remained with Davidson as a reliable support until the beginning of 1856. Thomas Goodwin was a glowing example of how a sick-berth man could help make a medical establishment. Goodwin was Smart's loyal attendant aboard *Diamond* at Balaclava, assisting Smart during operations, dispensing medicines and at times watching over up to 70 patients simultaneously. He had previously been a dispensary assistant in Manchester and now aspired to train as a dresser. 'Young men of his stamp deserve encouragement to enter the service in the capacity he did,' Smart reflected.[40] In light of this, Liddell found Goodwin a dispensary post at the Yarmouth hospital. Deas identified another deserving man whom he encountered in the Black Sea. John Brown, 18 years in the navy and six years a dependable sick-berth man aboard *Rodney*, was capable of bearing greater responsibilities. Brown could dispense medicines and was particularly attentive in his care for the sick. Such men, the surgeon on *Rodney* remarked, 'are rarely met with in the service'.[41] Deas himself had been well served for 11 years by one attendant, John Naylor, who, although not so well educated as Brown, had been a stalwart in every sick-bay where Deas had worked. Deas had left him on *Sanspareil*, he remarked to Liddell in September 1855; as an honest, zealous and careful man, Naylor deserved better.

Exemplary as men like Meadows, Goodwin, Brown and Naylor had proved to be, Liddell was nonetheless convinced that the future of hospital nursing lay with women. Yet though the navy had cause to be grateful for the dedication of some who had been matrons at its hospitals in recent decades, given its experience with the often drunk, dishonest and dissolute wives and widows of seamen who had worked alongside the pensioners and labourers at Haslar and East Stonehouse for generations, this was not an idea likely to gather immediate or widespread support. Too often such women had been given work at the home hospitals as an unwelcome necessity or as covert welfare in port towns. Yet Liddell seemed aware that times were changing. Nightingale with the army and MacKenzie with the navy at Therapia had demonstrated the worth of committed and competent women, while the British public had embraced the notion that the contribution of their followers, and that of other women who had gone out to the Crimea, had been both vital and praiseworthy. In 1856 Nightingale came back from the war a national heroine; she had altered perceptions of the place of women in society. Even before her return Liddell had become a member of the Nightingale Fund Council for nurses' training and in London he asked for assistance in introducing her protégés into naval establishments.

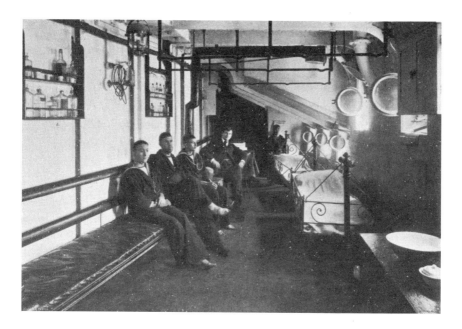

10. Sick-bay aboard 1880s warship.

Liddell's views, however, represented more than simply the acclaim afforded to those who had tended the nation's wounded. Changing attitudes reflected both shifts in Victorian society and the emergence of specific roles for women in an expanding workforce. Social change was obvious through urbanization and the growth of a large middle class. It was also calculated that by 1860 there was a surplus of about half a million women in Britain, for many of whom the option of raising families was unlikely to arise. Whether as individuals they sought careers, the truth was that increasing numbers would have to earn a living and, within the middle classes, would have to find a means of doing so distinct from the field, factory and domestic service where girls and women from the lower orders had traditionally toiled. Since the 1840s teacher training had been one outlet for such aspirations. Opportunities in clerical and commercial work were beginning, although in 1861 there were only 279 female clerks in England and Wales compared with 92,000 men.[42] For the daughters of many middle class and comfortable artisan families, however, nursing was becoming an acceptable alternative. Nightingale had enhanced its image. Its development nevertheless predated her exploits at Scutari.

Organized nursing evolved from religious orders and from the work

of women inspired by Christian conviction who had entered rudimentary hospital training from the 1830s onwards. Until this time nursing
entailed no qualification. Although private nursing for wealthy families
had provided some women with reasonable incomes in the early nineteenth
century, systematic provision dated from 1848 when Anglican Sisters of
Mercy formed St John's House in London. High Church sympathies led
Lydia Sellon to set up her own sisterhood at Devonport in the same year. St
John's House offered a two-year training in hospitals and for work in private
homes. It provided staff to undertake nursing at a number of London institutions; at King's College Hospital, for instance, it contracted for nursing
and catering services for many years after 1856. It did so at the Charing
Cross Hospital until 1889. By the 1860s St John's House was also supplying 4,000 meals per day for poor outpatients from King's and visiting their
homes as required. Yet there was no large pool of nursing talent from which
the navy's hospitals could draw. Since home care was widely regarded as
preferable to hospital admission until the late nineteenth century the
number of hospital beds in England and Wales, excluding workhouse infirmaries for the destitute, remained small, rising from about 4,000 in 1800
to only 12,000 in 1861. Before the 1860s fewer than 1,000 among the 25,000
trained and untrained women who nursed worked in a hospital.[43]

Liddell conceded that in the immediate future there would not be sufficient numbers of career women to satisfy demand. That, however, did not
prevent him from passing a damning judgement on the practices which
Burnett had tolerated for so long. Presenting proposals to the Board of
Admiralty early in January 1856, he observed that a complete change was
required. Surveying all naval hospitals, he confronted the Board with an
inescapable conclusion: nursing was 'so defective that one can hardly imagine that the selection of an able and responsible body of nurses should have
been so long delayed'.[44] His short-term remedy was hiring women of good
character; he added that society must divest itself of its preconception 'that
plain, ill-dressed, aged women are more moral or orderly in their habits and
life than young, well-dressed nurses'.[45] The work required a cheerful countenance in the face of repetitious and trying duties. That was not a quality
augmented by the passage of time. Acknowledging too that the issue of
cost was bound to arise, Liddell admitted at once that his scheme would
require paying a wage of more than the current five shillings a week. But it
was not just a matter of money. In the past, women entering naval hospitals
had been searched at the gates; in June 1854 Eliza Brown was specifically

employed to do this at Haslar for an additional payment of two shillings a week.[46] The reason was commendable: to prevent alcohol being smuggled in. Most women found it degrading, however, and Liddell advised that the practice would have to stop. Looking to the future, professional women would also need to be free from naval regulations or the authority of executive officers. They would be selected by the principal medical officer according to their abilities to nurse and only he would judge their behaviour, allocate their leave or, if necessary, administer punishment. Expense, regulations and the availability of suitably qualified women aside, there were, however, two further obstacles which stood in the way of Liddell's plan. One was the almost uniformly held view that it would be inappropriate for women to work in venereal wards, which, given the high incidence of venereal admissions to naval hospitals, meant that many less suitable men would still be needed. The second damper on Liddell's thinking was that the professional women whom he most sought were not always amenable to working in military establishments.

No one expressed that idea more clearly than Jane Shaw-Stewart, niece of Rear-Admiral Sir Houston Stewart and an experienced nurse who was both friend and admirer of Nightingale from their time in the Crimea. Shaw-Stewart had visited the Therapia hospital after arriving in the Bosphorus in 1854 and worked for the army at Scutari until moved to the general hospital at Balaclava. She eventually took over as superintendent of the women who nursed at Balaclava, remaining there until the army closed the facility in June 1856. Headstrong, hard working, devoted to patients and strict about regulations and staff discipline, she was, as one helper recalled, 'the only lady who went to the East in all respects really capable of a nurse's duties'.[47] Thereafter she retained firm views both on the importance of professional nursing and on the qualities required of dedicated women. Unfortunately for Liddell, Shaw-Stewart believed that hospitals for the armed services would always be different in character from civilian establishments and consequently were inherently ill suited to employ respectable women. Her advice for the navy, as conveyed to Nightingale, was: 'Let there be as few women, and those few as efficient and as respectable as can be. Let all that can really be done by men, be so done.'[48] Still in 1859 she was advising the War Office to defer the appointment of women nurses to the army hospital at Netley, although, when invited, she agreed to take charge there until her resignation in 1868. Sadly in want of support in 1856, therefore, Liddell's problem was to judge how his views about women nursing at Haslar, East

Stonehouse and Chatham might be received.

Presenting more details to the Board on 19 January 1856, Liddell proposed that those employed should be paid £20 per annum, with two gowns, two bonnets and one cloak allowed at a recurring cost of £2-5-10d. Provisions money would amount to 9d per day, making the overall annual cost of a nurse £35-10-6d. Male nurses for the venereal wards would be engaged on a daily basis at a notional annual cost of £45-4-6d. These were arrangements which the Admiralty had recently sanctioned for work among the pensioners at Greenwich. The Board seemed to favour some experiment, although it soon became clear that Liddell had not thought of everything when Edward Hilditch, by 1857 Inspector at East Stonehouse, asked whether he would be permitted to employ women for nightwatching. Hospital labourers had once been used for this but that practice had been discontinued on the grounds that they could not perform their sometimes arduous day jobs and then be relied upon to be alert throughout the hours of darkness. There was a lack of staff to provide night cover in both medical and surgical wards, particularly since two night nurses, as traditionally assigned to each, were no longer judged to be sufficient. Patients excited from the effects of alcohol withdrawal while undergoing treatment often had to be physically restrained: this was a task for strong men. Liddell had to concede the point. He replied that women might be used in an emergency but that, given the nature of nightwatching, male nurses should always be preferred. However, after studying Hilditch's accounts Liddell wanted to know where the costs ascribed to nightwatching had come from. The wards at Haslar covered their annual night attendance for £12 and even its lunatic asylum managed on £36. Why, therefore, at East Stonehouse was the figure £130 a year? Paying nurses specifically for night duties was no doubt appreciated by all recipients and relieved the regular nurses from a generally unwelcome task, yet over the years it 'seems to have grown into a system at Plymouth that does not exist at other hospitals'.[49] Embarrassed by another disguised expense in the Medical Department's accounts having come to light, Liddell ordered that rather than be allowed extra night cover Hilditch should cut back in this area. In any case, using women was no solution since they would need to be paid at the same rate as men.

By the 1850s the problems of the navy's home hospitals went far beyond the quality of nursing care. Haslar and East Stonehouse were generally well run but both were now a century old and the ravages of time were beginning to tell. At Haslar, physical deterioration was obvious. Outhouses and storerooms were overrun with rats and the cellars of most buildings reeked of the many cats kept on site. Smoking chimneys made cooking nigh impossible. Much of the institution's fresh water supply was lost through leaking pipes. Its drains stank. The roofs and windows let in rain which soaked the building and rotted the furniture. Many door locks and hinges were also broken. But though procedures for improving basic maintenance were put in place in 1845 and superficially the building was put into a state of better repair, Haslar remained essentially unaltered. The hospital was still lit by candles; indeed, the installation of gas lighting in 1854 was its first major modernization.[50] Years of peace had left the medical and administrative routines of the two great hospitals relatively undisturbed. Cholera in Plymouth tested the resources of East Stonehouse in 1849 but it emerged from the crisis with credit. At Haslar, however, the scarlatina epidemics in 1853 and 1854 strained arrangements to breaking point.

When Burnett went down to Portsmouth to assess the crisis at Haslar in 1854 he found the medical wards full and scarlatina patients spilling over into areas temporarily hived off from the asylum. The surgical department still had two wards but these had to be kept free in case of severe accidents. The only other areas which could be converted quickly for medical purposes were some old wards which had long been used for stores and the manufacture of bedding and other equipment. Perhaps another 100 men could be squeezed in if all space was maximized, Burnett surmised, but the best hope of managing the epidemic was by fitting up the nearby hulk *Menelaus* to receive 150 mostly convalescent patients. Since they would sleep in hammocks, *Menelaus* would not require a great deal of work and might soon be ready to take her first transfers.

Given Haslar's boast to be able to take above 2,000 cases in an emergency, it was a poor advertisement that when faced with a combined admission of 690 patients and 108 lunatics in April 1854 it struggled to meet demand. Antiquated facilities in part explained why the hospital's difficulties could not be met by simply drafting in more medical and nursing staff, but an even more obvious factor seemed to be the way in which so much of the building had been taken out of medical service. As stores and equipment had accumulated, so unused wards were allocated to the agent and steward as repositories. Burnett saw no solution to this but to erect two corrugated iron structures on either side of the porters' lodge and along the inside of the front wall in order to take supplies. This would then liberate much of the hospital for its intended purpose, adding about 200 beds.

The only alternative was to relocate the asylum, thereby incorporating the lunatics' accommodation into the main site. But Burnett begged the Board not to move those mentally ill from the comfortable and befitting facilities which they currently enjoyed: aside from the disturbance it would cause, it would not be the most economical option. Putting up corrugated iron 'can be effected <u>very rapidly</u> and at considerable less expense than any building of brick'.[51] In the meantime he asked the Board to refuse to allow ships entering the English Channel to bring their sick and invalids up to Portsmouth but to land them at Plymouth where the East Stonehouse hospital was still able to take them.

While clearing out some ward areas long used as workshops, erecting a couple of corrugated iron storage sheds and ordering a few dozen convalescents to sling their hammocks in *Menelaus* would doubtless see Haslar through in 1854, Burnett was mindful that these were not lasting solutions. Portsmouth needed a properly fitted hospital ship moored permanently close by, which would be capable of taking at least 200 patients as an overflow from Haslar. Inside the hospital grounds, too, Burnett wanted to construct accommodation for up to 300 men in two new buildings. This increased capacity would meet any wartime needs, he assured the Admiralty. Modernizing the navy's largest hospital would not be cheap; on top of building costs would come those of introducing new steam-laundry and drying facilities in 1855 which were essential even to provide for existing numbers. But the list did not stop there. In 1855, just weeks before he retired, Richardson reported that the drains had collapsed.

Richardson had noticed increasing numbers of gastro-enteric fever cases in Haslar's wards. The origin was obviously local but given the hospital's healthy site, good ventilation and, at least until 1853, the absence of overcrowding, it was hard to identify the exact source. Years before he had reported that sewerage was becoming a problem. The expense of replacing the original system, though, had ensured that nothing was done. By the early 1850s the flow had come to depend upon sending a couple of men up the drains every fortnight to rake down the night soil. Building nearby had interfered with the hospital's drainage. Somewhere in Gosport a ditch cut when constructing fortifications had intercepted the town's outlet which meant that deposits of effluent and other decomposing organic material regularly flooded the vicinity. In summer the smell from this became offensive and the hospital suffered accordingly. Neither the Board of Ordnance nor the local parish authority, however, would accept responsibility for the

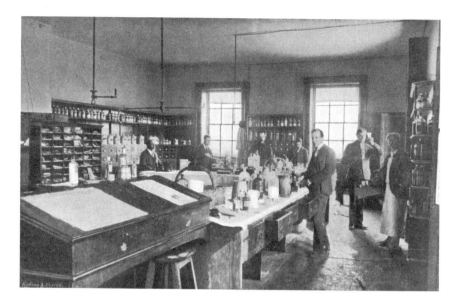

11. The dispensary at Haslar: 1890s.

necessary repair. In neighbouring Alverstoke increasing population and new housing also affected the hospital. Waste from these developments flowed into nearby Haslar lake which was, in consequence, gradually being transformed into an open cesspool. After so many years of neglect there was no escaping that Haslar's drains had to be rebuilt. In 1855 new 12-inch stoneware pipes were laid inside the old brick sewers. The direction of discharge was also altered: the new pipe-work took sewage directly to the sea.

With gas installed in 1854, new drainage in 1855 and plans afoot for building and laundry improvements, Haslar was undoubtedly changing. But Liddell still considered that it made a gloomy impression when he made his first inspection in August 1855. Several of the wards and the adjoining cabins used by nurses were sorely in need of painting. Outside the wards, doors in corridors and staircases were also in bad decorative order. Attending to this would 'remove the patched, broken and discoloured appearance of the woodwork'.[52] A hospital should be light, clean and cheerful, he remarked, believing as he did, perhaps a little naively, that this was how the navy's other establishments were maintained. But whatever its first impression on visitors, efforts made during the war were producing some effects. Russell, as agent, asked Liddell to authorize a store sufficient for 1,000 patients in August 1855. Haslar could now take that many, excluding lunatics, he continued, and more capacity would probably result from plans to convert rooms currently used by the museum curator, the store matron and as an assistant surgeons' mess into medical wards. East Stonehouse, though busy in the winter of 1854, saw out the war relatively undisturbed. Visiting in December 1856, Liddell was impressed with its good accommodation, contented patients and ample space for any emergency. For the time being, and with a review of its nursing provision underway, the Royal Navy could at least make the case that its home hospitals were performing as the nation expected.

෬

In July 1914 Director-General Sir Arthur May addressed an assembly of medical students at Edinburgh University. The navy was short of medical officers, he conceded, but the service did not deserve the low esteem in which most young doctors seemed to hold it. Whatever shortcomings might have existed 30 years previously had now been put to right. May did not disguise the navy's embarrassment. In 1904 the Admiralty had been allowed an establishment of 594 medical officers, which by 1913 had to provide for a navy of 122,500 men. Yet with the size of the fleet increased to over 147,000 and a further 56,000 employed in dockyards and civil establishments in 1914, there were only 525 medics on the active list. Recruitment had fallen to its lowest levels. The audience listened politely but dispersed unimpressed.[53] Men holding rank equivalent to the old surgeons' mate had to be brought back to help dress wounds, treat sores and ulcers, and thereby ensure that sufficient cover could be made available for smaller vessels; most were third- or fourth-year students. The Great War thus found the navy resorting to the same measures that Burnett had grudgingly introduced 60 years before when student-dressers had been despatched to the Baltic.

Were the students right to find May unconvincing? May had tried to show how improvements had taken place since the 1880s when, perhaps, the service could have been justly criticized for its general inefficiency and for hospitals which, in terms of equipment, care and organization, had fallen behind the times. Its image in 1914 remained, though, that of a career which offered few advantages. What made this image hard to refute, as so often in the nineteenth century, were comparisons which could be drawn with the army where there appeared to be no shortage of suitable applicants. In July 1914 the army had 240,000 men attended by 982 medics. May knew that the navy's reputation in the universities and medical schools had always been poor; only recently the dean of medicine at Edinburgh had lauded the army for its superior avenues for advancement and medical specialization – a distinction subsequently reinforced, albeit in the hope of rectifying matters, by the British Medical Association. May glossed over the benefits conferred by the army just as he glossed over the widely held view that the navy's career structure was outdated, its hospitals afforded little opportunity to enhance expertise, its pay was poor and that complaints about inadequate accommodation on board ship could still be heard. Even when keeping up its strength by resorting to temporary measures the army was quicker off the mark. In 1913 the Admiralty learnt that the Royal Army Medical Corps was already signing up students to be dressers in an emergency, promising them the title of probationary lieutenant.

During his time as Director-General between 1908 and 1913 Porter tried to address this failure to recruit by setting up a medical consultative board to consider how a career in the navy might be made more attractive. He confided in February 1912 that he was 'horribly short of surgeons'. With well-trained sick-berth staff also in short supply it was, he concluded, 'the tightest squeeze I have yet had'.[54] A year later he showed the Board of Admiralty medical recruitment statistics for the first four months of 1913. The army had received 44 candidates for 20 vacancies. The Indian medical service had filled 12 commissions from among 28 applicants. Meanwhile the navy's 25 available openings had elicited only 17 responses, three of which were worthless. The consultative board urgently recommended an increase in pay, especially for junior surgeons. It also wanted medical officers to be given disciplinary control over sick-berth staff in shore establishments, charge of invaliding panels and cabins on warships according to rank alongside executive officers. Naval surgeons should also be allowed private practice in the same way that this perk was extended to their army colleagues, and a quarterly journal should be created for the naval service, with some pecuniary allowance for its editor, along the same lines as the *Journal of the Royal Army Medical Corps*. Finally, senior medical officers should replace executive officers in running overseas hospitals, as they had superseded the old Captains-Superintendent at home hospitals 40 years earlier. Some concessions were made at the Admiralty but a widespread pay increase was not forthcoming. A request that the Director-General's salary, pension entitlement and terms of employment should be brought into line with those of his army counterpart was likewise declined.[55]

It was harsh to characterize the naval medical service in 1914 as one where almost nothing had changed in half a century. Liddell had set in train developments in nursing and Richardson had brought home to the Admiralty that its hospitals were desperately in need of investment. Regarding the former, in 1883 a committee set up to investigate the limitations of nursing and sick-berth care emphatically condemned the traditional system of care by pensioners, the disabled and those otherwise unqualified. Most seamen were already aware of these shortcomings, as Admiral Reginald Bacon graphically recalled in 1925. Admitted as a midshipman first to Malta hospital and then to Haslar in 1882, he still remembered his constant hunger combined with appalling levels of personal attendance and soon came to understand why so many officers were reluctant to be sent to any naval hospital.[56] Opinions on a female nursing establishment remained divided, although by the mid-1880s Liddell's dream of 30 years before was slowly becoming a reality.

Much had changed in Britain since the 1850s. In short, the participation of women in the workplace had been transformed, as widespread education qualified many to fill the ever growing opportunities in offices, schools and healthcare. The invention of the typewriter in 1868 led to a revolution in clerical routine. In 1881 there were 6,420 female clerks in England and Wales; the number rose to 125,000 by 1911. Banking, retailing, insurance, communications services and large companies all required their labour. By 1911, 51,000 women were employed in the civil service and local government alone. Even in 1875 less than half the 23,656 elementary school teachers were men; thereafter the number of women teachers rose steadily to 172,000 by 1901. Nursing was likewise an expanding occupation for young women and now becoming fashionable among the class of girl which Liddell had most wished to encourage. There were 35,000 female nurses employed in England and Wales in 1881. In 1891 the total was 53,000. By the turn of the century the figure was 63,000, more than one-third of whom could be categorized as trained. Hospital training was a growth industry from the early 1880s. The Nightingale School set up at St Thomas's in 1860 had, in one way or another, been widely emulated. Increasing numbers of the sick were being cared for in hospitals, with many institutions advertising their excellent nursing regimes. Nursing had acquired status. Whereas the training contracts enforced by the Nightingale School in the early 1860s resembled a relationship between mistress and servant, the terms on which young women entered hospitals in the 1880s indicated admission to a profession. Gone were the days when nurses had been treated as little more than housemaids. By 1890 places for probationers at leading hospitals were heavily oversubscribed; St Thomas's admitted 50 every year and alone had trained 2,000 by 1903. An experienced sister might earn £50 per annum, with higher levels for supervisors and matrons. For those independent-minded daughters of the middle classes who were prepared to undergo the rigours of its training, and for those from poorer, albeit respectable families who aspired to advance in the social hierarchy, nursing, whether in hospitals or in the developing area of district nursing, had much to offer.[57]

Although the navy had proved hesitant in the face of Liddell's representations after 1856 the army had been more innovative regarding women. In 1861 a female army nursing service was established at Woolwich where Jane Shaw-Stewart supervised six nurses. Women were on the staff when the army opened its vast hospital at Netley in 1863; their pay and conditions were commensurate with those nursing in civilian institutions. In its regulations, however, the army acknowledged the difficulties which Liddell also faced: army sisters neither worked with venereal cases nor, until 1885, were they allowed to undertake night duties. Women also meant higher costs. Whereas male orderlies could undertake a range of fetching, carrying and other general duties, women were clearly less equipped for heavy work, often needed servants and separate accommodation, and saw themselves as specialist health providers. In consequence, their recruitment was slower than it might otherwise have been. As late as 1880 the army employed only about a dozen female nurses.

Revised regulations in 1885 extended opportunities beyond Netley and Woolwich: all army hospitals with above 100 beds now used women and even that size restriction was removed in 1893. In 1890 there were 60 nursing sisters working in 16 military hospitals in Britain and overseas. In 1882, 14 women went out to South Africa with the army in the aftermath of the Zulu War. A team from Netley was likewise sent to support the Egyptian campaign in 1882; between 1882 and 1885 about 35 women served in Egypt and the Sudan. By 1898 the army could boast 72 female nurses; it was, nevertheless, still taking on ten male orderlies for every one of them. The Boer War proved to be the catalyst for a rapid acceleration in recruitment. In October 1899 the army medical department had 12 women in South Africa; by March 1900 the figure was 800. Whatever reservations may have lingered were swept away by necessity. The creation of the Queen Alexandra's Imperial Military Nursing Service in 1902 recognized the contribution of so many volunteers. Its initial establishment of 228 women had been raised to 420 by 1905.[58]

Small though the numbers of women in army service remained until the beginning of the twentieth century, it was broadly conceded that their introduction had been successful and that Netley, from the 1860s onwards, offered high standards of nursing care. The 1883 naval committee which re-examined nursing provision could not ignore the army's favourable example. It agreed that qualified women should join its hospitals: after 1884, therefore, the navy employed professional staff, comprising carefully selected matrons who would superintend trained nursing sisters. Matrons, termed head sisters, should be at least 30 and nursing sisters at least 25 years of age, and the initial complement was for a matron and eight sisters at Haslar and a matron and five sisters at East Stonehouse. In 1887 the Melville appointed its new head sister. In 1889 nursing sisters went out to Malta, in 1896 they joined the staff at the Dartmouth Royal Naval College and in 1902 two were sent, at the surgeon's request, to the hospital at Hong Kong. By 1900 the navy had three head sisters and 28 others.[59]

Under regulations drawn up in 1884 nursing sisters were civilians and not subject to naval discipline. That remained so until 1977. Their duties and conduct were comprehensively stipulated, however, and included instruction for the sick-berth staff with whom they worked. Nursing in the armed forces could be lonely. Turnover was high, as the army discovered in the late 1890s when it transpired that fewer than half those who joined in 1893 had stayed for even five years. Nor was it an easy life, as Porter discovered in 1886 when introduced to two of the sisters recently sent to East Stonehouse. 'At first they had been put up in boxes like those of the young surgeons,' Porter heard. Senior medical staff then 'gave them the cold shoulder', until eventually they won over all opposition. Porter was enthusiastic, although by 1891 seemed less sure that the service could become an attractive career for young women. Seeing the burden which the Malta hospital imposed upon its nursing staff, he concluded that 'these women have a heavy time of it'. The same was true in South Africa in February 1899 when Porter noticed three nursing sisters being sent up to the army base at Ladysmith. It was isolated and even the soldiers were reportedly unhappy there. As for the women, 'these sisters will have to live under canvas, a rough sort of life for them'.[60] Work aboard hospital ships in the tropics could be unpleasant too. This began in 1898 when four sisters were sent out on *Malacca* to deal with 1,000 cases of malaria off West Africa. But the story was not simply one of heroism in the face of initial hostility and uncomfortable surround-

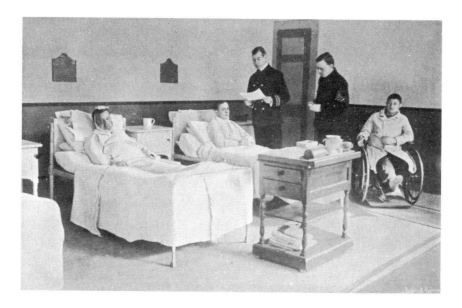

12. Surgical ward at the Melville: 1890s.

ings. Women at Dartmouth in the late 1890s proved to be a great annoyance, 'always wanting to shirk work and place it on the maidservants'.[61] Welcome as nursing sisters were in most naval establishments by the end of the century, they were not a panacea for all that was wrong.

Neglect, economies and slavish routine were held by many medical officers to characterize the way in which the Royal Navy still ran its shore establishments both at home and abroad. That said, May could reasonably claim in 1914 that some issues had been addressed. A medical school had been created at Haslar in 1881 which put the standard of naval medical training on a par with that which had existed for the army at Netley since the 1860s. In 1885 Haslar acquired a distinctive new water tower, a new deep well and a further modernization of its sewerage system. Its kitchens were refurbished in 1887 and many of its ward blocks were rebuilt between 1894 and 1896. Modern operating theatres were introduced in 1897; by 1904 well over 1,000 surgical operations were being performed annually at Haslar compared with only 15 trivial procedures in 1869.[62] Similar improvements could be claimed for East Stonehouse. A church was built inside the grounds in 1883, disinfectors were installed in the hospital in 1892 and the operating theatre updated between 1898 and 1904. The antiquated laundry, dating from 1808, was overhauled in 1899 when the mangling and work-

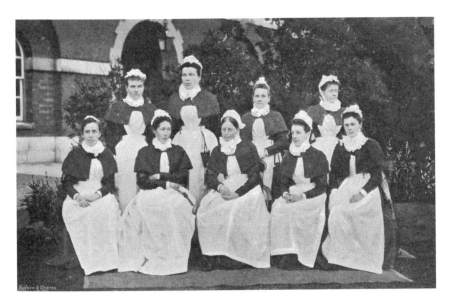

13. Post-1884 nursing sisters at Haslar.

rooms were reconstructed. Nine of the hospital blocks were refurbished between 1900 and 1906 with fireproof floors put in and bathing annexes added to each ward. Separate officers' accommodation was erected in 1900. A unit for infectious diseases, to take 50 patients, was built at the same time, as were quarters for nursing sisters and a new building to house the dispensary and hospital stores. In 1906 electricity superseded the old gas lighting and facilities for mental patients were completed. Open-air huts were provided for tuberculosis cases in 1908. East Stonehouse could even boast electric lifts in all its hospital blocks after 1912.[63] The home hospitals appeared to have entered the modern age. At Chatham, meanwhile, a new and expanded naval hospital was acquired in 1905 when the original Melville site was given over to the Royal Marines.

The Admiralty certainly believed that progress was being made. In addition to inquiring into sick-berth provision and how to improve knowledge of tropical diseases, the Board assured Porter in 1899 that 'we are also doing what money will allow to bring up the hospitals to something approaching modern ideas'.[64] A laboratory was opened at Haslar in 1899, making possible bacteriological research. Further advances there at the start of the twentieth century included new blocks for medical officers and nursing sisters in 1901, new hospital accommodation for naval officers in 1904 and the installation

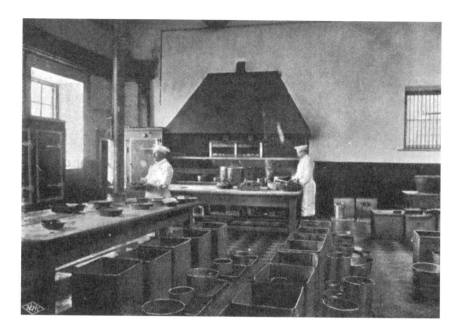

14. Post-1887 kitchens at Haslar.

of electric lighting in 1905. By this time Haslar certainly had an impressive staff establishment. The Inspector was assisted by two Deputy-Inspectors, a total of ten surgeons of varying degrees of seniority and six dispensers. The head sister had 14 women under her. Beyond the other specific offices of ward-master, storekeeper and cashier, chaplain and Inspector's secretary the institution employed 107 other staff, half of them in the general categories of labourers or servants to the medical officers.

Yet pre-eminent among naval hospitals as it was, and impressive to outsiders as its gradual upgrading might have appeared, Haslar was not a happy place to work. With a naval captain in overall command before the 1870s medical officers had generally found a common grievance. With no executive officer to blame for the way in which the hospital was run after 1870, however, personal and professional antagonisms increasingly soured the atmosphere. The problem lay, as often as not, with the manner in which Inspectors exercised their newly acquired administrative author-ity. Porter remembered James Watt Reid, Inspector in 1879–80, as 'that eminent shifter', and the medical school, for the foundation of which Reid had subsequently grabbed the credit, as nothing more than 'a sham and a fraud'.[65] Watt Reid had never intended it to be anything more; the medical school served its real purpose when it enabled his ambition to become Director-General to be realized in 1880. Porter also knew a great deal about the loathsome regime of Inspector Doyle Shaw between 1889 and 1892. Shaw was 'an ignorant pompo', Porter confided in 1890. When new medics joined the institution they were addressed by Shaw glorifying his own achievements while holding up his sleeve and exclaiming: 'these are an admiral's stripes'. It was all 'sickening twaddle'.[66] Shaw owed his position, and his retention of it, to his influence with the Director-General, Sir James Dick. Meanwhile Haslar was in chaos, with everyone hoping that Shaw would leave. Porter's opinion of Haslar had not altered by 1900 when he discovered that he was likely to be sent as Deputy-Inspector and realized that he lacked the necessary influence to get the appointment changed. The Inspector then was Richard Coppinger, 'a Jesuit with a system of espionage through police and other underlings', Porter discovered, who, at least on one occasion, seemed worryingly preoccupied with the lingerie issued to the nursing sisters.[67]

But were other naval hospitals run more smoothly? East Stonehouse certainly came in for criticism in 1891 after a surgeon was summarily removed because he needed outside help for an operation which he ought to have been able to complete unaided. Malta in 1890, like Haslar, seemed to be in a state of administrative disarray. Financial cutbacks dominated almost every area of the hospital's work. Seamen were reluctant to be sent there, patients were restricted to barely half the proper diet and the authority of medical staff was undermined by some issues of staff management having passed into the hands of the head sister. 'Even the charwoman has been dismissed,' Porter noted with astonishment when his ship put in there, 'and the stewards have to scrub the corridors & etc.' At the Cape in 1898 he was equally appalled when visiting Simon's Bay. 'This hospital here is prehistoric beyond words,' he concluded. Everywhere was evidence of neglect, either because Commanders-in-Chief had known or cared nothing about medical facilities or because medical officers over many years had been too cowed to remonstrate against the substandard conditions in which they had to work.[68] On a distant station the good will of the Commander-in-Chief remained essential for getting anything done.

Simon's Bay summed up so much that was unbearable for many in the medical service by the turn of the century. Doctors were too often in awe of executive officers drawn from distinguished naval families, while the

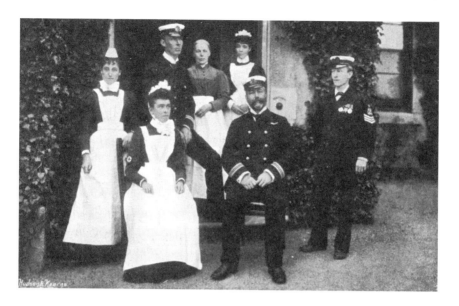

15. James Porter and staff at *Britannia*: 1897.

Medical Department lacked the public profile which might help to make it otherwise. Porter was prepared to concede that the exclusivity of the navy's officer corps had advantages: some medics were undoubtedly drawn to naval service because 'our executives are, if nothing else, at least gentlemen'. But the drawback was that by being so beholden and thereby often restrained in the proper practice of their profession, too many good men rejected or later left the service. This left it overly dependent on applications from 'waifs and strays, principally Irish, undesirably both medically and socially', Porter wrote disparagingly in 1890. Proper naval uniforms, though demanded by all medical staff in the early nineteenth century, had, it transpired, done nothing to increase the respect paid to surgeons throughout the fleet. Giving doctors distinctive lace and stripes only emphasized the fact that they were a sub-species of naval officer. Albeit too late by 1891, Porter wondered whether medical officers would fare better if they wore civilian clothes like chaplains and instructors rather than a uniform which he felt was 'destructive of self-respect by making men seem to be something which when put to the test they are not'.[69] The rot, however, started at the top. Those who ran the Admiralty still gave little thought to the men who literally had to pick up the pieces when the guns started firing.

In fact no one was spared criticism when Porter found time for private correspondence. The Queen took no interest in the navy, he asserted. She had always favoured the army, though as far as medical officers were concerned it probably made no difference since the medical Director-General of neither service, nor any honorary surgeons or physicians, were given a place in her funeral pageant. At the 1897 Jubilee no medals were awarded to any naval medic other than those serving on royal yachts. At the top of the service few knighthoods were handed out, he complained bitterly in 1899. 'The executives have to submit to an occasional bone being slung at the dogs, and they don't care what dog gets it.'[70] He was still arguing this point at the Admiralty before he retired in 1913. Only 16 medical officers on the active list of 527 then held any decoration whereas in the army 125 out of a total of 1,081 had been decorated. Was it any wonder that there were problems with recruitment? But Porter equally never spared a succession of Directors-General from his invective. Too many had been happy to enjoy their lives as senior Admiralty functionaries rather than champion the cause of medical colleagues.

After 1855 no Director-General served even half the length of Burnett's tenure nor acquired Burnett's standing. Liddell, admittedly, was an energetic man of reforming instincts who held the post for nine years. Alexander Armstrong was also long serving between 1869 and 1880. Watt Reid was Director-General for the following seven years, to be succeeded by James Dick between 1887 and 1898. Experience on the Board helped, but where the appointment was a poor one to begin with longevity in office was unlikely to make things much better. Michael Cowan and Dick were near contemporaries. 'Dick has been too much of a toady throughout his administrative career,' Cowan recalled in 1895.[71] This was a view which Porter shared. Years later, when Porter was embroiled in arguments with the First Lord, Winston Churchill, he recalled how Churchill's father had pared back expenditure on the navy's medical establishment in the 1880s 'willingly aided by ignorant Dick'.[72] In 1896 Dick failed to petition the Admiralty for more surgeons despite increases in the size of the navy. Henry Norbury was so economical as Director-General in 1901 that even the Board became frustrated: it 'could never get him to make suggestions because of the expense'.[73] Few were sorry when he retired in 1904.

Nevertheless costs were not at the root of everything. There was a pervasive culture which upheld precedent and tradition and placed little faith in ideas for change. The dead hand of seniority played its part in fostering such attitudes: promotion, especially to senior grades, too often owed little to ability and almost everything to the requisite years of service. For Porter, nothing exemplified the static practices of the service more than the Blane Medal which, he predicted accurately, he would never win. The prize had been awarded down the generations for journals written out in a clear hand where the style of compilation and presentation weighed more than the content. He revelled in the story of how Timotheus Haran, who became Inspector at East Stonehouse in 1886, had won the medal in 1875, having occupied the wardroom table aboard ship with books and journals for a whole year while writing 'goodness knows what day after day with patience and care, forming every letter, erasing smudges, making red ink lines'.[74] The tale might have seemed less significant had Porter not witnessed the effects of such inertia when with the 500 men of the naval brigade in South Africa. Warfare had changed: the naval medical service had not, it seemed, changed with it.

The British lost almost twice as many men from disease as from battle during the Boer War. Most, of course, were in the army, but being ashore at camp sites and when on the move the navy was exposed to unsanitary conditions, sickness, a lack of ambulance wagons and problems of supply as well as to enemy fire. Naval surgeons were in the front line, at field hospitals, at dressing stations, in hospital trains, with stretcher bearers, at base hospitals and on hospital ships. Two-tiered carriages on hospital trains were something new for naval medics: Porter found their rigid bed fixings quite unsuitable once in motion. The upper tier needed to be slung, as if a hammock, he reported. The lower tier needed rubber mountings to absorb the shock. In the field, wounded men were not collected promptly and, when survivors were gathered, too often they were all taken to the same place while other receiving stations stood idle. The general in command at Modder River in December 1899 did not seem to know where his three field hospitals were even five hours after the battle had ended. The truth was, Porter wrote home, 'the Boers are as well off medically as we are'. But, as a seasoned naval surgeon, he showed his experience when faced with a shambles. These were army arrangements and therefore 'nothing to do with me. I quietly worked away at the first collecting station.'[75]

It was also the army's fault that a number of surgeons and sick-berth staff sent out for the naval brigade were held back at Simon's Bay at the beginning of 1900, which meant that the brigade was short of medical cover. At the same time, sisters sent up to the Modder River camp absorbed more resources to make them comfortable than the need for their services merited. Porter reported the bread ration as a health hazard and lamented the standards of hygiene all around. Back in London the Director-General, Norbury, appeared to be administering a different war; 'You see more wounded in half an hour than probably he had in all his campaigns,' Porter concluded.[76] By April 1900 two of his three sick-berth stewards had collapsed from fever while of the brigade's original 33 stretcher bearers only 11 were still standing. Yet ships offshore were crammed with men, he observed. Why had the brigade been sent no replacements? In a complaint reminiscent of those from the Crimea, Porter explained how he had been forced to draw upon marines from the ranks and blue-jackets from the gun crews. Against that background, assurances from the Board that medical reforms in the navy were progressing well, that medical chests were being updated and that hospitals and equipment were becoming more efficient were not convincing. Money was supposed to be available for whatever the Medical Department needed. Understandably, that was why Porter was sure that the blame lay with Norbury for never asking.

Porter's widely acknowledged success in South Africa owed much to good fortune and to the ability to improvise upon which the naval medical service prided itself. In any case, as in the Crimea, it was the army which came under scrutiny while the navy took comfort from a small job reasonably well done. There were even moments of optimism – as when Field Marshal Lord Roberts inspected and then addressed medical staff with the naval brigade near Bloemfontein in March 1900. Roberts specifically asked to meet the stretcher bearers who duly stepped forward accompanied by the three surgeons in charge. He then thanked Porter and all his men for their gallantry amid danger and the professional manner in which all had acquitted themselves. Roberts, of course, was there to maintain morale, yet Porter much appreciated the gesture. Even with the war still raging Porter sensed that the navy's medics would come out of it with credit. 'The days of back seat for medical services are, I believe, over,' he predicted cheerfully.[77] Needless to say, he should have known better. In 1912, when Churchill withdrew £4,000 promised for new stretchers, Porter was furious that his department had been betrayed. The Japanese, American and Greek navies already had this equipment and in any war the Royal Navy's deficiency would be keenly felt. But, as so often, the grievance went further than simply economy: the Director-General had not even been consulted in advance.

Stretchers might have been a trivial issue over which to express so much

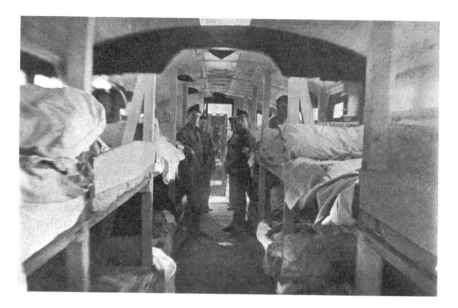

16. Naval brigade wounded aboard an ambulance train: South Africa 1899.

resentment had they not been in an area where Porter had always taken a particular interest – the sick-bay. The 1883 committee had envisaged a total complement of 396 sick-berth staff for the Royal Navy, of whom 223 would be afloat and 173 in hospitals and sick quarters ashore, while it set in motion programmes to promote training in hygiene, first aid, dispensing, nursing care and sick-room cookery – all of which, alongside the introduction of nursing sisters and greater knowledge of tropical medicine, Porter regarded as major advances.[78] There were, however, few expectations of rapid improvement. When the Deputy-Inspector at Bermuda reported two of his old hospital attendants to be worthless in 1886 he found the executive officer responsible at best disinterested. In 1890 Porter sent one useless helper aboard *Scout* to the Malta hospital in the hope that a pulmonary disorder would prevent any return, while another man detailed to work for him was usually polishing the ship's brass. Norbury, for all his limitations as Director-General, cared about this issue too. Norbury always remembered the diligence and skill of his sick-berth steward when ashore in 1879 during the Zulu War.[79] In 1900 he arranged warrant rank for head ward-masters – the most senior sick-berth officers at Haslar and East Stonehouse. Porter had the opportunity to carry these reforms further after 1908 and, despite his difficulties with Churchill, was acknowledged to have done much to improve conditions for all employed in routine care and nursing. After announcing his retirement Porter received a touching tribute from the head ward-master at Haslar, thanking the Director-General for all that he had done for this otherwise forgotten branch of naval service.

Yet for the audience which May was addressing during his recruitment drive in 1914, patchy improvements since the 1880s were not enough to overcome stereotypical perceptions. To that extent, the navy paid the price for neglecting grievances voiced for a century past. It had become a matter of trust. Wardroom rank for assistant surgeons, sanctioned in 1805, was not attained in practice until 1855; this stain upon the character of highly educated young men was not soon forgotten. Having no cabins, again after the navy had promised to make provision, likewise rankled with assistants. Station commanders had seldom favoured the idea but, while there were practical considerations, quite why appropriate cabins for all medical staff were still being offered as an inducement as late as 1914 was hard to explain. The title of assistant surgeon was abolished in 1873, whereupon the status of senior surgeons was acknowledged by the prefixes staff or fleet. But that did not remove other slights which surgeons of all ranks felt they still endured. Not until 1914 did medics join courts martial as equals to executive officers and only then were they granted the professional privilege of patient confidentiality.

In the late nineteenth century captains might still impose their own medical evaluations or disregard a surgeon's opinion which did not suit them. At Malta in 1891 *Temeraire's* commanding officer refused to face up to the fact that his midshipmen had picked up typhoid when allowed ashore at Smyrna. He would not accept that young gentlemen could be laid low by a bacillus usually found among ordinary seamen. A few months later Porter was ignored when sailors on *Scout* went down with diarrhoea. It was obviously due to the issue of rotten bread, yet, although he was the only man on board who had any training in or knowledge of hygiene, executive officers never invited his opinion. In South Africa in 1900 his advice to move the brigade camp to a healthier site was rejected by the commanding officer on the grounds that since no sickness had yet appeared therefore none was likely. A year later he was horrified when the admiral decided to put *Monarch* into Cape Town dock. The docks were overrun with rats, plague was rumoured to be out of control in the vicinity and specific medical advice to avoid the area had already been given. Porter expressed the customary surgeons' lament: on the one hand the admiral acknowledged his indispensable services while, on the other, 'when my precious advice does not square with his preconceived ideas it is not at all appreciated'.[80]

Pay, inevitably, remained a sore point whether as an absolute figure or in comparison with army levels. Beyond that, by the mid-nineteenth century the differential between the pay scales of surgeons and assistants and those for executive officers had also gradually widened in favour of the latter. Of course, men who joined the navy knew in advance that they would never be rich: in financial terms, as Michael Cowan advised the young Porter in 1886, the necessary calculation was between a certain and uncertain future. Nevertheless whatever regulations might allow, there were always some chances to earn a little extra. Cowan recalled how one old colleague at Bermuda made 'not a little' money from unofficial practice outside his dockyard duties. 'I think I got some small gifts in my day,' Cowan added modestly. Work done for a grateful patient privately 'does not involve sending in a bill'.[81]

Profitable opportunities among the population living around an overseas hospital, however, were small comfort to surgeons who found themselves on ships infested with rats and cockroaches, homesick, and where their few possessions were in constant danger from flooding. Not only that, but among shore appointments abroad there was still a distinct order of preference. 'Malta the best,' Cowan reflected in 1880, 'Bermuda next best or possibly Jamaica, and worst of all Hong Kong.'[82] The belief that patronage and chance played the greatest parts in advancement survived into the twentieth century. Despite encouragement from Louis Battenberg, his former Commander-in-Chief when in the Mediterranean, Porter had all but written off his prospects by 1899. When Norbury offered him the Simon's Bay hospital early in 1900 Porter turned it down, calculating that his only chance of reaching higher levels lay with the uncertainties of war. He was right. 'South Africa has indeed served you well,' one old friend reminded Porter in 1908. 'I told you there were always immense possibilities of picking up something on that station.'[83] But though he argued throughout his career that too much in the navy turned on favouritism, Porter still managed to reach the top. Perhaps the service was never quite as insensitive to talent as so many disgruntled members down the generations claimed.

But if defects were still evident before the First World War, so too were the attractions of a life spent so much abroad with the world's foremost naval power. Modest as material rewards might be, a naval uniform still represented mastery of the seas for the public at home, and though politicians might hold the purse strings tight they would never deny the nation's debt to those who tended the imperial fleet. 'They have an unanswerable claim to the consideration of their country,' the First Lord, Sir John Pakington, reminded the House of Commons when introducing the naval estimates for 1859–60. No body of men discharged their duties in nobler or more gallant fashion.[84] In 1862 Milroy similarly praised the naval medical service: 'In no branch of the profession can abler and more enlightened men be found.'[85] Some joined from family tradition; it was a way of life and not unnaturally the navy drew those eager to follow a trodden path. Others were drawn, as always, to the exceptional, exotic and sometimes exciting opportunities which the navy alone could provide. 'Queer how distorted visions become about professions outside those we happen to be stuck to,' Porter mused in 1898. There were better openings for promising young doctors than a life in the navy, he continued, 'but then it looks all roses to them'.[86]

Perhaps what distinguished naval surgeons had changed little since Burnett's youth when he had been present at Nelson's great battles. The glue which held the corps together was comradeship. Edward Cree felt this deeply when the crew of *Rattlesnake* assembled to cheer him off to his new ship in 1843. Despite uncertainty about his future, Porter felt the same in 1899. He could never consider his life misspent in the service. He looked back then on 20 years characterized by 'the strong bonds born of the stark naked intimacy of ship and service life'.[87] Needless to say, an understanding wife was an indispensable asset. Porter found his in 1886. As a struggling junior posted to the Bermuda hospital he had fallen for the Deputy-Inspector's daughter. Worried that Michael Cowan had harboured hopes for a more favourable match, Porter asked parental consent apologetically in light of his modest origins, poor pay and lack of any connections. He need not have fretted. Cowan's children were brought up to a lifestyle dominated by ships, hospitals and long family separations. 'Depend upon it,' Cowan replied graciously: 'Lutie knew when she accepted you what she was to look forward to.'[88]

Notes

Introduction

1. J. Keevil, *Medicine and the Navy 1200–1900*, vol. I, *1200–1648* (London, 1957), and vol. II, *1649–1714* (London, 1958).
2. C. Lloyd and J. Coulter, *Medicine and the Navy 1200–1900*, vol. III, *1714–1815* (London, 1961), and vol. IV, *1815–1900* (London, 1963).
3. N. Cantlie, *A History of the Army Medical Department*, 2 vols. (London, 1974).
4. An area of economic activity most recently explored in G. Bannerman, *Merchants and the Military in Eighteenth-Century Britain: British Army Contracts and Domestic Supply, 1739–1763* (London, 2008).
5. Y. Akiyama, 'Trained Cooks and Healthy Boys: Reforming the Mess in the Royal Navy before the First World War', *Mariner's Mirror* 94 (2008), pp 420–431. The place of both army and navy in promoting health, diet and even cookery in late nineteenth-century Britain is explained in Y. Akiyama, *Feeding the Nation: Nutrition and Health in Britain before World War One* (London, 2008). Changing routines and conditions on the lower deck in the early twentieth century are chronicled in C. McKee, *Sober Men and True: Sailor Lives in the Royal Navy 1900–1945* (London, 2002).
6. Martin to Porter, 20 January 1915, Papers of Sir James Porter, National Maritime Museum (NMM), Greenwich, MS 85/088.
7. J. Shepherd, *The Crimean Doctors: A History of the British Medical Services in the Crimean War* (Liverpool, 1991), vol. II, p 633.

Chapter 1. The Age of Cook and Nelson

1. G. Milroy, *The Health of the Royal Navy Considered in a letter addressed to the Rt. Hon. Sir John S. Pakington, Bart. M.P.* (London, 1862), p 1.
2. Figures are from D. Pope, *Life in Nelson's Navy* (London, 1997), p 131; and N. Blake and R. Lawrence, *The Illustrated Companion to Nelson's Navy* (London, 1999), p 94.

3.   J. Watt, 'Surgeons of the Mary Rose: The Practice of Surgery in Tudor England', *Mariner's Mirror* 69 (1983), pp 3–19. The standard work for this period remains Keevil, *Medicine and the Navy,* vol. I.

4.   S. Jenkinson, 'John Woodall, Surgeon, Royal Navy 1569–1643', *Journal of the Royal Naval Medical Service* 26 (1940), pp 107–116; and R. Williamson, 'John Woodall and his Book, "The Surgeon's Mate"', *Journal of the Royal Naval Medical Service* 11 (1925), pp 190–192. Woodall's career and the early Stuart navy are also discussed in Keevil, *Medicine and the Navy,* vol. I, pp 177–226.

5.   D. Stewart, 'Surgeon-General James Pierce, R.N.', *Journal of the Royal Naval Medical Service* 36 (1950), pp 214–225. Keevil also analyses his career in *Medicine and the Navy,* vol. II.

6.   Yonge's career is examined in E. Harper, 'The Sailor's Surgeon', *Journal of the Royal Naval Medical Service* 65 (1979), pp 35–37. See also Keevil, *Medicine and the Navy,* vol. II.

7.   S. Jenkinson, 'John Moyle, Surgeon, Royal Navy', *Journal of the Royal Naval Medical Service* 38 (1952), pp 1–7. See also Keevil, *Medicine and the Navy,* vol. II.

8.   Conditions for surgeons in the late seventeenth and early eighteenth centuries are succinctly explained in R. Allison, 'Sea Surgeons', *Journal of the Royal Naval Medical Service* 27 (1941), pp 125–137.

9.   Surgeons' Petition *c.*1780, reproduced in J. Hattendorf, R. Knight, A. Pearsall, N. Rodger and G. Till (eds), *British Naval Documents 1204–1960* (London, 1993), pp 537–538.

10.   Cook's voyages are discussed in Lloyd and Coulter, *Medicine and the Navy,* vol. III, pp 303–319; and in R. Williamson, 'Captain James Cook, R.N., F.R.S., and his Contribution to Medical Science', *Journal of the Royal Naval Medical Service* 14 (1928), pp 19–22. See also C. Lloyd, 'Cook and Scurvy', *Mariner's Mirror* 65 (1979), pp 23–28. Relevant extracts from A. Kitson, *Captain James Cook R.N., F.R.S.: The Circumnavigator* (London, 1907) appeared as 'Abstract from "Captain James Cook" by Kitson (1907)', *Journal of the Royal Naval Medical Service* 26 (1940), pp 329–335. The most recent biography is D. O'Sullivan, *In Search of Captain Cook: Exploring the Man through his Own Words* (London, 2008). Cook's exploits were witnessed and recorded by W. Ellis, *An Authentic Narrative of a Voyage Performed by Captain Cook and Captain Clerke, in His Majesty's Ships Resolution and Discovery during the years 1776, 1777, 1778, 1779, and 1780* (London, 1782).

11.   Selections from Lind's works are reproduced in C. Lloyd, *The Health of Seamen* (London, 1965), pp 2–130. Lind's contribution to naval medicine has

been thoroughly investigated over many years, beginning with H. Rolleston, 'James Lind: Pioneer of Naval Hygiene', *Journal of the Royal Naval Medical Service* 1 (1915), pp 181–190. His career is analysed in Lloyd and Coulter, *Medicine and the Navy*, vol. III, pp 296–303; and D. Thomas and E. Bardolph, 'Prevention of Scurvy in the Royal Navy', *Journal of the Royal Naval Medical Service* 84 (1998), pp 107–109. See also H. Whiteside, 'Some Problems (Old and New) of the Seafaring Doctor', *Journal of the Royal Naval Medical Service* 17 (1931), pp 1–5; J. Glass, 'James Lind, M.D. Eighteenth-Century Naval Medical Hygienist', *Journal of the Royal Naval Medical Service* 35 (1949), pp 1–20, 68–86; and R. Hughes, 'James Lind and the Cure of Scurvy: An Experimental Approach', *Medical History* 19 (1975), pp 342–351.

12. Blane's career, like that of Lind, has been extensively covered since H. Rolleston, 'Sir Gilbert Blane: An Administrator of Naval Medicine and Hygiene', *Journal of the Royal Naval Medical Service* 2 (1916), pp 72–81; and S. Jenkinson, 'Biography of Sir Gilbert Blane (1749–1834)', *Journal of the Royal Naval Medical Service* 23 (1937), pp 293–301. Blane's work is referred to throughout Lloyd and Coulter, *Medicine and the Navy*, vol. III, and sections of it are reproduced in Lloyd, *Health of Seamen*, pp 132–211.

13. W. Wright, 'Ageing in the Royal Navy', *Journal of the Royal Naval Medical Service* 48 (1962), pp 199–204.

14. Rolleston, 'Sir Gilbert Blane', p 76. Aside from the extensive discussions of diet, medical treatments, hygiene and ventilation aboard ships during the eighteenth century contained in Lloyd and Coulter, *Medicine and the Navy*, vol. III, there are informative surveys of conditions and health hazards at sea in G. Southwell-Sander, 'The Development of Naval Preventive Medicine', *Journal of the Royal Naval Medical Service* 43 (1957), pp 54–74; and R. James, 'A Naval Surgeon's Log, 1781–1783', *Journal of the Royal Naval Medical Service* 19 (1933), pp 221–240. More recent is J. Bowden-Dan, 'Diet, Dirt and Discipline: Medical Developments in Nelson's Navy. Dr. John Snipe's Contribution', *Mariner's Mirror* 90 (2004), pp 260–272.

15. Selections from Trotter's publications are reproduced in Lloyd, *Health of Seamen*, pp 214–316. His career has also been evaluated in most scholarship concerned with the cure of scurvy and medical conditions at sea since the work of H. Rolleston, 'Thomas Trotter M.D.', *Journal of the Royal Naval Medical Service* 5 (1919), 412–419. See, for example, I. Porter, 'Thomas Trotter, M.D., Naval Physician', *Medical History* 7 (1963), pp 155–164. Likewise that of Gillespie since T. Gillespie, 'The Diet and Health of Seamen in the West Indies at the End of the Eighteenth Century – Some Remarks on the Work

of Leonard Gillespie, M.D.', *Journal of the Royal Naval Medical Service* 37 (1951), pp 187–192. The achievements of both Trotter and Gillespie are covered in Lloyd and Coulter, *Medicine and the Navy*, vol. III. Senior naval officers at this time, however, also had a role to play in overcoming scurvy, as explained in B. Vale, 'The Conquest of Scurvy in the Royal Navy 1793–1800: A Challenge to Current Orthodoxy', *Mariner's Mirror* 94 (2008), pp 160–175.

16. Outlines of the Greenwich Hospital's history in the eighteenth century are provided in R. Bornmann, 'Doctors at Greenwich', *Journal of the Royal Naval Medical Service* 57 (1971), pp 145–149; and Lloyd and Coulter, *Medicine and the Navy*, vol. III, pp 196–206.

17. Craven to Owen, 19 May 1812, Haslar Hospital Records, National Archives (NA), London, ADM305/41. There is much information available about Haslar's early history in Lloyd and Coulter, *Medicine and the Navy*, vol. III, pp 207–260; Anon, 'Haslar', *Journal of the Royal Naval Medical Service* 39 (1953), pp 59–62; and W. Tait, *A History of Haslar Hospital* (Portsmouth, 1906). An interesting contemporary account is given in Lind to Dick, 3 September 1758, reproduced in R. Stockman, 'James Lind and Scurvy', *Journal of the Royal Naval Medical Service* 13 (1927), pp 81–98; and another by George Pinckard, 23 October 1795, reproduced in 'Puellae Porti Magni', *Journal of the Royal Naval Medical Service* 89 (2003), pp 73–75.

18. Lord Dundonald, *Observations on Naval Affairs* (London, 1847), p 19.

19. Henderson to Wood, 25 January 1836, Admiralty Records, NA, ADM97/140. The early history of the East Stonehouse hospital is told in A. Hurford, 'The Early History of Plymouth Hospital', *Journal of the Royal Naval Medical Service* 21 (1935), pp 40–47, 138–151, 249–252; and R. Johnson, 'The Diary of the First Governor of Plymouth Hospital', *Journal of the Royal Naval Medical Service* 2 (1916), pp 191–199. Lloyd and Coulter devote a chapter to it in *Medicine and the Navy*, vol. III, pp 261–290. See also P. Pugh, 'History of the Royal Naval Hospital, Plymouth', *Journal of the Royal Naval Medical Service* 58 (1972), pp 78–94, 207–226.

20. St Vincent to Baird, 27 August 1813, Papers of Sir William Parker, NMM, PAR/167/A.

21. Burnett to Graham, 12 March 1833, letterbooks of Sir William Burnett, NA, ADM105/70.

22. Craven to Curtis, 18 December 1810, Haslar Hospital Records, ADM305/41.

23. Craven to Bickerton, 17 January 1815, Haslar Hospital Records, ADM305/41.

24. T. Trotter, *A Review of the Medical Department in the British Navy with a Method of Reform proposed in a Letter to the Rt. Hon. the Earl of Chatham,*

First Lord of the Admiralty (London, 1790).

25. Quoted in Lloyd and Coulter, *Medicine and the Navy,* vol. III, p 31.

26. Conditions for seamen, diseases, instruments, drugs and the practice of naval medicine in the era of the French wars are covered in J. Goddard, 'An Insight into the Life of Royal Naval Surgeons during the Napoleonic War', *Journal of the Royal Naval Medical Service* 77 (1991), pp 205–222; and 78 (1992), pp 27–36. See also R. Hill, 'A Retrospective View of Naval Medical Conditions', *Journal of the Royal Naval Medical Service* 6 (1920), pp 1–12; J. Keevil, 'Ralph Cuming and the Interscapulo-Thoracic Amputation in 1808', *Journal of the Royal Naval Medical Service* 36 (1950), pp 63–72; N. Baldock, 'Health in the Royal Navy during the Age of Nelson: The Institute of Naval Medicine', *Journal of the Royal Naval Medical Service* 86 (2000), pp 60–63; J. Watt, 'Surgery at Trafalgar', *Mariner's Mirror* 91 (2005), pp 266–283; and J. Watt, 'Health in the Royal Navy during the Age of Nelson: Nelsonian Medicine in Context', *Journal of the Royal Naval Medical Service* 86 (2000), pp 64–71. J. Laffin, *Surgeons in the Field* (London, 1970), pp 99–115 also provides a good outline regarding disease and injuries at sea in this period. The origins of better care in cockpits and designated sick-bays are described in P. Goodwin, 'Health in the Royal Navy during the Age of Nelson: The Development of the Sick Berth 1740–1815 and its Relation to H.M.S. *Victory*', *Journal of the Royal Naval Medical Service* 86 (2000), pp 81–84; N. Blake, *Steering to Glory: A Day in the Life of a Ship of the Line* (London, 2005), pp 90–95; and G. Dickenson, 'The Origin of the Sick Berth Staff, Royal Navy', *Journal of the Royal Naval Medical Service* 13 (1927), pp 161–173. Hygiene improvements, victualling and ventilation are described in Lloyd and Coulter, *Medicine and the Navy,* vol. III, pp 70–93; T. Shaw, 'Ventilation in H.M. Ships from the Earliest Times to the Present Day', *Journal of the Royal Naval Medical Service* 12 (1926), pp 175–201; and W. Simpson, 'Progress of Hygiene in the Navy and its Effect on the Health of the Sailors', *Journal of the Royal Naval Medical Service* 1 (1915), pp 300–314. The most recent work covering all aspects of a sailor's life in the late eighteenth and early nineteenth centuries is R. Adkins and L. Adkins, *Jack Tar: Life in Nelson's Navy* (London, 2008).

27. The career of Harness is analysed in S. Jenkinson, 'Biographical Memoir of Dr. John Harness', *Journal of the Royal Naval Medical Service* 23 (1937), pp 2–14.

28. Tait, *History of Haslar,* pp 104–106.

29. Change in the navy after the French wars is discussed in C. Bartlett, *Great Britain and Sea Power 1815–1853* (Oxford, 1963); and A. Lambert, 'Preparing

for the Long Peace: The Reconstruction of the Royal Navy 1815–1830', *Mariner's Mirror* 82 (1996), pp 41–54. See also B. Greenhill and A. Giffard, *Steam, Politics and Patronage: The Transformation of the Royal Navy 1815–54* (London, 1994). For a contemporary political account see C. Wood, *State of the Navy* (London, 1839).

30. The reforms of the early 1830s are outlined in Graham memorandum, 6 December 1831, reproduced in Hattendorf et al (eds), *British Naval Documents*, pp 646–650. See also Bartlett, *Great Britain and Sea Power*, pp 49–53; R. Hamilton, *Naval Administration: The Constitution, Character and Functions of the Board of Admiralty, and of the Civil Departments it Directs* (London, 1896), pp 106–108; R. Morriss, *Cockburn and the British Navy in Transition: Admiral Sir George Cockburn 1772–1853* (Exeter, 1997), p 144; and R. Morriss, *Naval Power and British Culture 1760–1850: Public Trust and Government Ideology* (Aldershot, 2004). The subsequent work of the Medical Department is indicated in Burnett to Ashley, 12 March 1835, Burnett letterbook, ADM105/70. There are biographical sketches of Burnett by H. Rolleston, 'Sir William Burnett: The First Medical Director-General of the Royal Navy', *Journal of the Royal Naval Medical Service* 8 (1922), pp 1–10; and S. Jenkinson, 'Sir William Burnett', *Journal of the Royal Naval Medical Service* 26 (1940), pp 3–15. The starting point for these was a piece published in *The Lancet*, 16 November 1850. Burnett's career is summarized in Lloyd and Coulter, *Medicine and the Navy*, vol. IV, pp 2–6.

31. Burnett to Ward, 28 December 1847, ADM105/39.

32. Journal entry, 8 January 1853. Reproduced in J. Bockstoce (ed), *The Journal of Rochfort Maguire 1852–1854: Two Years at Point Barrow, Alaska, aboard HMS Plover in the search for Sir John Franklin* (London, 1988), vol. I, p 151; Burnett memorandum, 3 June 1851, Burnett letterbook, ADM105/68. Goldner's supplies and storage problems generally are discussed in Lloyd and Coulter, *Medicine and the Navy*, vol. IV, pp 96–106. The destruction of condemned stores at Portsmouth in the early 1850s is mentioned in L. Stephens, *History of the Naval Victualling Department and its Association with Plymouth* (Plymouth, 1996), chapter 9, p 1. Ships destined for the Arctic in 1819 had 'a large quantity of Messrs. Donkin and Hall's preserved meats and soups supplied'. A. Fisher, *A Journal of a Voyage of Discovery to the Arctic Regions in His Majesty's Ships Hecla and Griper in the Years 1819 and 1820* (London, 1821), pxi. One officer with the expedition also remarked in a letter dated 12 November 1819 on 'a considerable supply of Donkin's preserved meat, of concentrated vegetable soup, vinegar, lime-juice, wine, beer &etc'. An Offi-

cer of the Expedition, *Letters Written during the Late Voyage of Discovery in the Western Arctic Sea* (London, 1821), p 51. 'Preserved meats, according to Donkin's invention, in consequence of their portability and excellence' still featured prominently in provisions for Antarctic exploration 20 years later when in 1839 Gamble and Cooper were separately listed among six suppliers of preserved meats, concentrated soups and vegetables. Sir James Ross, *A Voyage of Discovery and Research in the Southern and Antarctic Regions, during the years 1839–43* (London, 1847), vol. I, pp xix–xx.

33. Burnett memorandum, 11 June 1832, ADM97/133.
34. Burnett memoranda, 25 January, 7 April 1841, Burnett letterbook, ADM105/72.
35. Fossett memorandum, 10 February 1851, ADM97/191.
36. Liddell memoranda, 14 January, 31 March 1856, ADM97/225. Comparative office loads for 1830 and 1850 are from minutes by Fossett and MacLaurin on Parker to Burnett, 8 December 1851, ADM97/195; while those for 1853–54 and 1854–55 are from Fossett memorandum, 5 April 1855, ADM97/213.
37. Burnett memorandum, 26 July 1854, ADM97/213.
38. Budget figures are from Burnett memoranda, 11 January 1833, ADM97/134; 13 January 1834, Burnett letterbook, ADM105/70.
39. Burnett memorandum, 26 April 1839, Burnett letterbook, ADM105/72.
40. Burnett memoranda, 13, 26 April 1839, Burnett letterbook, ADM105/72.
41. Burnett memorandum, 20 July 1833, ADM97/134.

Chapter 2. Surgeons at Sea in the Early Nineteenth Century

1. Report by Burnett, 23 February 1846, ADM105/38. Figures regarding recruitment and comparisons with the army are from Burnett memorandum, 6 March 1834, Burnett letterbook, ADM105/70; *The Lancet*, 15 January 1848, p 80; and Burnett memorandum, 19 December 1837, Burnett letterbook, ADM105/71.
2. Burnett to Richmond, 19 August 1841, Papers of the Duke of Richmond (Goodwood Papers), West Sussex Record Office, Chichester, 1619.
3. Burnett memorandum, 2 December 1852, Burnett letterbook, ADM105/68.
4. Dillon to Stilwell, 11 February 1841, Papers of Henry Willan, in the temporary keeping of the author, HW4/1/1; Cowan to John Cowan, 22 April, 30 May, 3 August, 31 October 1854; Papers of Michael Cowan (preserved among the papers of Sir James Porter), NMM, PTR/1.
5. Burnett memorandum, 24 May 1848, ADM105/39.
6. Cowan to John Cowan, 3 July 1856, Cowan Papers, PTR/1. Figures relating to

the number of medical officers, their pay and pension rates are from Burnett to Graham, 14 June 1831, Papers of the Earl of Minto, NMM, ELL/245; and Burnett to Grey, 23 January 1835, ADM97/137. Pay for surgeons and assistants is discussed in Lloyd and Coulter, *Medicine and the Navy*, vol. IV, pp 11–20. Data specific to the years 1817–30 are available in Parliamentary Accounts and Papers (P.P.) (1830), XVIII.

7. Arguments and statistics regarding commutation are elaborated in Burnett memorandum, 23 December 1833, and Burnett to Berkeley, 15, 20 May 1834, Burnett letterbook, ADM105/70.

8. Accounts of this exist in the letters of William Dent and are discussed in L. Woodford (ed), *A Young Surgeon in Wellington's Army* (Woking, 1976); and L. Woodford, 'A Medical Student's Career in the Early Nineteenth Century', *Medical History* 14 (1970), pp 90–95. Medical provision and reform in the army are comprehensively covered in Cantlie, *A History of the Army Medical Department*. Military losses in the West Indies are analysed in M. Duffy, *Soldiers, Sugar and Seapower: The British Expeditions to the West Indies and the War against Revolutionary France* (Oxford, 1987), pp 326–367. See also J. Laffin, *Surgeons in the Field* (London, 1970).

9. Detailed comparisons between army and navy pay were made in Burnett to Graham, 14 June 1831, Minto Papers, ELL/245; Burnett memorandum, 25 January 1836, Burnett letterbook, ADM105/71; enclosure in Burnett to Richmond, 14 July 1838, Goodwood Papers, 1584; and Burnett memorandum, 17 March 1855, ADM97/218.

10. Burnett memorandum, 14 December 1837, Burnett letterbook, ADM105/71.

11. Report by Burnett, 23 February 1846, ADM105/38.

12. Burnett to Richmond, 14 July 1838, Goodwood Papers, 1584.

13. Diary, 17 August 1844, Papers of Sir Thomas Cochrane, National Library of Scotland, Edinburgh, MS 2601.

14. Bayne to Burnett, 29 September 1837, ADM97/143.

15. Journal of Robert Guthrie, 22 September 1828, NMM, JOD/16.

16. Report by Burnett, 23 February 1846, ADM105/38. Surgeon Alexander Mackay recorded his satisfaction in 1860 when medical officers were permitted to wear the distinctive marks of the executive officers with whom they ranked on their uniforms. Diary of Alexander Mackay, 6, 5 July 1860, Royal Naval Museum, Portsmouth. Grievances regarding status are discussed in S. Jenkinson, 'The Medical Officers', *Journal of the Royal Naval Medical Service* 35 (1949), pp 87–90; and R. Allison, 'One Hundred Years of Commissioned Rank', *Journal of the Royal Naval Medical Service* 29 (1943), pp 83–90. The

most exhaustive contemporary expression of dissatisfaction appeared as a 28-page pamphlet from A Naval Medical Officer, *An Exposition of the Case of the Assistant Surgeons of the Royal Navy* (London, 1849). Earlier an article 'Brutal Treatment of Naval Assistant Surgeons', dated December 1847 and attributed to An Assistant Surgeon, R.N., was published in *The Lancet*, 15 January 1848, pp 80–81.

17. Baring to Hornby, 31 January 1849, Papers of Sir Francis Baring (Northbrook Papers), ING Baring, London, NP/5/1/3/6.

18. Minute by Burnett on Palmer to Admiralty, 30 June 1854, ADM97/212.

19. Burnett memorandum, 30 December 1850, ADM105/39.

20. McIlroy to Victualling Commissioners, 13 December 1830, ADM97/52.

21. Burnett memorandum, 16 May 1849, ADM97/182.

22. Robertson to Burnett, 3 August 1853, ADM97/205.

23. Cowan to John Cowan, 3 August 1854 and 19 June 1862, Cowan Papers, PTR/1. Alexander Mackay also records timely visits to Somerset House to advance his claim for promotion to Deputy-Inspector. Mackay diaries, 5 and 6, 1 August 1859 and 13 April 1860.

24. Burnett memorandum, 1 July 1852, ADM105/39; Bryson memorandum 27 June 1853, ADM97/204; Burnett memorandum, 31 October 1854, ADM105/39; Minute by Liddell on Tucker to Milne, 22 May 1856, ADM97/227.

25. Dolling to Burnett, 15 May 1847, ADM97/171; minute by Burnett on Lithgow to Burnett, 24 November 1852, ADM97/200; Burnett to Layton, 20 October 1852, ADM97/200; Burnett memorandum, 11 August 1854, ADM97/214.

26. Report on *Belleisle*, 9 March to 31 March 1859, ADM102/850.

27. Burnett memorandum, 5 June 1852, Burnett letterbook, ADM105/68.

28. Crellin to Burnett, 10 August 1846, ADM97/169.

29. Barrow to Burnett, 28 January 1842, ADM97/28.

30. Minute by Burnett on Conyngham to Burnett, 24 May 1839, ADM97/147.

31. Story to Preston, 4 September 1852, enclosed in Preston to Burnett, 4 September 1852, ADM97/199.

32. Milne to Baring, 22 November 1851, Northbrook Papers, NP5/1/3/11.

33. Hawes to Admiralty, 12 January 1854, ADM97/207.

34. Burnett memorandum, 29 June 1838, Burnett letterbook, ADM105/71.

35. Campbell to Burnett, 2 May 1850, ADM97/187.

36. Fossett memorandum, 7 May 1845, ADM97/163.

37. Minute by Bryson on Crawford to Burnett, 10 September 1851, ADM97/194.

38. Minute by Burnett on Taylor to Burnett, 30 June 1853, ADM97/205.

39. Mackay diary, 4, 1 May 1858 and 3, 20 March 1856.

40. Burnett memorandum, 13 December 1851, Burnett letterbook, ADM105/68.

41. Statistics relating to disease and mortality and the medicines carried at sea are analysed in N. Baldock, 'Doctor's Orders No. 9 – or 10 Green Bottles Skulking in the Hulk?', *Journal of the Royal Naval Medical Service* 86 (2000), pp 157–162; and E. James, 'Naval Health and the Environment', *Journal of the Royal Naval Medical Service* 51 (1965), pp 201–207. Sea diseases and mortality are also discussed in Lloyd and Coulter, *Medicine and the Navy*, vol. IV, pp 198–212.

42. Henning to Burnett, 20 April 1851, ADM97/192.

43. J. Winton, *Hurrah for the Life of a Sailor: Life on the Lower Deck of the Victorian Navy* (London, 1977), p 24. The struggle in the early nineteenth century to limit alcohol consumption in the navy is thoroughly covered in D. Marjot, 'Aspects of Alcohol and Service Medicine', *Journal of the Royal Naval Medical Service* 53 (1967), pp 113–136.

44. Carruthers to Burnett, 15 September 1844, ADM97/161.

45. Journal of Maurice West, 24 November 1842, NMM, JOD/167.

46. Loney to Burnett, 12 March 1853, ADM97/204.

47. Brien to Burnett, 4 February 1848, ADM97/175.

48. Clarke to Burnett, 16 April 1852, ADM97/197.

49. McArthur to Burnett, 7 December 1838, ADM97/146.

50. The case of *Eclair* is thoroughly investigated in R. Musson, 'A Memory of the "Eclair"', *Journal of the Royal Naval Medical Service* 37 (1951), pp 125–133. A comprehensive contemporary study was published by G. King, *The Fever at Boa Vista in 1845–6 unconnected with the Visit of the 'Eclair' to that Island* (London, 1852). Fever in the navy is more widely analysed in S. Dudley, 'Yellow Fever, as seen by the Medical Officers of the Royal Navy in the Nineteenth Century', *Journal of the Royal Naval Medical Service* 19 (1933), pp 151–165. See also Lloyd and Coulter, *Medicine and the Navy*, vol. IV, pp 173–196. Problems posed by cholera are examined in R. Taylor, 'Cholera and the Royal Navy 1817–1867', *Journal of the Royal Naval Medical Service* 83 (1997), pp 147–156.

51. Parker to Baring, 17 September 1849, Northbrook Papers, NP5/1/3/1.

52. Journal of Alexander Bryson, 28 June 1831 to 24 February 1832, ADM101/88/3. There is a sketch of Bryson, his research and publications regarding fevers in S. Jenkinson, 'Alexander Bryson', *Journal of the Royal Naval Medical Service* 25 (1939), pp 99–108. Bryson was Director-General between 1864 and 1869. His career is outlined in Lloyd and Coulter, *Medicine and the Navy*, vol. IV, pp 7–9.

53. Journal of John Sole, 1 July 1855 to 20 December 1856, ADM101/99/7.

54. Methven to Burnett, 23 January 1838, ADM97/144.

55. Lambert to Burnett, 7 February 1839, ADM97/146.

56. Veitch to Burnett, 20 August 1844, ADM97/163.

57. Journal of William Aitken, 1 January to 19 October 1827, ADM101/88/2.

58. Codrington to his brother, November 1827, reproduced in Lady Bourchier (ed), *Memoir of the Life of Admiral Sir Edward Codrington* (London, 1873), vol. II, p 88.

59. MacPherson's account of the battle is reproduced in H. Baynham, *From the Lower Deck: The Old Navy 1780–1840* (London, 1969), pp 144–168. His description of the cockpit is also quoted in Winton, *Hurrah for the Life of a Sailor*, p 36.

60. West journal, 17 January 1844, JOD/167.

61. Quoted in M. Levien, *The Cree Journals: The Voyages of Edward H. Cree, Surgeon R.N. as related in his Private Journals, 1837–1856* (Exeter, 1981), p 166.

62. Bankier to Burnett, 22 April 1846, ADM97/168.

63. Journal of William Jones, 1 October 1847 to 30 September 1848, ADM101/114/3.

64. Journal of William Guland, 1 January to 20 July 1853, ADM101/125/2.

65. Aitken journal, 1 January to 9 October 1827, ADM101/88/2.

66. Journal of Thomas Spencer Wells, 1 January to 31 December 1852, ADM101/109/3. There is a brief study of his career in J. Shepherd, 'Spencer Wells – Surgeon R.N.', *Journal of the Royal Naval Medical Service* 56 (1970), pp 252–259.

67. Goodridge to Burnett, 20 April 1847, ADM97/171.

68. Diary of Henry James, 30 November 1836, quoted in E. Festing (ed), *Life of Commander Henry James R.N.* (London, 1899), p 275.

69. Mackay diary, 4, 1 May 1858.

70. Guthrie journal, 23 May 1830, JOD/16.

71. Aitken journal, 1 January to 19 October 1827, ADM101/88/2.

Chapter 3. Opportunity and Adventure

1. Bell to White, 17 October 1830, ADM97/53; and Prentice to Burnett, 28 October 1849, ADM97/184.

2. Jones to Burnett, 1 January 1840, ADM97/150.

3. Gairdner to Burnett, 22 April 1832, ADM97/132.

4. Bynoe's career is revealed in J. Keevil, 'Bejamin Bynoe (1804–1865): Surgeon of HMS *Beagle*', *Journal of the Royal Naval Medical Service* 35 (1949), pp 251–268.

5. Burnett to Richmond, 9 August 1843, Goodwood Papers, 1651.

6. Mackay diary, 2, 8 December 1855. Simpson's *Essay on the Eskimos of North-western Alaska* is published as Appendix VII in Bockstoce, *The Journal of Rochfort Maguire*, vol. II, pp 501–550.

7. Richardson was Inspector at Haslar between 1838 and his retirement in 1856. His life and career are extensively covered in H. Rolleston, 'Sir John Richardson', *Journal of the Royal Naval Medical Service* 10 (1924), pp 161–172; and D. Stewart, 'Sir John Richardson, Surgeon, Physician, Sailor, Explorer, Naturalist, Scholar', *Journal of the Royal Naval Medical Service* 22 (1936), pp 181–187. An early journal is reproduced in C. Stuart-Houston, *Arctic Ordeal: The Journal of John Richardson, Surgeon-Naturalist with Franklin 1820–1822* (Gloucester, 1984). There are full biographies by J. McIlraith, *Life of Sir John Richardson* (London, 1868); and R. Johnson, *Sir John Richardson: Arctic Explorer, Natural Historian, Naval Surgeon* (London, 1976). An outline of his career, as those of other surgeon-naturalists, can be found in Lloyd and Coulter, *Medicine and the Navy*, vol. IV, pp 69–80.

8. J. Hooker (ed), *Voyage of the Erebus and Terror: Zoology* (London, 1844). The section on fish was compiled by Richardson. Hooker's medical colleagues on the 1839–43 expedition were surgeons Robert McCormick and John Robertson and assistant surgeon David Lyall. Ross acknowledged their contributions to the zoological, botanical and geological research undertaken in his *A Voyage of Discovery and Research in the Southern and Antarctic Regions*, vol. I, pp xlvi–xlvii, in consequence of which he claimed that several thousand genera of flora from the southern hemisphere had been added to scientific catalogues.

9. R. Hinds (ed), *The Botany of the Voyage of HMS Sulphur under the Command of Sir Edward Belcher during the years 1836–42* (London, 1844). Published in two volumes, Richardson again contributed the material relating to fish.

10. Huxley's research is recorded, evaluated and his observations reproduced in J. Huxley (ed), *T.H. Huxley's Diary of the Voyage of HMS Rattlesnake* (London, 1935).

11. W. Baikie, *Narrative of an Exploring Voyage up the Rivers Kwo'ra and Bi'nue (commonly known as the Niger and Tsádda) in 1854* (London, 1856). Baikie's earlier work was *Historia Naturalis Orcadensis* (Edinburgh, 1848). There is a short study of Baikie by S. Jenkinson, 'Dr. Baikie, M.D., Surgeon, R.N., Naturalist, Traveller, Philologist', *Journal of the Royal Naval Medical Service* 29 (1943), pp 203–207.

12. Adams to Burnett 22 November 1847, ADM97/174; Burnett memorandum, 30 December 1850, ADM105/39. Adam's monumental edition was published as

The Zoology of the Voyage of HMS Samarang; under the Command of Captain Sir Edward Belcher during the years 1843–1846 (London, 1850), with Richardson supplying the chapter on fish. Adams subsequently published, in three volumes and jointly with H. Adams, *The Genera of Recent Mollusca* (London, 1858).

13. This last case is described in G. Loch, *The Closing Events of the Campaign in China: The Operations in the Yang-tsze-Kiang; and Treaty of Nanking* (London, 1843), pp 91–92.

14. Journal of William Kay, 1843–1847, NMM, LOG/N/T/12.

15. Minute by Burnett on Hawes to Burnett, 8 August 1847, ADM97/172; and memorandum by Burnett, 20 July 1848, ADM105/39.

16. Burnett memorandum, 20 July 1848, ADM105/39.

17. Collier to Auckland, 23 February, and Baring to Collier, 24 April 1849, Northbrook Papers, NP5/1/3/4.

18. Described in Levien, *The Cree Journals*, p 122.

19. Mackay diary, 2, 18 January 1855.

20. British intervention in the Spanish civil war is outlined in Bartlett, *Great Britain and Sea Power*, pp 96–98; and discussed in K. Bourne, *Palmerston: The Early Years 1784–1841* (London, 1982), pp 553–555. Details of military activity are best covered in F. Duncan, *The English in Spain; or, the Story of the War of Succession between 1834 and 1840* (London, 1877); and E. Holt, *The Carlist Wars in Spain* (London, 1967). A great deal of medical information regarding the auxiliary legion is contained in R. Alcock, *Notes on the Medical History and Statistics of the British Legion of Spain, comprising the results of Gun-shot Wounds, in relation to Important Questions of Surgery* (London, 1838). See also R. Carr, *Spain 1808–1975* (Oxford, 1982), pp 155–209; and E. Christiansen, *The Origins of Military Power in Spain 1800–1854* (Oxford, 1967). By February 1837 the British government had forwarded arms, stores, tents and hospital supplies to support the Queen of Spain worth £468,878, with further materials to the value of £68,200 advanced to the British auxiliary legion. Naval stores provided amounted to £969 for the Spanish government and £763 for the legion. Military medical stores for the Spanish army had been allowed totalling £572. P.P. (1837), XL.

21. Browne to Burnett, 15 June 1836, ADM97/140.

22. Browne to Burnett, 16 July 1836, ADM97/140.

23. Quoted in Holt, *The Carlist Wars*, p 135. Some of Hay's correspondence relating to events at Pasajes and Fuenterrabia was published in P.P. (1836), XXXVIII.

24. Browne to Burnett, 19 August 1836, ADM97/140.

25. Watson to Burnett, 18 December 1836, ADM97/141.

26. Browne to Burnett, 21 March 1837, ADM97/141. Hay's correspondence relating to cooperation between British sailors and marines and the army of the Queen of Spain and to the unsuccessful attack on Hernani in March 1837 was published in P.P. (1837), XXXIX.

27. Browne to Burnett, 3 September 1837, ADM97/143.

28. The Eastern crisis and British involvement is discussed in Bartlett, *Great Britain and Sea Power*, pp 128–148; Bourne, *Palmerston*, pp 568–620; and P. Padfield, *Rule Britannia: The Victorian and Edwardian Navy* (London, 1981), pp 87–94. There is also a great deal of detail about military and naval activity in H. Williams, *The Life and Letters of Admiral Sir Charles Napier* (London, 1917).

29. Journal of Charles Wilkinson, 30 August, 1 September 1840, NMM, JOD/51.

30. Wilkinson journal, 9 September 1840, JOD/51.

31. Wilkinson journal, 12 September 1840, JOD/51.

32. Wilkinson journal, 20, 29 October 1840, JOD/51.

33. Wilkinson journal, 1–4 November 1840, JOD/51. See also E. Napier, *The Life and Correspondence of Admiral Sir Charles Napier KCB, from Personal Recollections, Letters and Official Documents* (London, 1862) vol. II, pp 114–115.

34. Burnett memorandum, 23 December 1840, Burnett letterbook, ADM105/72.

35. Accounts of this action can be found in Levien, *The Cree Journals*, p 166; see also Reid to Burnett, 1 September 1845, ADM97/165. For the background to the navy's campaign against piracy in Eastern seas see Padfield, *Rule Britannia*, pp 98–106; and G. Fox, *British Admirals and Chinese Pirates 1832–1869* (London, 1940).

36. Carpenter to Burnett, 29 December 1851, ADM97/196; and Bruce to Baring, 1 January 1852, Northbrook Papers, NP/5/1/3/3.

37. Kelsall to Burnett, 7, 10 September 1842, ADM97/156.

38. Culhane to Burnett, 2 March 1852, ADM97/197.

39. Pritchett to Burnett, 23 May 1837, ADM97/142. The campaign to stop the African slave trade is described in R. Howell, *The Royal Navy and the Slave Trade* (London, 1987); L. Bethell, *The Abolition of the Brazilian Slave Trade: Britain, Brazil, and the Slave Trade Question 1807–1869* (Cambridge, 1970); W. Ward, *The Royal Navy and the Slavers: The Suppression of the Atlantic Slave Trade* (London, 1969); and Winton, *Hurrah for the Life of a Sailor*, pp 237–252. See also Bartlett, *Great Britain and Sea Power*, pp 269–270; and Padfield, *Rule Britannia*, pp 109–125. Palmerston's determination to end the traffic is

outlined in Bourne, *Palmerston*, pp 622–625. For a more recent account see M. Hunter, 'The Hero Packs a Punch: Sir Charles Hotham, Liberalism and West Africa, 1846–1850', *Mariner's Mirror* 92 (2006), pp 282–299.

40. Campbell to Wood, 28 April 1838, reproduced in Hattendorf et al (eds), *British Naval Documents*, pp 626–628.

41. Pritchett to Burnett, 17 June 1842, ADM97/156. Sickness off West Africa is discussed in P. Aubrey, 'Climate and Health in West African Waters 1825–1870', *Journal of the Royal Naval Medical Service* 40 (1954), pp 84–88.

42. Burton to Burnett, 29 September 1853, ADM97/206; and Bruce to Admiralty, 14 October 1852, ADM97/200.

43. Fanshawe to Baring, 15 July 1850, Northbrook Papers, NP5/1/3/5.

44. Anderson to Burnett, 8 January 1853, ADM97/202.

45. McIlroy to Thomas McIlroy, 1 July 1841, Journal of John McIlroy, NMM, LBK/41.

46. McIlroy to Thomas McIlroy, 23 March 1842, LBK/41.

47. McCrae to Burnett, 16 August 1847, ADM97/173.

48. Journal of Henry Piers, 28 December 1850, NMM, JOD/102; Journal of David Lyall, 16 February 1852 to 15 May 1854, ADM101/87/8; Journal of Abraham Bradford, 28 February 1850 to 9 October 1851, ADM101/117/3. Polar voyages are outlined in Lloyd and Coulter, *Medicine and the Navy,* vol. IV, pp 107–123. Piers's journal is extensively reproduced and discussed in A. Savours, 'The Diary of Assistant Surgeon Henry Piers, HMS Investigator, 1850–54', *Journal of the Royal Naval Medical Service* 76 (1990), pp 33–38. Entertainments and other communal ice-bound activities were described on 12 November 1819 by An Officer of the Expedition, *Letters*, p 51; and in T. Collinson (ed), *Journal of H.M.S. Enterprise, on the Expedition in Search of Sir John Franklin's Ships by Behring Strait 1850–55* (London, 1889), pp 247, 391–397.

49. William Domville's scientific lectures to an attentive crew are recorded in G. M'Dougall, *The Eventful Voyage of H.M. Discovery Ship Resolute to the Arctic Regions in Search of Sir John Franklin and the Missing Crews of H.M. Discovery Ships Erebus and Terror, 1852, 1853, 1854* (London, 1857), pp 342–343, 347–349. He also gives an account of the crew's theatrical abilities on pp 158–162, 178–181, 343–346. Schooling aboard *Fox* in the Arctic in 1857 is described in F. M'Clintock, *Fate of Sir John Franklin: The Voyage of the Fox in the Arctic Seas in Search of Franklin and his Companions* (London, 1881), pp 46–47.

50. S. Osborn, *Stray Leaves from an Arctic Journal; or, Eighteen Months in the Polar Regions, in Search of Sir John Franklin's Expedition, in the years 1850–51* (London, 1852), p 34.

51. Bradford journal, 28 February 1850 to 9 October 1851, ADM101/117/3. In 1819 Alexander Fisher, surgeon accompanying *Hecla* and *Griper* to the Arctic, noted that 'antiscorbutics, of different kinds, were also provided, such as lemon-juice, sour-crout, essence of spruce and essence of malt and hops'. Fisher, *A Journal of a Voyage of Discovery to the Arctic Regions*, pxi. Fisher had accompanied Ross as assistant surgeon to explore Baffin Bay and to search for a North West passage in 1818. The consequences of an inadequate supply of antiscorbutics are described by George McDiarmid, surgeon with *Victory* in the Arctic between 1829 and 1833. His problems treating frostbite and 17 serious scurvy cases by 1832 were written up in his surgeon's report published in Sir John Ross, *Appendix to the Narrative of a Second Voyage in Search of a North-West Passage and of a Residence in the Arctic Regions during the years 1829, 1830, 1831, 1832, 1833* (London, 1835), pp cxvii–cxxvii.

52. Piers journal, 15 March 1851, 16 February 1852, JOD/102. Captain Richard Collinson compiled data concerning the health, diet and clothing of the crews of *Enterprise* (1851–52), *Investigator* (1852–53) and *Resolute* (1853) while in the Arctic, cited, with average monthly sick-lists aboard *Enterprise* for 1852, 1853 and 1854, in Collinson (ed), *Journal of H.M.S. Enterprise*, pp 250, 398–401.

53. Journal of John Robertson, 3 February 1848 to 26 November 1849, ADM101/99/4.

54. Piers journal, 23 October 1851, JOD/102.

55. Osborn, *Stray Leaves from an Arctic Journal*, pp 201, 225–226.

56. Journal of William Domville, Kellett order book entry, 21 October 1852, and memorandum by Domville, 6 August 1854, NMM, JOD/67.

57. Piers journal, 25 December 1851, JOD/102.

58. Domville journal, 26 December 1852, JOD/67.

59. Journal of John Holman, 22 February to 25 October 1854, ADM101/112/7.

60. Journal of John Ricards, 21 April 1852 to 30 September 1853, ADM101/113/1; and Lyall journal, 16 February 1852 to 15 May 1854, ADM101/87/8. Captain Francis M'Clintock, setting out for the Arctic on *Fox* in 1857, also took 'as much of Messrs. Allsopp's stoutest ale as we could find room for.' M'Clintock, *Fate of Sir John Franklin*, p 6.

61. Piers journal, 9, 22 October and 3 November 1851, JOD/102.

Chapter 4. Home Hospitals

1. The 1830 regulations are listed in Keevil, 'Ralph Cuming', p 66.

2. Rae to Burnett, 16 October 1852, ADM97/200.

3. The introduction of chloroform is discussed in P. Glew, 'Singular Experiences: The Early History of Anaesthesia in the Royal Navy 1847 to 1854', *Journal of the Royal Naval Medical Service* 83 (1997), pp 42–44.

4. Burnett memorandum, 4 June 1835, Burnett letterbook, ADM105/70.

5. Burnett memorandum, 21 October 1833, Burnett letterbook, ADM105/70.

6. Figures are from Burnett memorandum, 4 June 1835, Burnett letterbook, ADM105/70.

7. Rae to Burnett, 3 March 1848, ADM97/175.

8. Rae to Burnett, 3 March 1848, ADM97/175.

9. Dickson to Burnett, 23 November 1837, ADM97/143.

10. Burnett memorandum, 4 June 1835, Burnett letterbook, ADM105/70.

11. Scott to Burnett, 21 August 1835, ADM97/138.

12. The libraries at Haslar and East Stonehouse are discussed in M. Lattimore, 'Early Naval Medical Libraries, Personal and Corporate', *Journal of the Royal Naval Medical Service* 69 (1983), pp 107–111, 156–160.

13. Burnett memorandum, 28 November 1832, Burnett letterbook, ADM105/70.

14. Naval museums are discussed in C. Parsons, 'Haslar Museum', *Journal of the Royal Naval Medical Service* 71 (1985), pp 117–120. See also memoranda by Burnett, 30 December 1841 and 28 November 1842, Burnett letterbook, ADM105/73.

15. Burnett memorandum, 21 October 1833, Burnett letterbook, ADM105/70.

16. Minute by Burnett on Drummond to Burnett, 4 December 1848, ADM97/179.

17. Millar to Burnett, 17 January 1854, ADM97/207. The work of Millar and Kay during the 1849 cholera epidemic in Plymouth is explained in D. McLean, *Public Health and Politics in the Age of Reform: Cholera, the State and the Royal Navy in Victorian Britain* (London, 2006), pp 120–126.

18. Problems with the midwifery funds are revealed in Evans to Liddell, 18 April 1838, and Little to Admiralty, 3 June 1845, ADM97/163; and Miller to Burnett, 27 April 1846, ADM97/167.

19. Rae to Burnett, 27 March 1851, ADM97/191.

20. Minute by Bryson on Clark to Burnett, 4 February 1855, ADM97/217.

21. Reports on Wounded Officers, 31 December 1857, ADM105/32.

22. Burnett memorandum, 21 October 1833, Burnett letterbook, ADM105/70.

23. Burnett memorandum, 20 March 1833, Burnett letterbook, ADM105/70.

24. Burnett to Richmond, 4 February 1845, Goodwood Papers, 1669.

25. Burnett memorandum, 22 September 1832, Burnett letterbook, ADM105/70.

26. Toon to Burnett, 9 December, and Burnett memorandum, 16 December 1845, ADM97/165.

27. Rae to Burnett, 3 March 1848, ADM97/175.

28. Burnett memorandum, 5 February 1848, ADM97/175.

29. Richardson to Burnett, 13 March 1854, ADM97/216.

30. Dundas to Burnett, 14 March 1854, ADM97/216.

31. Rae to Burnett, 3 March 1848, ADM97/175.

32. Burnett memorandum, 23 October 1832, Burnett letterbook, ADM105/70.

33. Varlo to Burnett, 20 October 1848, ADM97/178; and Varlo to Burnett, 28 February 1849, ADM97/181.

34. Hope-Johnstone to Admiralty, 7 May 1853, ADM97/203.

35. Drummond to Burnett, 6 July 1854, ADM97/212.

36. Irvine to Burnett, 26 April, and memorandum by Burnett, 5 May 1845, ADM97/163.

37. Burnett memorandum, 13 February 1851, Burnett letterbook, ADM105/68.

38. Drummond to Burnett, 26 January 1852, ADM97/195; and Evans to Dundas, 18 January 1854, ADM97/207.

39. Burnett memorandum, 21 October 1833, Burnett letterbook, ADM105/70.

40. Griffin to Barrow, 18 November, and Mortimer to Chetham, 25 November 1839, ADM97/148. Griffin's assertions were, however, given some credibility nearly 70 years later when Sir John Richardson's son recalled his boyhood residence at Haslar. In a sketch of Anderson's regime and the benefits thereby brought to the asylum, he remembered how 'several rough attendants were discharged', and, when reflecting on the violence which had previously characterized the behaviour of some inmates, concluded that this was 'not surprising after so much brutal treatment'. J. Richardson, 'A Visit to Haslar, 1916', *Journal of the Royal Naval Medical Service* 2 (1916), p 334.

41. Burnett memorandum, 9 December 1843, Burnett letterbook, ADM105/73.

42. Report by Wilson, 31 March 1854, ADM97/210.

43. Stuart to Dacres, 29 December 1856, ADM97/230.

44. Mackay diary, 4, 6 August 1858.

Chapter 5. Hospitals Abroad

1. Journal of John Gibson, 18 August 1829 to 31 December 1830, ADM101/115/4.

2. Evans to Burnett, 23 March 1847, ADM97/171.

3. Minute by Liddell on Hardinge to Dundas, 9 January 1857, ADM97/230. Details of staffing levels and pay at overseas hospitals are enclosed in Burnett memorandum, 11 October 1852, Burnett letterbook, ADM105/68.

4. For the Malta hospital see O. Brownfield, 'Royal Naval Hospital, Malta', *Journal of the Royal Naval Medical Service* 35 (1949), pp 245–251; and J. Falconer-

Hall, 'The Royal Naval Hospitals, Malta', *Journal of the Royal Naval Medical Service* 13 (1927), p 253. It is also mentioned in Lloyd and Coulter, *Medicine and the Navy,* vol. IV, pp 247–254; and in Shepherd, 'Spencer Wells', pp 252–259.

5.   Burnett memorandum, 6 October 1838, Burnett letterbook, ADM105/72.

6.   Salmon to Liddell, 25 November 1856, ADM97/229.

7.   Cowan to his mother, 30 January 1856, Cowan Papers, PTR/1.

8.   C. Sloane-Stanley, *Reminiscences of a Midshipman's Life from 1850 to 1856* (London, 1893), p 234.

9.   Stewart to Liddell, 23 August 1855, ADM97/221.

10. Stewart to Burnett, 7 July 1852, ADM97/198.

11. Watson to Burnett, 25 March 1854, ADM97/210.

12. Wingate-Johnston to Burnett, 28 September 1850, ADM97/189.

13. Festing (ed), *Life of Commander Henry James*, p 166.

14. Burnett memorandum, 24 February 1841, Burnett letterbook, ADM105/72.

15. Watson to Burnett, 22 November 1852, ADM97/202.

16. Linton to Burnett, 8 January 1836, ADM97/139.

17. Linton to Burnett, 6 November 1835, ADM97/139; and Linton to Burnett, 16 June 1839, ADM97/147.

18. Minute by Burnett on Fossett memorandum, 7 May 1845, ADM97/163.

19. Minute by Burnett on Stewart to Burnett, 7 January 1848, ADM97/175; and Wingate-Johnston to Burnett, 11 October 1852, ADM97/199.

20. Jones to Clifton, 24 August 1829, ADM97/89. Lloyd and Coulter provide some information about the Bermuda hospital in *Medicine and the Navy,* vol. IV, pp 254–256.

21. Burnett memorandum, 22 February 1844, Burnett letterbook, ADM105/73; and Lindsay to Burnett, 3 January 1844, ADM97/160.

22. Burnett memorandum, 30 June 1841, Burnett letterbook, ADM105/73.

23. Hilditch to Burnett, 20 June 1850, ADM97/188.

24. Baring to Harvey, 30 April 1849, Northbrook Papers, NP5/1/3/6. For discussion of these enquiries into naval costs see Bartlett, *Great Britain and Sea Power*, pp 294–303.

25. More O'Ferrall to Baring, 24 March 1849, Northbrook Papers, NP5/1/3/8.

26. Baring to Milne, 29 June 1849, Northbrook Papers, NP5/1/3/7.

27. Minute by Burnett on Trevelyan to Baring, 11 July 1849, ADM97/182.

28. Baring to Dundonald, 28 September, and Dundonald to Baring, 18 October 1849, Northbrook Papers, NP5/1/3/4.

29. Padfield, *Rule Britannia*, pp 84–85.

30. Burnett memorandum, 11 October 1852, Burnett letterbook, ADM105/68.

31. Burnett memorandum, 22 March 1853, Burnett letterbook, ADM105/68.

32. Burnett memorandum, 4 June 1849, ADM97/182.

33. The different arrangements made at Valparaiso are cited in the Journal of John Cunningham, 19, 20 May 1824, NMM, JOD/21; Clavell to Rouse, 8 August 1844, letterbook of John Clavell, NMM, LBK/28; and West to Burnett, 29 November 1849, ADM97/186.

34. Martin to Baring, 8 October 1851, Northbrook Papers, NP5/1/3/7.

35. Warden to Milne, 4 June 1852, ADM97/200.

36. Huxley diary, 31 December 1848, reproduced in Huxley (ed), *T.H. Huxley's Diary*, pp 146–147.

Chapter 6. *Minden* on the China Coast

1. J. Wilson, *Medical Notes on China* (London, 1846), p viii. Wilson's *Statistical Report on the Health of the Navy 1830–1836* was published in P.P. (1840), XXX. Earlier he had published *Memoirs of West Indian Fever constituting brief notices regarding the Treatment, Origin and Nature of the Disease commonly called Yellow Fever* (London, 1827). Wilson had been a surgeon since 1822, winning the Blane Medal in 1833. When his statistical research at Somerset House was completed in 1840 Wilson was attached for a year as an additional surgeon to Greenwich Hospital before being promoted to Inspector in December 1841. In addition to *Medical Notes* he also published *Outlines of Naval Surgery* in 1846.

2. The origins and course of the war are thoroughly covered in P. Fay, *The Opium War 1840–1842* (Chapel Hill, 1975); J. Beeching, *The Chinese Opium Wars* (London, 1975); B. Inglis, *The Opium War* (London, 1976); and G. Graham, *The China Station: War and Diplomacy 1830–1860* (Oxford, 1978). Medical aspects of the war are discussed in D. McLean, 'Surgeons of the Opium War: The Navy on the China Coast, 1840–42', *English Historical Review* 121 (2006), pp 487–504.

3. Auckland to Elliot, 27 November and 20, 28 December 1840, Papers of the Earl of Auckland, British Library (BL), London, add.mss. 37715. For the disaster on Chusan see also McLean, 'Surgeons of the Opium War', p 497; and Cantlie, *A History of the Army Medical Department*, vol. I, pp 477–478.

4. Quoted in Levien, *The Cree Journals*, pp 86, 89. Entries for 29 May, 19, 21 June 1841.

5. Minto to Elliot, 4 June 1840, Minto Papers, ELL/234.

6. Burnett memoranda, 15 February and 7 August 1841, Burnett letterbook,

ADM105/72.

7. Allan to Burnett, 30 September 1842, ADM97/156. Details of the Macao hospital are also contained in Journal of James Allan, 15 June 1841 to 30 June 1842, ADM101/108/1.

8. Burnett memoranda, 1 October 1841, ADM97/22; and 2 October 1841, ADM97/27.

9. Quoted in Levien, *The Cree Journals*, p 93. Entry for 1 October 1841.

10. Quoted in Levien, *The Cree Journals*, p 113. Entry for 22 August 1842.

11. Parker to Ellenborough, 31 August 1842, quoted in A. Phillimore, *The Life of Admiral of the Fleet Sir William Parker* (London, 1879) vol. II, p 499.

12. A. Cunynghame, *An Aide-de-Camp's Recollections of Service in China, a Residence in Hong Kong, and Visits to other Islands in the Chinese Seas* (London, 1844), vol. I, p 260.

13. Baker to his mother, November 1842, Papers of Wyndham Baker, National Army Museum (NAM), London, 6312–212.

14. Journal of Edward Cree, 2 October 1842, NMM, MS 86/083.

15. Burnett memorandum, 4 February 1843, Burnett letterbook, ADM105/73.

16. Hope to Parker, 9–12 September 1842, Papers of Charles Hope, NMM, HPE/3.

17. Wilson, *Medical Notes*, pp 29–30; Log of *Minden* 3 December 1841 to 21 October 1842, ADM53/864.

18. Wilson's statistical analysis is explained in *Medical Notes*, pp 49–53.

19. Hope to Parker, 19 April and 7 May 1843, Hope Papers, HPE/3.

20. Wilson, *Medical Notes*, pp xii, 123.

21. Wilson, *Medical Notes*, p 142.

22. Wilson to Burnett, 2 October 1843, ADM97/160; Wilson, *Medical Notes*, p 142.

23. Cochrane to Cockburn, 11 October 1843, Cochrane Papers, MS 2607.

24. Parker to Burnett, 8 September 1843, ADM97/160.

25. Journal of Chilley Pine, 10 March 1841, NAM, 6807/262/4.

26. Cochrane to Pringle, 29 September 1842, Cochrane Papers, MS 2607.

27. Arguments over what to do with *Minden* are expressed in Cochrane to Cockburn, 11 October 1843, Cochrane Papers, MS2607; Burnett memorandum, 26 October 1843, Burnett letterbook, ADM105/73; and Cockburn to Parker, 6 February 1844, Parker Papers, PAR/155b.

28. Wilson, *Medical Notes*, p 171.

29. Wilson, *Medical Notes*, pp 195–196.

30. Wilson, *Medical Notes*, pp 201, 223.

31. Cochrane to ships' captains, 14 February 1845, Papers of Richard Collinson, NMM, CLS/4.

32. Mackay diary, 1, 27 December 1853. Mackay also provided the sketch of Bankier.

33. Bankier to Burnett, 30 March 1849, ADM97/182.

34. Austen to Baring, 7 May 1851, Northbrook Papers, NP5/1/3/3.

35. Keown to Burnett, 26 January 1854, ADM97/209.

36. Mackay diary, 1, 21 May 1854.

Chapter 7. Baltic and Crimea

1. Stewart to Burnett, 23 August 1853, ADM97/205.

2. Mackay to Burnett, 25 August 1853, ADM97/205.

3. Mackay to Burnett, 5 September 1853, ADM97/205.

4. Rees to Burnett, 23 November 1953, ADM97/206.

5. British diplomacy and the unfolding of the international crisis leading to war are analysed in a vast literature, among the most recent of which are J. Sweetman, *The Crimean War* (Oxford, 2001); W. Baumgart, *The Crimean War 1853–1856* (London, 1999); and D, Goldfrank, *The Origins of the Crimean War* (London, 1994). See also R. Ffrench-Blake, *The Crimean War* (London, 1971); and A. Barker, *The Vainglorious War 1854–56* (London, 1970).

6. Naval action in the war is likewise extensively covered, in particular by A. Lambert, *The Crimean War; British Grand Strategy, 1853–1856* (Manchester, 1990); and B. Greenhill and A. Giffard, *The British Assault on Finland 1854–1855: A Forgotten Naval War* (London, 1988). For a contemporary account see Sir H. Douglas, *Remarks on the Naval Operations in the Black Sea and the Siege of Sebastopol* (London, 1855). Burnett's directions to surgeons of the fleet on the outbreak of war were published in *The Lancet*, 29 April 1854.

7. Rees to Burnett, 19 August 1854, ADM97/214. Cholera and fevers in the fleet and among soldiers in the Black Sea in 1854 are discussed in Shepherd, *The Crimean Doctors*, vol. I, pp 73–109. See also Lloyd and Coulter, *Medicine and the Navy,* vol. IV, pp 141–144.

8. Milroy, *The Health of the Royal Navy Considered*, pp 23–24. Milroy attached significance to the fact that no officer aboard *Britannia* died, which he implicitly attributed to their higher standards of personal sanitation.

9. Deas to Burnett, 22 August 1854, ADM97/214.

10. Burnett memoranda, 22 April, 17 June and 31 July 1854, ADM105/39. Official statistics for the numbers, requirements and deficiencies of surgeons and assistants for May and July 1854 were published in P.P. (1854), XLII.

11. Graham to Dundas, 25 October 1854, reproduced in D. Bonner-Smith and A. Dewar (eds), *Russian War, 1854. Baltic and Black Sea Official Correspondence* (London, 1943), pp 417–418. Much of Napier's correspondence is reproduced in Napier, *The Life and Correspondence of Admiral Sir Charles Napier*. See also P. Napier, *Black Charlie: A Life of Admiral Sir Charles Napier K.C.B. 1787–1860* (Norwich, 1995). Medical provision in the Baltic fleet in 1854 is discussed in Shepherd, *Crimean Doctors*, vol. I, pp 94–101.

12. Medical and Surgical Report of HMS *Belleisle*, 8 to 30 June 1854, ADM102/850. See also log of *Belleisle*, ADM53/5209.

13. Dickson to Burnett, 18 May 1854, ADM97/212.

14. McKechnie to Burnett, 16 July 1854, ADM97/213.

15. Quoted in Levien, *The Cree Journals*, p 246.

16. McKechnie to Burnett, 9 January 1855, ADM97/216; and memorandum by Fossett, 1 February 1855, ADM97/217.

17. Richardson to Burnett, 18 November 1854, ADM97/215.

18. Graham to Milne, 21 September 1854, Papers of Alexander Milne, NMM, MLN/165/5.

19. Davidson to Burnett, 2, 7 March and 5 April 1854, ADM97/210.

20. Davidson to Burnett, 7 April 1854, ADM97/210; and Davidson to Burnett, 8 May 1854, ADM97/218.

21. Rees to Burnett, 10 June 1854, ADM97/218.

22. Burnett to Richards, 24 November 1854, ADM97/215.

23. Medical provision for the army, casualty figures and transport for the wounded after the battle of Alma are described in Shepherd, *The Crimean Doctors,* vol. I, pp 126–142. Details of the experiences of Pearce and Smith are contained in their report to Deas, 5 October 1854, P.P. (1854–55), IX, part 1. Between 22 and 28 September 1854, 2,705 sick and wounded were conveyed the 300 miles from Balaclava to Scutari of whom 319 died on the voyage. Conditions in the military hospitals are vividly revealed in Florence Nightingale's correspondence, reproduced in S. Goldie (ed), *'I Have Done My Duty': Florence Nightingale in the Crimean War 1854–56* (Manchester, 1987). See also F. Robinson, *Diary of the Crimean War* (London, 1856).

24. Reynolds to Burnett, 5 October 1854, ADM97/216; and Deas to Burnett, 27 September 1854, P.P. (1854), IX, part 1.

25. Mackay to Burnett, 23 October, and Donovan to Burnett, 19 October 1854, ADM97/215. See also log of *Agamemnon*, 17 October 1854, NMM, LOG/N/A/24.

26. Christie to Milne, 10 June and 27 September 1854, Milne Papers, MLN/156/1.

27. Journal of Howard Banks, 1 July 1854 to 30 June 1855, ADM101/122/5.

28. Deas to Burnett, 30 August 1854, ADM97/214; and Deas to Burnett, 31 October 1854, ADM97/215.

29. Burnett to Hair, 31 October 1854, Goodwood Papers, 1779.

30. Deas to Burnett, 21 January 1855, ADM97/217.

31. Burnett memorandum, 3 January 1855, ADM105/39. Recruitment is investigated in C. Penn, 'The Medical Staffing of the Royal Navy in the Russian War, 1854–6', *Mariner's Mirror* 89 (2003), pp 51–58.

32. Cowan to his mother, 23 March 1855, Cowan Papers, PTR/1. Shepherd, *The Crimean Doctors,* vol. I, p 158, confirms that in three months, October to December 1854, a total of 7,682 sick and wounded were transported from Balaclava to hospitals on the Bosphorus of whom 549 died *en route.* The figure 7,941 for the combined months December 1854 and January 1855 is from Christie to Milne, 2 February 1855, reproduced in J. Beeler (ed), *The Milne Papers: The Papers of Admiral of the Fleet Sir Alexander Milne, Bt., K.C.B., (1806–1896)* (Aldershot, 2004), vol. I, pp 547–548.

33. Davidson to Burnett, 9 November 1854, P.P. (1854–55), IX, part 1.

34. Boxer to Admiralty, 25 December 1854, Papers of Edward Boxer, NMM, MS 86/057.

35. Milne to Stirling, 29 January 1855, reproduced in Beeler (ed), *Milne Papers,* p 543.

36. Davidson to Burnett, 1 March 1855, ADM97/218. Davidson rose to become Inspector at East Stonehouse between 1868 and 1873, assuming full control of the hospital in 1870 when the post of Captain-Superintendent was abolished.

37. Deas to Burnett, 29, 30 January 1855, ADM97/217.

38. Boxer to Lyons, 1 June 1855, Boxer Papers, MS 86/057. The number of transports under Admiralty hire had risen from 100 in June 1854 to 216 by April 1855.

39. Christie to Milne, 8 January 1855, reproduced in Beeler (ed), *Milne Papers,* p 533.

40. Deas to Liddell, 21 May 1855, ADM97/220. There is a succinct survey of medical provision for the naval brigade and marines at Balaclava in Shepherd, *The Crimean Doctors,* vol. I, pp 330–335; vol. II, pp 492–498. The work of the Sanitary Commission is outlined in Shepherd, *The Crimean Doctors,* vol. II, pp 395–401.

41. Medical and Surgical Report of HMS *Belleisle,* 26 May to 30 June 1855, ADM102/850.

42. Carruthers to Liddell, 31 May 1855, ADM97/220.

43. Sabben to Burnett, 22 January 1855, P.P. (1854–55), IX, part 1.

44. Medical and Surgical Report of HMS *Belleisle*, 26 May to 30 June 1855, ADM102/850.

45. Naval operations in the Baltic are analysed in Lambert, *The Crimean War*. Correspondence between Dundas and the Admiralty concerning the 1855 Baltic campaign is reproduced extensively in D. Bonner-Smith (ed), *Russian War, 1855. Baltic: Official Correspondence* (London, 1944). Medical provision in the Baltic fleet in 1855 is discussed in Shepherd, *The Crimean Doctors*, vol. II, pp 539–547.

46. Wallace to Liddell, 10 September 1855, ADM97/222.

47. Minute by Burnett on Yorke to Osborne, 3 February 1855, ADM97/217.

48. Liddell memorandum, 20 September 1855, ADM97/222.

49. Liddell memorandum, 6 December 1855, ADM97/223.

50. Drummond to Admiralty, 21 June 1855, ADM97/220.

51. Burnett memorandum, 28 March 1855, ADM97/218.

52. Salmon to Liddell, 12 June 1855, ADM97/220.

53. Salmon to Liddell, 20 June 1855, ADM97/220.

54. Liddell memorandum, 13 July 1855, ADM97/221.

55. Minute by Burnett on Deas to Burnett, 14 February 1855, ADM97/217.

56. Salmon to Liddell, 11 December 1855, ADM97/223. Salmon was later Inspector at Haslar, assuming full control between 1870 and 1873 after the post of Captain-Superintendent was abolished.

57. Edward Cree was witness to many of these actions, as recorded in Levien, *The Cree Journals*, pp 248–266. Correspondence between Lyons and the Admiralty regarding operations in the Black Sea is reproduced extensively in A. Dewar (ed), *The Russian War, 1855. Black Sea: Official Correspondence* (London, 1945).

58. Deas to Liddell, 21 May 1855, ADM97/220. Some of the correspondence relating to the harbour at Balaclava between February and July 1855, including Boxer's regulations for the port issued from *Diamond* on 6 March, was published in P.P. (1854–55), XXXIV.

59. A. Parry (ed), *The Admirals Fremantle* (London, 1971), pp 179–181.

60. Medical Report on the Transport Service by Costello, 28 August, 1856, ADM97/228.

61. Deas to Liddell, 3 July 1855, ADM97/221.

62. Keppel to Lyons, 29 July 1855, letterbook of Henry Keppel, NMM, HTN/57.

63. MacKenzie's work at Therapia is best covered in R. Huntsman, M. Bruin and D. Holttum, 'Light before Dawn: Naval Nursing and Medical Care during

the Crimean War', *Journal of the Royal Naval Medical Service* 88 (2002), pp 5–27. See also M. Penney, 'Letters from Therapia', *Blackwood's Magazine* 275 (1954), pp 413–421. Shepherd outlines MacKenzie's time in his description of the Therapia hospital in *The Crimean Doctors,* vol. II, pp 549–554. Nursing by women during the Crimean War, albeit overwhelmingly with the army, is dealt with in A. Summers, *Angels and Citizens: British Women as Military Nurses 1854–1914* (London, 1988), pp 29–66; and S. Bingham, *Ministering Angels* (London, 1979), pp 32–57.

64. Deas to Lyons, 15 October 1855, ADM97/223.

65. Deas to Liddell, 21 August 1855, ADM97/222.

66. Deas to Liddell, 29 September 1855, ADM97/222. Smart, whose first assignment had been as one of the five acting assistant surgeons sent out to China when the Far Eastern squadron had been short of medics in 1841, was awarded the Blane Medal in 1857 and retired from a distinguished career as Inspector at Haslar in 1877.

67. Deas to Liddell, 8 October 1855, ADM97/222; and Deas to Liddell, 2 November 1855, ADM97/223.

68. R. Brooks, *The Long Arm of Empire: Naval Brigades from the Crimea to the Boxer Rebellion* (London, 1999), p 26.

69. Liddell memorandum, 2 August 1855, ADM97/221. The hospital's muster book of admissions is preserved as ADM102/849.

70. Davidson to Liddell, 29 March 1856, ADM97/226. MacKenzie had been obliged to return home on account of her health in November 1855.

71. The extensive official investigations of the army and navy during the war were published as *Report and Evidence of the Select Committee on the Army before Sebastopol,* P.P. (1854–55), IX. Army medical provision was exhaustively examined in *Report upon the State of the Hospitals of the British Army in the Crimea and Scutari,* P.P. (1854–55), XXXIII; and in *Medical and Surgical History of the British Army which Served in Turkey and the Crimea during the War against Russia in the years 1854–55–56,* P.P. (1857–58), XXXVIII.

72. Figures are from Milroy, *The Health of the Royal Navy Considered,* p 51; Shepherd, *The Crimean Doctors,* vol. II, pp 554–556; and Liddell memorandum, 24 March 1857, ADM97/230. See also Lloyd and Coulter, *Medicine and the Navy,* vol. IV, pp 148–152. For the army see J. Sweetman, *War and Administration: The Significance of the Crimean War for the British Army* (Edinburgh, 1984). Medical Statistical Returns for the Baltic and Black Sea Fleets during the Years 1854 and 1855 were published in P.P. (1857), IX.

73. Deas to Liddell, 21 August 1855, ADM97/222.

74. Liddell to Jenkins, 13 December 1855, ADM97/223.
75. Cowan to his mother, 31 August and 12 October 1855, Cowan Papers, PTR/1.
76. Deas to Liddell, 17 December 1855, ADM97/224.
77. Journal of George Mackay, 1 August 1854 to 9 September 1855, ADM101/81/3.

Chapter 8. Modernization and 1914

1. Mackay diary, 2, 19 May 1855.
2. Burnett to Hair, 20 October 1854, Goodwood Papers, 1779. Figures for naval increases are from Bartlett, *Great Britain and Sea Power*, pp 339–340.
3. Journal of John Sabben, 5 June 1854 to 30 June 1855, ADM101/120/5.
4. Journal of Edward Heath, 1 January to 31 December 1855, ADM101/96/2.
5. Cotton to Liddell, 28 July 1856, ADM97/227.
6. Deas to Liddell, 10 July, and Smart to Baird, 17 August 1856, Papers of William Baird, NMM, BGY/B/5.
7. Among the most comprehensive contemporary accounts of the navy and changes occurring in the decades following the Crimean War are R. Main, *The British Navy in 1871* (London, 1871); and Sir T. Brassey, *The British Navy: Its Strength, Resources, and Administration* (London, 1882).
8. Naval brigades from the Crimea onwards are investigated in Brooks, *The Long Arm of Empire*. For a contemporary record see H. Norbury, *The Naval Brigade in South Africa during the years 1877–78–79* (London, 1880). The circumstances in which William Maillard won his Victoria Cross in 1898 are described in A. O'Connor, 'Surgeon William Job Maillard, V.C., M.D., R.N.', *Journal of the Royal Naval Medical Service* 50 (1964), pp 64–70; and in a similarly entitled, though unattributed piece in the 1956 volume (42) of the same journal, pp 106–108. More recent is J. Wickenden, 'A Note on William Job Maillard: Marking the 100th Anniversary of his Death', *Journal of the Royal Naval Medical Service* 89 (2003), pp 9–10.
9. Main, *The British Navy in 1871*, pp 6–7.
10. Porter to Lutie Porter, 8 October 1899, Porter Papers, PTR/6/2.
11. Statistics are cited in Lloyd and Coulter, *Medicine and the Navy,* vol. IV, pp 270–271. Simpson also analyses statistics in 'Progress of Hygiene', p 313.
12. Burnett memorandum, 25 June 1847, ADM97/171.
13. Journal of Robert Bernard, 1 January to 31 December 1851, ADM101/111/1.
14. Burnett memorandum, 25 January 1847, ADM97/171; and Burnett to Richmond, 19 October 1854, Goodwood Papers, 1779.
15. Journal of William Graham, 1 July 1852 to 30 June 1853, ADM101/124/4. The revised schedule of medicines is referred to in Burnett memorandum, 12

January 1852, Burnett letterbook, ADM105/68.

16. E. Pollard, 'Diary of a Medical Officer on Active Service with the Royal Marines in Egypt in 1882', *Journal of the Royal Naval Medical Service* 22 (1936), p 135.

17. Porter to Lutie Porter, 29 November 1899, Porter Papers, PTR/6/2. Porter was writing after the battle at Graspan (Enslin) on 25 November at which the naval brigade took heavy losses. Marine captain W.T.C. Jones described the dead and wounded as 'little brown patches dotted over the veldt'. He also recorded how 'many that day owed their lives to Fleet Surgeon Porter and his stoker stretcher-bearers, who had followed close in rear of the firing line and had done their work under the hottest fire'. T. Jeans (ed), *Naval Brigades in the South African War 1899–1900* (London, 1901), pp 32–33.

18. Ward to Ogle, 12 November 1846, Papers of Sir Charles Ogle, NMM, LBK/32.

19. Parker to Dundas, 18 November 1849, Northbrook Papers, NP5/1/3/1.

20. See Akiyama, *Feeding the Nation*, pp 144–172. Improvements were recorded in the Journal of Alexander Rattray, reproduced in 'Extract from the Journal of a Medical Officer 1865–1866', *Journal of the Royal Naval Medical Service* 22 (1936), pp 51–61; and later in *Report of the Committee into Naval Rations* (1901), reproduced in Hattendorf et al (eds), *British Naval Documents*, pp 969–972. Simpson, 'Progress of Hygiene', provides a comprehensive contemporary survey.

21. Punishments are explained in more detail in Winton, *Hurrah for the Life of a Sailor*, pp 68–70, 178; and E. Rasor, *Reform in the Royal Navy: A Social History of the Lower Deck 1850–1880* (Connecticut, 1976), pp 38–61. See also Laffin, *Surgeons in the Field*, pp 116–123.

22. Slade to Eden, 5 February 1852, Northbrook Papers, NP5/1/3/9.

23. Burnett to Cochrane, 26 July 1854, Cochrane Papers, MS 2294.

24. Porter to Lutie Porter, 15 May 1898, Porter Papers, PTR/5.

25. Journal of Thomas Dunn, 1 October 1846 to 7 October 1847, ADM101/100/4; and Dundas memorandum, 2 November 1849, Northbrook Papers, NP5/1/3/4. This problem in the late nineteenth century is dealt with in Rasor, *Reform in the Royal Navy*, pp 80–86.

26. Bernard journal, 1 January to 31 December 1851, ADM101/111/1.

27. Milroy, *The Health of the Royal Navy Considered*, pp 61–62.

28. Journal of John Nihill, 1 January to 14 September 1852, ADM101/94/3.

29. Parker to Gage, 31 May 1846, reproduced in Phillimore, *The Life of Parker*, vol. III, pp 53–54.

30. Journal of John Dunlop, 11 January 1851 to 17 June 1852, ADM101/121/2.
31. Drummond to Pilcher, 2 May 1853, ADM97/204.
32. Rae to Burnett, 18 June 1853, ADM97/204; Richardson to Burnett, 31 October 1853, ADM97/206; and Liddell memorandum, 10 December 1856, ADM97/229.
33. Venereal afflictions in the late nineteenth century are discussed in Lloyd and Coulter, *Medicine and the Navy,* vol. IV, pp 198–201; and Rasor, *Reform in the Royal Navy,* pp 87–100. The statistical record of infections for the period 1860–1875 is collated, with variations between different ports shown in P.P. (1877), LII.
34. Lloyd and Coulter, *Medicine and the Navy,* vol. IV, pp 201–204.
35. Brassey, *The British Navy,* vol. V, p 179.
36. Grigor to Burnett, 23 January 1855, ADM97/217.
37. Mackay diary, 7, 11 April 1861; and Deas to Burnett, 20 March 1855, ADM97/219.
38. Liddell memorandum, 16 January 1857, ADM97/230.
39. Osborne memorandum: Admiralty Order Circular 300, 11 August 1857, ADM97/230.
40. Smart to Deas, 5 September 1855, ADM97/222.
41. Kinnear to Deas, 6 September 1855, ADM97/222.
42. C. Maggs, *The Origins of General Nursing* (London, 1983), pp 49–51.
43. M. Baly, *Florence Nightingale and the Nursing Legacy* (London, 2nd ed, 1997), p 72; Maggs, *Origins of General Nursing,* pp 6–8.
44. Liddell memorandum, 7 January 1856, ADM97/224. Naval nursing in the eighteenth and nineteenth centuries is explored in Dickenson, 'The Origin of the Sick Berth Staff, Royal Navy'.
45. Liddell memorandum, 7 January 1856, ADM97/224. The navy's experience of women working in its hospitals is sketched in K. Harland, 'A Short History of Queen Alexandra's Royal Naval Nursing Service', *Journal of the Royal Naval Medical Service* 70 (1984), pp 59–64.
46. Courtney memorandum, 23 June 1854, General Order Book, Haslar Hospital Records, ADM305/40.
47. J. Williams (ed), *The Autobiography of Elizabeth Davis, a Balaclava Nurse* (London, 1857), vol. II, p 137.
48. Shaw-Stewart to Nightingale, 16 March 1857, Papers of Florence Nightingale, BL, add.mss. 45774. Shaw-Stewart's career and views regarding nursing and the peculiarity of military hospitals are elaborated in Summers, *Angels and Citizens,* pp 73–92.

49. Minute by Liddell on Hilditch to Liddell, 22 March 1857, ADM97/231.

50. Early improvements at Haslar are mentioned in Lloyd and Coulter, *Medicine and the Navy,* vol. IV, pp 227–230, 236. See also C. Parsons, 'The Modernisation of Haslar', *Journal of the Royal Naval Medical Service* 72 (1986), pp 107–110; Tait, *A History of Haslar Hospital*; and Richardson, 'A Visit to Haslar, 1916'.

51. Burnett memorandum, 3 April 1854, ADM97/210.

52. Liddell memorandum, 8 August 1855, ADM97/221. It was still a joke within the medical service in the 1890s that Haslar had inscribed above its entrance: 'Abandon Hope All Ye Who Enter Here.' One recruit, fresh from medical school in 1894, observed how the 'begrimed, prison-like windows only added to the prevailing gloom'. T. Jeans, *Reminiscences of a Naval Surgeon* (London, 1927), p.2.

53. May's speech and recruitment problems by 1914 are reported in R. Allison, *The Surgeon Probationers* (Belfast, 1979); and R. Allison, 'Surgeon Probationers: The Young Medical Students who Served in the Royal Navy during the First Great War of 1914–1918', *Journal of the Royal Naval Medical Service* 62 (1976), pp 121–131.

54. Porter to Lutie Porter, 6 February 1912, Porter Papers, PTR/7/4.

55. Porter to Second Sea Lord, 7 May 1913, Porter Papers, PTR/7/3.

56. R. Bacon, *A Naval Scrap-Book: First Part 1877–1900* (London, 1925), pp 74–79.

57. Statistics regarding these expanding professional opportunities in the late nineteenth century are from Maggs, *Origins of General Nursing,* pp 4, 8, 46–47, 49–57; Baly, *Florence Nightingale and the Nursing Legacy,* pp 202, 217; B. Abel-Smith, *A History of the Nursing Profession* (London, 1960), pp 52, 57; and G. Bowman, *The Lamp and the Book: The Story of the Royal College of Nursing 1916–1966* (London, 1967), p 23.

58. The authoritative study of women entering military nursing is Summers, *Angels and Citizens.* See also Baly, *Florence Nightingale and the Nursing Legacy,* p III; and Bingham, *Ministering Angels.*

59. Harland, 'A Short History of Queen Alexandra's Royal Naval Nursing Service', pp 60–61; and Lloyd and Coulter, *Medicine and the Navy,* vol. IV, pp 66–68. The findings of the 1883 (Hoskins) committee enquiring into the training of sick-berth and nursing staff in naval hospitals appear in P.P. (1884), XVII.

60. Porter to Lutie Porter, 6 July 1886, Porter Papers, MS 85/088; Porter to Lutie Porter, 6 May 1891, Porter Papers, PTR/2; and Porter to Lutie Porter, 2 February 1899, Porter Papers, PTR/5.

61. Crocker to Porter, 21 May 1900, Porter Papers, PTR/6/2.

62. Improvements at Haslar between the 1880s and 1914 are surveyed in Lloyd and Coulter, *Medicine and the Navy,* vol. IV, pp 241–242; Tait, *A History of Haslar Hospital*, pp 26–57, 108–109; Parsons, 'The Modernisation of Haslar', p 107; and J. Holford, 'Some Highlights of Naval Medical History', *Journal of the Royal Naval Medical Service* 51 (1965), pp 54–55.

63. Hurford, 'The Early History of Plymouth Hospital', pp 251–252.

64. Moore to Porter, 5 March 1899, Porter Papers, PTR/5. The findings of the committee enquiring at that time into the training of medical officers, specifically at Haslar, were published in P.P. (1899), LV. Recollections by Surgeon Rear-Admiral T. Jeans suggest that improvement was a slow process. He stated that 'in 1894 naval hospitals lagged sadly behind civil hospitals'. Furthermore, 'surgery in the navy, then, was somewhat primitive, and an operation which would be termed a "major" one, today, a rarity'. Jeans, *Reminiscences*, p 5.

65. Porter to Lutie Porter, 27 September 1899, Porter Papers, PTR/5.

66. Porter to Lutie Porter, 16 October 1890, Porter Papers, PTR/2.

67. Porter to Lutie Porter, 25 June 1901, Porter Papers, PTR/7/1.

68. Porter to Lutie Porter, 5 January 1890, Porter Papers, PTR/2; and Porter to Lutie Porter, 19 January 1898, Porter Papers, PTR/5.

69. Porter to Lutie Porter, 12 March 1891, 13 March 1890, 25 August 1891, Porter Papers, PTR/2.

70. Porter to Lutie Porter, 3 July 1899, Porter Papers, PTR/5.

71. Cowan to Porter, 11 January 1895, Porter Papers, PTR/3. Looking back on his career in 1927 Jeans spoke highly of Porter as Director-General but believed, like Cowan and others in the service, that 'the Lords of the Admiralty do not care to have too self-willed an officer at the head of the Medical Department'. Jeans, *Reminiscences*, p 203.

72. Porter to Lutie Porter, 21 February 1912, Porter Papers, PTR/7/4.

73. Porter to Lutie Porter, 19 February 1901, Porter Papers, MS 85/088.

74. Porter to Lutie Porter, 30 October 1900, Porter Papers, PTR/6/2. Porter's criticisms notwithstanding, the findings of an official investigation into the rank, pay and position of naval medical officers were published in P.P. (1881), XXII.

75. Porter to Lutie Porter, 21, 27 December 1899, Porter Papers, PTR/6/2.

76. Porter to Lutie Porter, 8 February 1900, Porter Papers, PTR/6/2.

77. Porter to Lutie Porter, 23 March 1900, Porter Papers, PTR/6/2.

78. S. Clark, 'Farewell to the SBA', *Journal of the Royal Naval Medical Service* 70 (1984), p 6. Training for sick-berth staff after 1883 in comprehensively covered

in Akiyama, *Feeding the Nation*, pp 173–202.

79. Norbury, *The Naval Brigade in South Africa*, pp 249–250.
80. Porter to Lutie Porter, 4 March 1901, Porter Papers, MS 85/088.
81. Cowan to Porter, 17 March 1893, Porter Papers, MS 85/088. Nineteenth-century pay scales and differentials are listed in detail in M. Lewis, *The Navy in Transition 1814–1864: A Social History* (London, 1965), pp 212–213.
82. Cowan to John Cowan, 16 December 1880, Cowan Papers, PTR/1.
83. Cox to Porter, 12 April 1908, Porter Papers, PTR/7/3.
84. Hansard, CLII (1859), p 900.
85. Milroy, *The Health of the Royal Navy Considered*, pp 61–62.
86. Porter to Lutie Porter, 19 September 1898, Porter Papers, MS 85/088.
87. Porter to Lutie Porter, 18 September 1899, Porter Papers, PTR/5.
88. Cowan to Porter, 2 June 1886, Porter Papers, PTR/3.

Bibliography

Unpublished Material

1. Official Papers

(a) *At the National Archives, London*
Admiralty Records, ADM53/..., ADM97/..., ADM105/..., ADM114/...
Surgeons' Journals, ADM101/...
Hospital Ships' Logs, ADM102/..., ADM104/...
Letterbooks of Sir William Burnett, ADM105/68–73
Haslar Hospital Records, ADM305/...

(b) *At the National Maritime Museum, Greenwich*
Ships' Logs, LOG/...

2. Private Collections

(a) *At the National Maritime Museum, Greenwich*
Papers of William Baird
Papers of Edward Boxer
Papers of Richard Collinson
Papers of Charles Hope
Papers of Sir Alexander Milne
Papers of the Earl of Minto
Papers of Sir Charles Ogle
Papers of Sir William Parker
Papers of Sir James Porter (including the Papers of Michael Cowan)
Journal of Edward Cree
Journal of John Cunningham
Journal of William Domville
Journal of Robert Guthrie

Journal of William Kay
Journal of John McIlroy
Journal of Henry Piers
Journal of Maurice West
Journal of Charles Wilkinson
Letterbook of John Clavell
Letterbook of Henry Keppel

(b) *At the British Library, London*
Papers of the Earl of Auckland
Papers of Sir Charles Napier
Papers of Florence Nightingale

(c) *At the National Library of Scotland, Edinburgh*
Papers of Sir Thomas Cochrane

(d) *At the Royal Naval Museum, Portsmouth*
Diary of Alexander Mackay

(e) *At the National Army Museum, Chelsea*
Papers of Wyndham Baker
Papers of Chilley Pine

(f) *At the West Sussex Record Office, Chichester*
Papers of the Fifth Duke of Richmond (Goodwood Papers)

(g) *At the Plymouth and West Devon County Record Office, Plymouth*
Turnbull, A., *History of the Naval Medical Service from the Earliest Dates to the Present Time* (Manuscript, 1904)

(h) *At ING Baring, London*
Papers of Sir Francis Baring (Northbrook Papers)

(i) *In the temporary keeping of the author*
Papers of Henry Willan

Published Material

1. Documentary Sources

A Naval Medical Officer, *An Exposition of the Case of the Assistant Surgeons of the Royal Navy* (London, 1849)

Hansard

Illustrated London News

Journal of the Royal Naval Medical Service

The Lancet

Navy and Army Illustrated

The Navy List

Parliamentary Accounts and Papers

2. Secondary Sources

Abel-Smith, B., *A History of the Nursing Profession* (London, 1960)

Adams, A., *The Zoology of the Voyage of H.M.S. Samarang; under the Command of Captain Sir Edward Belcher C.B., F.R.A.S., F.G.S., during the years 1843–1846* (London, 1850)

Adams, H. and A. Adams, *The Genera of Recent Mollusca*, 3 vols. (London, 1858)

Adkins, R. and L. Adkins, *Jack Tar: Life in Nelson's Navy* (London, 2008)

Akiyama, Y., *Feeding the Nation: Nutrition and Health in Britain before World War One* (London, 2008)

___, 'Trained Cooks and Healthy Boys: Reforming the Mess in the Royal Navy before the First World War', *Mariner's Mirror* 94 (2008), pp 420–431

Alcock, R., *Notes on the Medical History and Statistics of the British Legion of Spain, Comprising the Results of Gun-Shot Wounds, in relation to Important Questions in Surgery* (London, 1838)

Allison, R., *The Surgeon Probationers* (Belfast, 1979)

___, 'Surgeon Probationers: The Young Medical Students who Served in the Royal Navy during the First Great War of 1914–1918', *Journal of the Royal Naval Medical Service* 62 (1976), pp 121–131

___, *Sea Diseases: The Story of a Great Natural Experiment in Preventive Medicine in the Royal Navy* (London, 1943)

___, 'One Hundred Years of Commissioned Rank', *Journal of the Royal Naval Medical Service* 29 (1943), pp 83–90

___, 'Sea Surgeons', *Journal of the Royal Naval Medical Service* 27 (1941), pp 125–137

Anon, 'Surgeon William Job Maillard, V.C., M.D., R.N.', *Journal of the Royal Naval Medical Service* 42 (1956), pp 106–108

___, 'Haslar', *Journal of the Royal Naval Medical Service* 39 (1953), pp 59–62

___, 'Editorial', *Journal of the Royal Naval Medical Service* 5 (1919), pp 319–320

Aubrey, P., 'Climate and Health in West African Waters 1825–1870', *Journal of the Royal Naval Medical Service* 40 (1954), pp 84–88

Bacon, R., *A Naval Scrap-Book: First Part 1877–1900* (London, 1925)

Baikie, W., *Narrative of an Exploring Voyage up the Rivers Kwo'ra and Bi'nue (commonly known as the Niger and Tsádda) in 1854* (London, 1856)

___, *Historia Naturalis Orcadensis: Zoology. Part I. Being a catalogue of the Mammalia and Birds hitherto observed in the Orkney Islands* (Edinburgh, 1848)

Baldock, N., 'Doctor's Orders No.9 – or 10 Green Bottles Skulking in the Hulk?', *Journal of the Royal Naval Medical Service* 86 (2000), pp 157–162

___, 'Health in the Royal Navy during the Age of Nelson: The Institute of Naval Medicine', *Journal of the Royal Naval Medical Service* 86 (2000), pp 60–63

Baly, M., *Florence Nightingale and the Nursing Legacy* (London, 1997)

Bannerman, G., *Merchants and the Military in Eighteenth-Century Britain: British Army Contracts and Domestic Supply, 1739–1763* (London, 2008)

Barford, J., 'How to Run a Sick Bay', *Journal of the Royal Naval Medical Service* 3 (1917), pp 353–360

Barker, A., *The Vainglorious War 1854–56* (London, 1970)

Bartlett, C., *Great Britain and Sea Power 1815–1853* (Oxford, 1963)

Baumgart, W., *The Crimean War 1853–1856* (London, 1999)

Baylen, J. and A. Conway (eds), *Soldier Surgeon: The Crimean War Letters of Dr. Douglas A. Reid 1855–1856* (Knoxville, Tennessee, 1968)

Baynham, H., *Before the Mast: Naval Ratings of the Nineteenth Century* (London, 1971)

___, *From the Lower Deck: The Old Navy 1780–1840* (London, 1969)

Beechey, F., *The Zoology of Captain Beechey's Voyage* (London, 1839)

Beeching, J., *The Chinese Opium Wars* (London, 1975)

Beeler, J. (ed), *The Milne Papers: The Papers of Admiral of the Fleet Sir Alexander Milne, Bt., K.C.B. (1806–1896)*, vol. I (Aldershot, 2004)

Belcher, E., *Narrative of the Voyage of H.M.S. Samarang during the years 1843–1846*, 2 vols. (London, 1848)

___, *Narrative of a Voyage Round the World, Performed in H.M.S. Sulphur, during the years 1836–1842, including details of the Naval Operations in China from December 1840 to November 1841*, 2 vols. (London, 1843)

Bethell, L., *The Abolition of the Brazilian Slave Trade: Britain, Brazil and the Slave Trade Question 1807–1869* (Cambridge, 1970)

Bingham, S., *Ministering Angels* (London, 1979)

Blake, N., *Steering to Glory: A Day in the Life of a Ship of the Line* (London, 2005)

Blake, N. and R. Lawrence, *The Illustrated Companion to Nelson's Navy* (London, 1999)

Bockstoce, J. (ed), *The Journal of Rochfort Maguire 1852–1854: Two Years at Point Barrow, Alaska, aboard HMS Plover in the search for Sir John Franklin*, 2 vols. (London, 1988)

Bonham-Carter, V. (ed), *Surgeon in the Crimea: The Experiences of George Lawson Recorded in Letters to his Family 1854–1855* (London, 1968)

Bonner-Smith, D. (ed), *Russian War, 1855. Baltic: Official Correspondence* (London, 1944)

___, and A. Dewar (eds), *Russian War, 1854. Baltic and Black Sea: Official Correspondence* (London, 1943)

Booker, J. *Maritime Quarantine: The British Experience, c.1650–1900* (Aldershot, 2007).

Bornmann, R., 'Doctors at Greenwich', *Journal of the Royal Naval Medical Service* 57 (1971), pp 145–149

Bourchier, Lady (ed), *Memoir of the Life of Admiral Sir Edward Codrington*, 2 vols. (London, 1873)

Bourne, K., *Palmerston: The Early Years 1784–1841* (London, 1982)

Bowden-Dan, J., 'Diet, Dirt and Discipline: Medical Developments in Nelson's Navy. Dr. John Snipe's Contribution', *Mariner's Mirror* 90 (2004), pp 260–272

Bowen, F., *History of the Royal Naval Reserve* (London, 1926)

Bowman, G., *The Lamp and the Book: The Story of the Royal College of Nursing 1916–1966* (London, 1967)

Brassey, T., *The British Navy: Its Strength, Resources, and Administration*, 5 vols. (London, 1882–83)

Brooks, R., *The Long Arm of Empire: Naval Brigades from the Crimea to the Boxer Rebellion* (London, 1999)

Brownfield, O., 'Royal Naval Hospital, Malta', *Journal of the Royal Naval Medical Service* 35 (1949), pp 245–251

Bryson, A., *An Account of the Origin, Spread, and Decline of the Epidemic Fevers of Sierra Leone* (London, 1849)

___, *Report on the Climate and Principal Diseases of the African Station* (London, 1847)

Burnett, W., *Reports and Testimonials respecting the Solution of Chloride of Zinc (Sir William Burnett's Disinfecting Fluid) as a means of destroying Deleterious Gases, or the Effluvia arising from Putrid Animal and Vegetable Substance, and preventing the spread of Infectious Diseases; – as an application to Ulcers with Foetid Discharges and as an agent for Purifying Hospitals or Chambers of the Sick; and for preserving Anatomical Preparations* (London, 1850)

___, *Reports on the Solution of Chloride of Zinc: as an agent for the Destruction of Deleterious gases, or the Effluvia arising from the Decomposition of Animal and Vegetable Substances; for Purifying the Wards of Hospitals or Sick Chambers; and for Preserving Anatomical Preparations* (London, 1848)

___, *A Practical Account of the Mediterranean Fever, as it appeared in the Ships and Hospitals of His Majesty's Fleet on that Station* (London, 1816)

Cantlie, N., *A History of the Army Medical Department*, vol. I (London, 1974)

Carr, R., *Spain 1808–1975* (Oxford, 1982)

Christiansen, E., *The Origins of Military Power in Spain 1800–1854* (Oxford, 1967)

Clark, S., 'Farewell to the SBA', *Journal of the Royal Naval Medical Service* 70 (1984), pp 3–8

Collinson, T. (ed), *Journal of H.M.S. Enterprise, on the Expedition in Search of Sir John Franklin's Ships by Behring Strait 1850–55* (London, 1889)

Colomb, P., *Memoirs of Admiral the Right Honourable Sir Astley Cooper-Key* (London, 1898)

Cunynghame, A., *An Aide-de-Camp's Recollections of Service in China, a Residence in Hongkong, and Visits to other Islands in the Chinese Seas*, 2 vols. (London, 1844)

Dewar, A. (ed), *The Russian War, 1855. Black Sea: Official Correspondence* (London, 1945)

Dewar, P., 'A Survey of Post Mortems, Malta Hospital 1829–1838 with special reference to the Cholera Epidemic of 1837', *Journal of the Royal Naval Medical Service* 55 (1969), pp 84–88

Dickenson, G., 'The Origin of the Sick Berth Staff, Royal Navy', *Journal of the Royal Naval Medical Service* 13 (1927), pp 161–173

Douglas, H., *Remarks on the Naval Operations in the Black Sea and the Siege of Sebastopol* (London, 1855)

Druett, J., *Rough Medicine: Surgeons at Sea in the Age of Sail* (New York, 2000)

Dudley, S., 'Yellow Fever, as seen by the Medical Officers of the Royal Navy in the Nineteenth Century', *Journal of the Royal Naval Medical Service* 19 (1933), pp 151–165

Duffy, M., *Soldiers, Sugar and Seapower: The British Expeditions to the West Indies and the War against Revolutionary France* (Oxford, 1987)

Duncan, F., *The English in Spain; or, the Story of the War of Succession between 1834 and 1840* (London, 1877)

Dundonald, Lord, *Observations on Naval Affairs* (London, 1847)

Eardley-Wilmot, S., *Life of Vice-Admiral Edmund, Lord Lyons* (London, 1898)

Ellis, W., *An Authentic Narrative of a Voyage Performed by Captain Cook and Captain Clerke, in His Majesty's Ships Resolution and Discovery during the years 1776, 1777, 1778, 1779, and 1780* (London, 1782)

Estes, J., *Naval Surgeon: Life and Death at Sea in the Age of Sail* (Canton, Massachusetts, 1998)

___, 'Naval Medicine in the Age of Sail: The Voyage of the *New York*, 1802–1803', *Bulletin of the History of Medicine* 56 (1982), pp 238–253

Falconer-Hall, J., 'The Royal Naval Hospitals, Malta', *Journal of the Royal Naval Medical Service* 13 (1927), pp 251–255

Fay, P., *The Opium War 1840–1842* (Chapel Hill, 1975)

Festing, E. (ed), *Life of Commander Henry James R.N.* (London, 1899)

Ffrench-Blake, R., *The Crimean War* (London, 1971)

Fisher, A., *A Journal of a Voyage of Discovery to the Arctic Regions in His Majesty's Ships Hecla and Griper in the years 1819 and 1820* (London, 1821)

Forbes, E., *The Zoology of the Voyage of HMS Herald under the Command of Captain Henry Kellett R.N., C.B., during the years 1845–51* (London, 1854)

Fortescue, J., *A History of the British Army*, vol. 12 (London, 1927)

Fox, G., *British Admirals and Chinese Pirates 1832–1869* (London, 1940)

Franklin, J., *Narrative of a Journey to the Shores of the Polar Sea, in the years 1819, 20, 21, and 22* (London, 1823)

___, *Narrative of a Second Expedition to the Shores of the Polar Sea in the years 1825, 1826 and 1827* (London, 1828)

Friedenberg, Z., *Medicine Under Sail* (Annapolis, 2000)

Gillespie, T., 'The Diet and Health of Seamen in the West Indies at the end of the Eighteenth Century – Some Remarks on the Work of Leonard Gillespie, M.D.', *Journal of the Royal Naval Medical Service* 37 (1951), pp 187–192

Glass, J., 'James Lind, M.D. Eighteenth Century Naval Medical Hygienist', *Journal of the Royal Naval Medical Service* 35 (1949), pp 1–20, 68–86

Glew, P., 'Singular Experiences: The Early History of Anaesthesia in the Royal Navy 1847 to 1854', *Journal of the Royal Naval Medical Service* 83 (1997), pp 42–44

Goddard, J., 'An Insight into the Life of Royal Naval Surgeons during the Napoleonic War', *Journal of the Royal Naval Medical Service* 77 (1991), pp 205–222; and 78 (1992), pp 27–36

Goldfrank, D., *The Origins of the Crimean War* (London, 1994)

Goldie, S. (ed), *'I Have Done my Duty': Florence Nightingale in the Crimean War*

1854–56 (Manchester, 1987)

Goodman, M., *Experiences of an English Sister of Mercy* (London, 1862)

Goodwin, P., 'Health in the Royal Navy during the Age of Nelson: The Development of the Sick Berth 1740–1815 and its Relation to H.M.S. *Victory*', *Journal of the Royal Naval Medical Service* 86 (2000), pp 81–84

Graham, G., *The China Station: War and Diplomacy 1830–1860* (Oxford, 1978)

Greenhill, B. and A. Giffard, *Steam, Politics and Patronage: The Transformation of the Royal Navy 1815–54* (London, 1994)

___, *The British Assault on Finland 1854–1855: A Forgotten Naval War* (London, 1988)

Haas, J., *A Management Odyssey: The Royal Dockyards, 1714–1914* (London, 1994)

Hamilton, R., *Naval Administration: The Constitution, Character and Functions of the Board of Admiralty, and of the Civil Departments it Directs* (London, 1896)

Harland, K., 'The Royal Naval Hospital at Minorca, 1711: An Example of an Admiral's Involvement in the Expansion of Naval Medical Care', *Mariner's Mirror* 94 (2008), pp 36–47

___, 'A Short History of Queen Alexandra's Royal Naval Nursing Service', *Journal of the Royal Naval Medical Service* 70 (1984), pp 59–64

Harper, E., 'The Sailor's Surgeon', *Journal of the Royal Naval Medical Service* 65 (1979), pp 35–37

Hattendorf, J., R. Knight, A. Pearsall, N. Rodger and G. Till (eds), *British Naval Documents 1204–1960* (London, 1993)

Hill, R., 'A Retrospective View of Naval Medical Conditions', *Journal of the Royal Naval Medical Service* 6 (1920), pp 1–12

Hinds, R. (ed), *The Botany of the Voyage of HMS Sulphur under the Command of Sir Edward Belcher, R.N., C.B., F.R.G.S., etc. during the years 1836–42* (London, 1844)

___, (ed), The *Zoology of the Voyage of HMS Sulphur under the Command of Sir Edward Belcher, R.N., C.B., F.R.G.S., etc. during the years 1836–42* (London, 1844)

Holford, J., 'Some Highlights of Naval Medical History', *Journal of the Royal Naval Medical Service* 51 (1965), pp 51–57

Holt, E., *The Carlist Wars in Spain* (London, 1967)

Hooker, J. (ed), *Voyage of the Erebus and Terror: Zoology* (London, 1844)

Howard-Jones, N., 'Cholera Therapy in the Nineteenth Century', *Journal of the History of Medicine and Allied Sciences* 27 (1972), pp 373–395

Howell, R., *The Royal Navy and the Slave Trade* (London, 1987)

Hughes, R., 'James Lind and the Cure of Scurvy: An Experimental Approach',

Medical History 19 (1975), pp 342–351

Hunter, M., 'The Hero Packs a Punch: Sir Charles Hotham, Liberalism and West Africa, 1846–1850', *Mariner's Mirror* 92 (2006), pp 282–299

Huntsman, R., M. Bruin and D. Holttum, 'Light before Dawn: Naval Nursing and Medical Care during the Crimean War', *Journal of the Royal Naval Medical Service* 88 (2002), pp 5–27

Hurford, A., 'The Early History of Plymouth Hospital', *Journal of the Royal Naval Medical Service* 21 (1935), pp 40–47, 138–151, 249–252

Huxley, J. (ed), *T. H. Huxley's Diary of the Voyage of HMS Rattlesnake* (London, 1935)

Inglefield, E., *A Summer Search for Sir John Franklin; with a Peep into the Polar Basin* (London, 1853)

Inglis, B., *The Opium War* (London, 1976)

James, E., 'Naval Health and the Environment', *Journal of the Royal Naval Medical Service* 51 (1965), pp 201–207

James, R., 'A Naval Surgeon's Log, 1781–1783', *Journal of the Royal Naval Medical Service* 19 (1933), pp 221–240

Jeans, T., *Reminiscences of a Naval Surgeon* (London, 1927)

___ (ed), *Naval Brigades in the South African War 1899–1900* (London, 1901)

Jenkins, I., 'The Royal Defence Medical College', *Journal of the Royal Naval Medical Service* 83 (1997), pp 113–115

Jenkinson, S., 'Extract from a Naval Scrapbook (Naval Hospitals)', *Journal of the Royal Naval Medical Service* 42 (1956), pp 120–122

___, 'John Moyle, Surgeon, Royal Navy', *Journal of the Royal Naval Medical Service* 38 (1952), pp 1–7

___, 'The Medical Officers', *Journal of the Royal Naval Medical Service* 35 (1949), pp 87–90

___, 'Dr. Baikie, M.D., Surgeon, R.N., Naturalist, Traveller, Philologist', *Journal of the Royal Naval Medical Service* 29 (1943), pp 203–207

___, 'Sir William Burnett K.C.B., K.C.H., M.D., F.R.S.', *Journal of the Royal Naval Medical Service* 26 (1940), pp 3–15

___, 'John Woodall, Surgeon, Royal Navy 1569–1643', *Journal of the Royal Naval Medical Service* 26 (1940), pp 107–116

___, 'Alexander Bryson', *Journal of the Royal Naval Medical Service* 25 (1939), pp 99–108

___, 'Biographical Memoir of Dr. John Harness', *Journal of the Royal Naval Medical Service* 23 (1937), pp 2–14

___, 'Biography of Sir Gilbert Blane (1749–1834)', *Journal of the Royal Naval*

Medical Service 23 (1937), pp 293–301

Jewitt, L., *A History of Plymouth* (London, 1873)

Johnson, R, 'The Diary of the First Governor of Plymouth Hospital', *Journal of the Royal Naval Medical Service* 2 (1916), pp 191–199

Johnson, R.E., *Sir John Richardson: Arctic Explorer, Natural Historian, Naval Surgeon* (London, 1976)

Keevil, J., *Medicine and the Navy 1200–1900*, vols. I and II (London, 1957 and 1958)

___, 'Ralph Cuming and the Interscapulo-Thoracic Amputation in 1808', *Journal of the Royal Naval Medical Service* 36 (1950), pp 63–72

___, 'Benjamin Bynoe (1804–1865): Surgeon of HMS *Beagle*', *Journal of the Royal Naval Medical Service* 35 (1949), pp 251–268

___, 'Robert McCormick, R.N.: The Stormy Petrel of Naval Medicine', *Journal of the Royal Naval Medical Service* 29 (1943), pp 36–62

Kemp, P., *The British Sailor: A Social History of the Lower Deck* (London, 1970)

Keppel, H., *A Sailor's Life under Four Sovereigns*, 3 vols. (London, 1899)

King, G., *The Fever at Boa Vista in 1845–6 unconnected with the Visit of the 'Eclair' to that Island* (London, 1852)

Kirby, P., *Sir Andrew Smith, M.D., K.C.B: His Life, Letters and Works* (Cape Town, 1965)

Kitson, A., *Captain James Cook R.N., F.R.S.: 'The Circumnavigator'* (London, 1907)

___, 'Abstract from "Captain James Cook" by Kitson (1907)', *Journal of the Royal Naval Medical Service* 26 (1940), pp 329–335

Laffin, J., *Surgeons in the Field* (London, 1970)

___, *Jack Tar: The Story of the British Sailor* (London, 1969)

Lambert, A., *Franklin: Tragic Hero of Polar Navigation* (London, 2009)

___, *Admirals: The Naval Commanders who Made Britain Great* (London, 2008)

___, 'Preparing for the Long Peace: The Reconstruction of the Royal Navy 1815–1830', *Mariner's Mirror* 82 (1996), pp 41–54

___, *The Crimean War; British Grand Strategy, 1853–1856* (Manchester, 1990)

___ (ed), 'Sir Henry Keppel's Account, Capture of Bomarsund, August 1854', in N. Rodger (ed), *The Naval Miscellany*, vol. V (London, 1984), pp 354–370

Lattimore, M., 'Early Naval Medical Libraries, Personal and Corporate', *Journal of the Royal Naval Medical Service* 69 (1983), pp 107–111, 156–160

Levien, M., *The Cree Journals: The Voyages of Edward H. Cree, Surgeon R.N. as related in his Private Journals, 1837–1856* (Exeter, 1981)

Lewis, M., *The Navy in Transition 1814–1864: A Social History* (London, 1965)

Lewis-Smith, F., 'A Short Account of the Royal Naval Medical Service', *Journal of the Royal Naval Medical Service* 15 (1929), pp 177–185

Lloyd, C., 'Cook and Scurvy', *Mariner's Mirror* 65 (1979), pp 23–28

___, *Mr. Barrow of the Admiralty: A Life of Sir John Barrow 1764–1848* (London, 1970)

___, *The Health of Seamen* (London, 1965)

___, and J. Coulter, *Medicine and the Navy 1200–1900*, vols. III and IV (London, 1961 and 1963)

Loch, G., *The Closing Events of the Campaign in China: The Operations in the Yang-tsze-Kiang; and Treaty of Nanking* (London, 1843)

Lysons, D., *The Crimean War from First to Last* (London, 1895)

McBride, W., '"Normal" Medical Science and British Treatment of Sea Scurvy, 1753–75', *Journal of the History of Medicine and Allied Sciences* 46 (1991), pp 158–177

M'Clintock, F., *Fate of Sir John Franklin: The Voyage of the Fox in the Arctic Seas in Search of Franklin and his Companions* (5th ed, London, 1881)

___, *Discovery of the Fate of Sir John Franklin and his Companions* (London, 1859)

MacDonald, J., *Feeding Nelson's Navy: The True Story of Food at Sea in the Georgian Era* (London, 2004)

McDonald, J., 'The Question of Quarantine in Britain during the Nineteenth Century', *Bulletin of the History of Medicine* 25 (1951), pp 22–44

M'Dougall, G., *The Eventful Voyage of H.M. Discovery Ship Resolute to the Arctic Regions in Search of Sir John Franklin and the Missing Crews of H.M. Discovery Ships Erebus and Terror, 1852, 1853, 1854* (London, 1857)

McIlraith, J., *Life of Sir John Richardson* (London, 1868)

McKee, C., *Sober Men and True: Sailor Lives in the Royal Navy 1900–1945* (London, 2002)

McLean, D., *Public Health and Politics in the Age of Reform: Cholera, the State and the Royal Navy in Victorian Britain* (London, 2006)

___, 'Surgeons of the Opium War: The Navy on the China Coast, 1840–42', *English Historical Review* 121 (2006), pp 487–504

MacLeod, R., *Public Science and Public Policy in Victorian England* (Aldershot, 1996)

___ (ed), *Government and Expertise: Specialists, Administrators and Professionals, 1860–1919* (Cambridge, 1988)

MacLeod, W., 'Outbreak of Yellow Fever, 1859. Extract from the Journal of Surgeon William MacLeod. R.N. HMS *Madagascar*, at Rio de Janeiro', *Journal of the Royal Naval Medical Service* 19 (1933), pp 186–200

McNeil, D., 'Medical Care aboard Australia-Bound Convict Ships, 1786–1840', *Bulletin of the History of Medicine* 26 (1952), pp 117–140

M'William, J., *Medical History of the Expedition to the Niger during the years 1841–2, Comprising an Account of the Fever which led to its Abrupt Termination* (London, 1843)

Maggs, C., *The Origins of General Nursing* (London, 1983)

Main, R., *The British Navy in 1871* (London, 1871)

Marjot, D., 'Aspects of Alcohol and Service Medicine', *Journal of the Royal Naval Medical Service* 53 (1967), pp 113–136

Masefield, J., *Sea Life in Nelson's Time* (London, 1905)

Mayne F., *The Book of Plymouth* (Plymouth, 1938)

Milroy, G., *The Health of the Royal Navy Considered in a letter addressed to the Rt. Hon. Sir John S. Pakington, Bart. M.P.* (London, 1862)

___, *The Cholera not to be Arrested by Quarantine: A brief historical sketch of the great Epidemic of 1817, and its Invasions of Europe in 1831–2 and 1847 with practical remarks on the Treatment, Preventive and Curative, of the Disease* (London, 1847)

Morriss, R., *Naval Power and British Culture 1760–1850: Public Trust and Government Ideology* (Aldershot, 2004)

___, *Cockburn and the British Navy in Transition: Admiral Sir George Cockburn 1772–1853* (Exeter, 1997)

Musson, R., 'A Memory of the "Eclair"', *Journal of the Royal Naval Medical Service* 37 (1951), pp 125–133

Napier, E., *The Life and Correspondence of Admiral Sir Charles Napier KCB, from Personal Recollections, Letters and Official Documents*, 2 vols. (London, 1862)

Napier, P., *Black Charlie: A Life of Admiral Sir Charles Napier KCB 1787–1860* (Norwich, 1995)

Norbury, H., *The Naval Brigade in South Africa during the years 1877–78–79* (London, 1880)

Northcote-Parkinson, C., *Britannia Rules: The Classic Age of Naval History 1793–1815* (London, 1977)

O'Connor, A., 'Surgeon William Job Maillard, V.C., M.D., R.N.', *Journal of the Royal Naval Medical Service* 50 (1964), pp 64–70

An Officer of the Expedition, *Letters Written during the Late Voyage of Discovery in the Western Arctic Sea* (London, 1821)

O'Sullivan, D. *In Search of Captain Cook: Exploring the Man through his Own Words* (London, 2008)

Osborn, S., *Stray Leaves from an Arctic Journal; or, Eighteen Months in the Polar Regions, in Search of Sir John Franklin's Expedition, in the years 1850–51* (London, 1852)

Padfield, P., *Rule Britannia: The Victorian and Edwardian Navy* (London, 1981)

Parkinson, R., *The Late Victorian Navy: The Pre-Dreadnought Era and the Origins of the First World War* (Woodbridge, 2008)

Parry, A. (ed), *The Admirals Fremantle* (London, 1971)

Parry, E., *Memoirs of Rear-Admiral Sir W. Edward Parry, Kt., F.R.S.* (London, 1857)

Parsons, C., 'The Modernisation of Haslar', *Journal of the Royal Naval Medical Service* 72 (1986), pp 107–110

___, 'Haslar Museum', *Journal of the Royal Naval Medical Service* 71 (1985), pp 117–120

Paul, R., 'The Institute of Naval Medicine', *Journal of the Royal Naval Medical Service* 73 (1987), pp 119–122

Penn. C., 'The Medical Staffing of the Royal Navy in the Russian War, 1854–6', *Mariner's Mirror* 89 (2003), pp 51–58

Penney, M., 'Letters from Therapia, 1855', *Blackwood's Magazine* 275 (1954), pp 413–421

Phillimore, A., *The Life of Admiral of the Fleet Sir William Parker Bart., G.C.B.*, 3 vols. (London, 1876, 1879 and 1880)

Pick, B., 'Extract from a Medical Officer's Journal in the Year 1866', *Journal of the Royal Naval Medical Service* 20 (1934), pp 51–63

___, 'Medical Department of the Navy in 1838', *Journal of the Royal Naval Medical Service* 19 (1933), pp 241–253

Pinckard, G., 'Puellae Porti Magni', *Journal of the Royal Naval Medical Service* 89 (2003), pp 73–75

Plumridge, J., *Hospital Ships and Ambulance Trains* (London, 1975)

Pollard, E., 'Diary of a Medical Officer on Active Service with the Royal Marines in Egypt in 1882', *Journal of the Royal Naval Medical Service* 22 (1936), pp 132–143

Pope, D., *Life in Nelson's Navy* (London, 1981)

Porter, I., 'Thomas Trotter, M.D., Naval Physician', *Medical History* 7 (1963), pp 155–164

Pugh, P., 'History of the Royal Naval Hospital, Plymouth' *Journal of the Royal Naval Medical Service* 58 (1972), pp 78–94, 207–226

Rae, J., *Narrative of an Expedition to the Shores of the Arctic Sea in 1846 and 1847* (London, 1850)

Rasor, E., *Reform in the Royal Navy: A Social History of the Lower Deck 1850–1880* (Connecticut, 1976)

Rattray, A., 'Extract from the Journal of a Medical Officer 1865–1866', *Journal of the Royal Naval Medical Service* 22 (1936), pp 51–61

Richardson, J., *The Polar Regions* (Edinburgh, 1861)

___, *The Last of the Arctic Voyages, being a narrative of the Expedition in HMS Assistance, under the command of Captain Sir Edward Belcher C.B., in search of Sir John Franklin, during the years 1852–53–54, with notes on the Natural History*, 2 vols. (London, 1855)

___, *Arctic Searching Expedition: a journal of a boat-voyage through Rupert's Land and the Arctic Sea, in search of the discovery ships under command of Sir John Franklin*, 2 vols. (London, 1851)

___, *Fauna Boreali-Americana or the Zoology of the Northern Parts of British America*, 4 vols. (London, 1829, 1831, 1836 and 1837)

Richardson, J.B., 'A Visit to Haslar, 1916', *Journal of the Royal Naval Medical Service* 2 (1916), pp 329–339

Richardson, R. (ed), *Nurse Sarah Anne: with Florence Nightingale at Scutari* (London, 1977)

Risse, G., 'Britannia Rules the Seas: The Health of Seamen, Edinburgh, 1791–1800', *Journal of the History of Medicine and Allied Sciences* 43 (1988), pp 426–446

Robinson, C., *Victorian Plymouth* (Plymouth, 1991)

Robinson, F., *Diary of the Crimean War* (London, 1856)

Rodger, N., *The Command of the Ocean: A Naval History of Britain 1649–1815* (London, 2004)

___, *The Admiralty* (Lavenham, Suffolk, 1979)

Rolleston, H., 'Sir John Richardson', *Journal of the Royal Naval Medical Service*, 10 (1924) pp 161–172

___, 'Sir William Burnett: The First Medical Director-General of the Royal Navy', *Journal of the Royal Naval Medical Service* 8 (1922), pp 1–10

___, 'Thomas Trotter M.D.', *Journal of the Royal Naval Medical Service* 5 (1919), pp 412–419

___, 'Sir Gilbert Blane: An Administrator of Naval Medicine and Hygiene', *Journal of the Royal Naval Medical Service* 2 (1916), pp 72–81

___, 'James Lind: Pioneer of Naval Hygiene', *Journal of the Royal Naval Medical Service* 1 (1915), pp 181–190

Ross, J., *Narrative of a Second Voyage in Search of a North-West Passage and of a Residence in the Arctic Regions during the years 1829, 1830, 1831, 1832, 1833* (London, 1835)

___, *Appendix to the Narrative of a Second Voyage in Search of a North-West Passage and of a Residence in the Arctic Regions during the years 1829, 1830, 1831, 1832, 1833* (London, 1835)

___, *A Voyage of Discovery made under the Orders of the Admiralty in His Majesty's Ships Isabella and Alexander for the purpose of Exploring Baffin's Bay, and Inquiring into the probability of a North-West Passage* (London, 1819)

Ross, J.C., *A Voyage of Discovery and Research in the Southern and Antarctic Regions, during the years 1839–43*, 2 vols. (London, 1847)

Savours, A., 'The Diary of Assistant Surgeon Henry Piers, HMS Investigator, 1850–54', *Journal of the Royal Naval Medical Service* 76 (1990), pp 33–38

Sharp, J. (ed), *Memoirs of the Life and Services of Rear-Admiral Sir William Symonds, Surveyor of the Navy from 1832 to 1847: with Correspondence and other Papers relative to the Ships and Vessels Constructed upon his Lines* (London, 1858)

Shaw, T., 'Ventilation in H.M. Ships from the Earliest Times to the Present Day', *Journal of the Royal Naval Medical Service* 12 (1926), pp 175–201

Shepherd, J., *The Crimean Doctors: A History of the British Medical Services in the Crimean War*, 2 vols. (Liverpool, 1991)

___, 'Spencer Wells – Surgeon R.N.', *Journal of the Royal Naval Medical Service* 56 (1970), pp 252–259

___, 'The Civil Hospitals in the Crimea (1855–1856)', *Proceedings of the Royal Society of Medicine* 59 (1966), pp 199–204

Sherwood, M., *After Abolition: Britain and the Slave Trade since 1807* (London, 2007)

Simpson, W., 'Progress of Hygiene in the Navy and its Effect on the Health of the Sailors', *Journal of the Royal Naval Medical Service* 1 (1915), pp 300–314

Sloane-Stanley, C., *Reminiscences of a Midshipman's Life from 1850 to 1856* (London, 1893)

Small, H., *Florence Nightingale: Avenging Angel* (London, 1998)

Smith, F., *Florence Nightingale: Reputation and Power* (New York, 1982)

Smith, G. (ed), *Physician and Friend: Alexander Grant* (London, 1902)

Snow, W., *Voyage of the Prince Albert in Search of Sir John Franklin: A Narrative of Every-Day Life in the Arctic Seas* (London, 1851)

Southwell-Sander, G., 'The Development of Naval Preventive Medicine', *Journal of the Royal Naval Medical Service* 43 (1957), pp 54–74

Stephens, L., *History of the Naval Victualling Department and its Association with Plymouth* (Plymouth, 1996)

Stewart, D., 'Surgeon-General James Pierce, R.N.', *Journal of the Royal Naval Medical Service* 36 (1950), pp 214–225

___, 'Sir John Richardson, Surgeon, Physician, Sailor, Explorer, Naturalist, Scholar', *Journal of the Royal Naval Medical Service* 22 (1936), pp 181–187

Stockman, R., 'James Lind and Scurvy', *Journal of the Royal Naval Medical Service*

13 (1927), pp 81–98

Stuart-Houston, C., *Arctic Ordeal: The Journal of John Richardson, Surgeon-Naturalist with Franklin 1820–1822* (Gloucester, 1984)

___ (ed), *To the Arctic by Canoe 1819–1821: The Journal and Paintings of Robert Hood, Midshipman with Franklin* (London, 1974)

Summers, A., *Angels and Citizens: British Women as Military Nurses 1854–1914* (London, 1988)

Sutherland, P., *Journal of a Voyage in Baffin's Bay and Barrow Straits, in the years 1850–51, performed by M. M. Ships Lady Franklin and Sophia, under the Command of Mr. William Penny, in Search of the Missing Crews of H.M. Ships Erebus and Terror*, 2 vols. (London, 1852)

Sweetman, J., *The Crimean War* (Oxford, 2001)

___, *War and Administration: The Significance of the Crimean War for the British Army* (Edinburgh, 1984)

Tait, W., *A History of Haslar Hospital* (Portsmouth, 1906)

Taylor, R., 'Cholera and the Royal Navy 1817–1867', *Journal of the Royal Naval Medical Service* 83 (1997), pp 147–156

Thomas, D., *Cochrane* (London, 1978)

Thomas, D. and E. Bardolph, 'Prevention of Scurvy in the Royal Navy', *Journal of the Royal Naval Medical Service* 84 (1998), pp 107–109

Tomlinson, C., *Winter in the Arctic Regions* (London, 1860)

Trewin, J., *Portrait of Plymouth* (London, 1973)

Trotter, T., *A Review of the Medical Department in the British Navy with a Method of Reform proposed in a Letter to the Rt. Hon. the Earl of Chatham, First Lord of the Admiralty* (London, 1790)

Vale, B., 'The Conquest of Scurvy in the Royal Navy 1793–1800: A Challenge to Current Orthodoxy', *Mariner's Mirror* 94 (2008), pp 160–175

Ward, W., *The Royal Navy and the Slavers: The Suppression of the Atlantic Slave Trade* (London, 1969)

Watson, W., 'Thomas Trotter: Naval Surgeon, 1793–1828', *Bulletin of the History of Medicine* 46 (1972), pp 131–149

___, 'An Edinburgh Surgeon of the Crimean War – Patrick Heron Watson (1832–1907)', *Medical History* 10 (1966), pp 166–176

Watt, J., 'Surgery at Trafalgar', *Mariner's Mirror* 91 (2005), pp 266–283

___, 'Health in the Royal Navy during the Age of Nelson: Nelsonian Medicine in Context', *Journal of the Royal Naval Medical Service* 86 (2000), pp 64–71

___, 'Surgeons of the Mary Rose: The Practice of Surgery in Tudor England', *Mariner's Mirror* 69 (1983), pp 3–19

West, A., *Memoir of Sir Henry Keppel: Admiral of the Fleet* (London, 1905)

Whiteside, H., 'Some Problems (Old and New) of the Seafaring Doctor', *Journal of the Royal Naval Medical Service* 17 (1931), pp 1–5

Wickenden, J., 'A Note on William Job Maillard: Marking the 100th Anniversary of his Death', *Journal of the Royal Naval Medical Service* 89 (2003), pp 9–10

Williams H., *The Life and Letters of Admiral Sir Charles Napier, K.C.B.* (London, 1917)

Williams, J. (ed), *The Autobiography of Elizabeth Davis, a Balaclava Nurse*, 2 vols. (London, 1857)

Williamson, R., 'Captain James Cook, R.N., F.R.S., and his Contribution to Medical Science', *Journal of the Royal Naval Medical Service* 14 (1928), pp 19–22

___, 'John Woodall and his Book, "The Surgeon's Mate"', *Journal of the Royal Naval Medical Service* 11 (1925), pp 190–192

Wilson, J., *Treatment of Cholera in the Royal Hospital, Haslar, during the months of July and August 1849, with remarks on the name and origin of the disease* (London, 1849)

___, *Medical Notes on China* (London, 1846)

___, *Outlines of Naval Surgery* (Edinburgh, 1846)

___, *Memoirs of West Indian Fever constituting brief notices regarding the Treatment, Origin, and Nature of the Disease commonly called Yellow Fever* (London, 1827)

Winton, J., *Hurrah for the Life of a Sailor: Life on the Lower Deck of the Victorian Navy* (London, 1977)

Wood, C., *State of the Navy* (London, 1839)

Woodford, L. (ed), *A Young Surgeon in Wellington's Army* (Woking, 1976)

___, 'A Medical Student's Career in the Early-Nineteenth Century', *Medical History* 14 (1970), pp 90–95

Wright, W., 'Ageing in the Royal Navy', *Journal of the Royal Naval Medical Service* 48 (1962), pp 199–204

Yexley, L., *The Inner Life of the Navy* (London, 1908)

Index

Toon, William, 91–93
Treasury, 54, 56, 117, 120–122
Trotter, Thomas, 6, 10, 87
tuberculosis, 42, 77, 135, 202, 206
Tucker, Alfred, 128, 138, 140, 143
Tucker, Douglas, 33

U
universities, 23–26, 28, 170–171, 196,
    198, 218
    Edinburgh University, 25, 218–219

V
vaccination, 6, 177, 207
Valparaiso, 124
Veitch, James, 76–77
Veitch, John, 44
venereal disease, 4, 14, 36, 39, 43–44,
    54, 75, 77–78, 84, 99, 140, 147, 183,
    205–206, 213–214, 221
Victoria, Queen, 182, 228
Victoria Cross, 201

W
Walcheren expedition, 28
Wallace, Robert, 180
Walling, Michael, 65
War Office, xi, xiii, 106, 213
Warden, Frederick, 125
Watson, John, 59

Weale, Mrs, 98–99
Webb, Samuel, 34
Weir, John, 11, 13
Wells, Samuel, 177
Wells, Sarah, 118
Wells, Thomas Spencer, 48
West, Maurice, 41, 46
Whipple, Dodwell, 65
Wilkinson, Charles, 61–64
Willan, Henry, 25
Wilson, John, 102–103, 128, 133–143,
    254
Wingate-Johnston, James, 114, 182
Wolrige, George, 45
Woodall, John, 2, 5
Woodcock, Alexander, 43
Woolwich, 20, 88–89, 205–206, 221;
    see also Royal Marines
Wright, Margaret, 98

Y
Yangtse river, 131–133, 135, 137, 141, 143;
    see also China War
Yokohama, 54
Yonge, James, 3

Z
Zanzibar, 67
zinc chloride, 43, 155–156, 202
Zulu War, 201, 221, 231